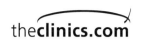

theclinics.com

OTOLARYNGOLOGIC CLINICS

OF NORTH AMERICA

Endoscopic Surgery of
the Orbit and
Lacrimal System

GUEST EDITORS
Raj Sindwani, MD, FACS, FRCS
and John J. Woog, MD, FACS

October 2006 • Volume 39 • Number 5

SAUNDERS

An Imprint of Elsevier, Inc.
PHILADELPHIA   LONDON   TORONTO   MONTREAL   SYDNEY   TOKYO

W.B. SAUNDERS COMPANY
A Division of Elsevier Inc.

1600 John F. Kennedy Boulevard, Suite 1800, Philadelphia, PA 19103–2899

http://www.theclinics.com

OTOLARYNGOLOGIC CLINICS	Volume 39, Number 5
OF NORTH AMERICA	ISSN 0030–6665
October 2006	ISBN 1-4160-3926-0

Editor: Joanne Husovski

The ideas and opinions expressed in *Otolaryngologic Clinics of North America* do not necessarily reflect those of the Publisher. The Publisher does not assume any responsibility for any injury and/or damage to persons or property arising out of or related to any use of the material contained in this periodical. The reader is advised to check the appropriate medical literature and the product information currently provided by the manufacturer of each drug to be administered to verify the dosage, the method and duration of administration, or contraindications. It is the responsibility of the treating physician or other health care professional, relying on independent experience and knowledge of the patient, to determine drug dosages and the best treatment for the patient. Mention of any product in this issue should not be construed as endorsement by the contributors, editors, or the Publisher of the product or manufacturers' claims.

Otolaryngologic Clinics of North America (ISSN 0030–6665) is published bimonthly by Elsevier Inc., 360 Park Avenue South, New York, NY 10010-1710. Months of issue are February, April, June, August, October, and December. Business and Editorial Offices: 1600 John F. Kennedy Blvd., Suite 1800, Philadelphia, PA 19103-2899. Customer Service Office: 6277 Sea Harbor Drive, Orlando, FL 32887-4800. Periodicals postage paid at New York, NY and additional mailing offices. Subscription price is $205.00 per year (US individuals), $370.00 per year (US institutions), $100.00 per year (US student/resident), $270.00 per year (Canadian individuals), $455.00 per year (Canadian institutions), $285.00 per year (international individuals), $455.00 per year (international institutions), $145.00 per year (international & Canadian student/resident). Foreign air speed delivery is included in all *Clinics'* subscription prices. All prices are subject to change without notice. **POSTMASTER:** Send address changes to *Otolaryngologic Clinics of North America*, Elsevier Periodicals Customer Service, 6277 Sea Harbor Drive, Orlando, FL 32887-4800. **Customer Service: 1-800-654-2452 (US). From outside the US, call 407-345-4000.**

Otolaryngologic Clinics of North America is also published in Spanish by McGraw-Hill Interamericana Editores S.A., P.O. Box 5-237, 06500 Mexico D.F., Mexico.

Otolaryngologic Clinics of North America is covered in *Index Medicus, Current Contents/Clinical Medicine, Excerpta Medica, BIOSIS, Science Citation Index,* and *ISI/BIOMED.*

Printed in the United States of America.

GUEST EDITORS

RAJ SINDWANI, MD, FACS, FRCS, Assistant Professor of Otolaryngology and Director of the Division of Rhinology and Sinus Surgery, Department of Otolaryngology-Head & Neck Surgery, Saint Louis University School of Medicine, Saint Louis, Missouri

JOHN J. WOOG, MD, FACS, Consultant in Eye Plastic, Lacrimal, and Orbital Surgery; Chair, Department of Ophthalmology Mayo Clinic; and Associate Professor, Mayo Clinic College of Medicine, Rochester, Minnesota

CONTRIBUTORS

DANIEL E. BUERGER, MD, Clinical Instructor, University of Pittsburgh; and Pittsburgh Oculoplastic Associates, Pittsburgh, Pennsylvania

DAVID G. BUERGER, MD, Clinical Instructor, University of Pittsburgh; and Pittsburgh Oculoplastic Associates, Pittsburgh, Pennsylvania

JOHN B. CHASTAIN, MD, Chief Resident, Department of Otolaryngology-Head and Neck Surgery, Saint Louis University School of Medicine, Saint Louis, Missouri

MICHAEL J. CUNNINGHAM, MD, Associate Professor of Otology and Laryngology, Harvard Medical School; and Surgeon in Otolaryngology, Massachusetts Eye and Ear Infirmary, Boston, Massachusetts

SAMER FAKHRI, MD, FRCSC, Assistant Professor of Otolaryngology, Director of Rhinology and Sinonasal Surgery, Department of Otolaryngology-Head and Neck Surgery, University of Texas Medical School at Houston, Houston, Texas

SUZANNE K. FREITAG, MD, Assistant Professor of Ophthalmology, Boston University School of Medicine; and Department of Ophthalmology, Boston Medical Center, Boston, Massachusetts

MORRIS E. HARTSTEIN, MD, Department of Ophthalmology, Saint Louis University School of Medicine, Saint Louis, Missouri

MITESH K. KAPADIA, MD, PhD, Assistant Professor of Ophthalmology, Tufts University School of Medicine; New England Eye Center, Tufts-New England Medical Center; and Department of Ophthalmology, Boston Medical Center, Boston, Massachusetts

AAYESHA M. KHAN, MD, Resident, Department of Otolaryngology-Head and Neck Surgery, Saint Louis University School of Medicine, Saint Louis, Missouri

PHILIP D. KOUSOUBRIS, MD, Neuroradiology Division, Department of Diagnostic Radiology, Lahey Clinic, Burlington, Massachusetts

H.B. HAROLD LEE, MD, Chief Resident Associate, Department of Ophthalmology, Mayo Clinic, Rochester, Minnesota

RALPH METSON, MD, Professor of Otology & Laryngology, Harvard Medical School; and Department of Otolaryngology, Massachusetts Eye and Ear Infirmary, Boston, Massachusetts

DALE R. MEYER, MD, FACS, Professor of Ophthalmology, Ophthalmic Plastic Surgery, Lions Eye Institute, Albany Medical Center, Slingerlands, New York

DAVID M. MILLS, MD, Instructor of Ophthalmology, Ophthalmic Plastic Surgery, Lions Eye Institute, Albany Medical Center, Slingerlands, New York

YASAMAN MOHADJER, MD, Department of Ophthalmology, Saint Louis University School of Medicine, Saint Louis, Missouri

KEVIN PEREIRA, MD, MS(ORL), Professor Of Otolaryngology and Pediatrics, Director of Pediatric Otolaryngology, Department of Otolaryngology-Head and Neck Surgery, University of Texas Medical School at Houston, Houston, Texas

STEVEN D. PLETCHER, MD, Assistant Professor, Department of Otolaryngology-Head and Neck Surgery, University of California San Francisco, San Francisco, California

I. RAND RODGERS, MD, Assistant Clinical Professor of Ophthalmology, Mount Sinai University, New York, New York; and Director, Ophthalmic Plastic and Facial Reconstructive Surgery, Northshore Long Island Jewish Medical Center, Manhasset, New York

DAVID A. ROSMAN, MD, MBA, Neuroradiology Division, Department of Diagnostic Radiology, Lahey Clinic, Burlington, Massachusetts

RAJ SINDWANI, MD, FACS, FRCS, Assistant Professor of Otolaryngology and Director of the Division of Rhinology and Sinus Surgery, Department of Otolaryngology-Head & Neck Surgery, Saint Louis University School of Medicine, Saint Louis, Missouri

STANLEY E. THAWLEY, MD, Associate Professor of Otolaryngology, Washington University School of Medicine, Saint Louis, Missouri

ANGELO TSIRBAS, MD, Assistant Professor, Department of Otolaryngology, Jules Stein Eye Institute, David Geffen School of Medicine at the University of California at Los Angeles, Los Angeles, California

MARK A. VARVARES, MD, Professor and Chairman, Department of Otolaryngology-Head and Neck Surgery, Saint Louis University School of Medicine, Saint Louis, Missouri

JOHN J. WOOG, MD, FACS, Consultant in Eye Plastic, Lacrimal, and Orbital Surgery; Chair, Department of Ophthalmology Mayo Clinic; and Associate Professor, Mayo Clinic College of Medicine, Rochester, Minnesota

PETER JOHN WORMALD, MD, Professor, Department of Otolaryngology, Woodville, Australia

RENZO A. ZALDÍVAR, MD, Chief Resident Associate, Department of Ophthalmology, Mayo Clinic, Rochester, Minnesota

CONTENTS

Otolaryngology and ophthalmology have a long and congenial professional relationship in the development of their mutual specialties over many years. In the early years they were one professional society, but later split into their separate specialties. Some problems involve both specialties because of the shared common anatomic area. These problems include: orbital complications of sinusitis, management of exopthalmus, silent sinus syndrome, lacrimal apparatus problems, tumor and trauma problems, optic nerve decompressioin, and complications of endoscopic sinus surgery. Both specialties have their own expertise to contribute to these common problems. In many cases it is in the best interest of the patient if both specialties consult and contribute their knowledge, experience, and techniques in these cases. Otolaryngologists and opthalmologists continue their long and mutually respected professional relationship.

Endoscopic approaches to the orbit take advantage of key anatomic relationships that arise from the fact that the sinonasal tract and orbit are contiguous structures separated by thin bone. For the most part, the orbit is surrounded by air-containing sinuses for much of the length of three of its four borders. Thus, a thorough understanding of both sinonasal and orbital anatomy is essential for safe and efficacious surgery in this complex region. The structural features of the lateral nasal wall and medial orbit are highlighted, and relevant aspects of orbital, lacrimal, and paranasal sinus anatomy are reviewed.

This article discusses the evaluation of specific lacrimal disorders and orbital trauma using CT, MRI, and other radiologic techniques.

The selection of the surgical approach to the orbit depends on the indication for surgery and the location, size, and extent of the lesion. For the anterior half of the orbit, anterior orbitotomy provides adequate exposure. For the posterior half, more extensive procedures with osteotomy are necessary. This article details the external approaches to the orbit. The traditional approaches for orbital decompression for Grave's ophthalmopathy are also described.

This article describes a stepwise system for evaluating the function of the lacrimal system. It discusses evaluation of the orbit with particular attention to thyroid eye disease and orbital fractures.

Graves' orbitopathy, also known as Graves' ophthalmopathy or thyroid eye disease, is a potentially progressive but generally self-limited autoimmune process associated with hyperthyroidism. It is the most common cause of proptosis and the most common orbital inflammatory disorder in adults.

The endoscopic transnasal approach is well suited for decompression of both the orbit and optic canal. High-resolution nasal endoscopes provide excellent visualization for bone removal along the orbital apex and skull base. Endoscopic orbital decompression has proved to be safe and effective for the treatment of patients with Graves' orbitopathy; however, the indications and outcomes for endoscopic decompression of the optic nerve remain controversial.

cluded in this latter group are dacryocystoceles or nasolacrimal duct cysts. The application of endoscopic sinus surgical techniques to children with persistent symptomatic nasolacrimal obstruction provides an alternative to external dacryocystorhinostomy that appears to be equally efficacious and concurrently allows for the potential correction of any predisposing intranasal pathology. Endonasal endoscopic dacryocystorhinostomy is best performed as a joint otolaryngologic–ophthalmologic procedure.

FORTHCOMING ISSUES

RECENT ISSUES

The Clinics are now available online!

Access your subscription at
www.theclinics.com

ELSEVIER
SAUNDERS

Otolaryngol Clin N Am
39 (2006) xi–xii

OTOLARYNGOLOGIC
CLINICS
OF NORTH AMERICA

Preface

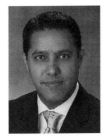
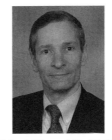

Raj Sindwani, MD, FACS, FRCS   John J. Woog, MD, FACS
Guest Editors

Advances in the field of endoscopic sinus surgery over the past 20 years have fostered the development of new approaches to the management of orbital and lacrimal disorders. With concurrent improvement in office examination techniques and imaging technology, clinicians with an interest in these disorders are now able to achieve increased precision in preoperative diagnosis and offer patients more refined, and minimally invasive options for treatment. Endosopic approaches to the orbit take exquisite advantage of key anatomic relationships that arise from the fact that the sinonasal tract and orbit are contiguous structures separated by very thin bone, and the techniques employed are well within the realm of the general otolaryngologist–ophthalmologist tandem. Successful surgical outcomes are predicated upon a thorough understanding of the relevant anatomy, meticulous surgical technique, and seamless cross-specialty collaboration.

We are personally indebted to our colleagues in the fields of otolaryngology, ophthalmology, and radiology for their generosity in sharing their insights and expertise, and hope that the collective experience shared within this unique issue of *Otolaryngologic Clinics of North America* will be helpful to the reader caring for patients with orbital and lacrimal problems.

Raj Sindwani, MD, FACS, FRCS
Department of Otolaryngology-Head and Neck Surgery
Saint Louis University School of Medicine
3635 Vista Avenue, 6th Floor FDT
Saint Louis, MO 63110, USA

E-mail address: Sindwani@slu.edu

John J. Woog, MD, FACS
Department of Ophthalmology
Mayo Clinic
200 First Street SW
Rochester, MN 55905, USA

E-mail address: Woog.John@mayo.edu

Otolaryngol Clin N Am
39 (2006) xiii

OTOLARYNGOLOGIC
CLINICS
OF NORTH AMERICA

Dedication

To my daughter, Sienna.
   Raj Sindwani, MD, FACS, FRCS

To my family.
   John J. Woog, MD, FACS

doi:10.1016/j.otc.2006.08.013   *oto.theclinics.com*

ELSEVIER
SAUNDERS

Otolaryngol Clin N Am
39 (2006) 845–853

OTOLARYNGOLOGIC
CLINICS
OF NORTH AMERICA

The Otolaryngologist–Ophthalmologist Relationship: An Historic Perspective

Stanley E. Thawley, MD

Department of Otolaryngology, Washington University School of Medicine, 660 S. Euclid Avenue, Campus Box 8115, Saint Louis, MO 63110, USA

There has been a long and close relationship between physicians who care for the eye and those with expertise in the areas of the ear, nose, and throat. One of the earliest recorded treatises concerning vision and hearing was by Hieronomi Fabricius of Aquapendente in the early 1600s. In England, in 1805, the London Infirmary for Curing Disease of the Eye and Ear was established and later became Moorfield's Hospital, currently a famous English hospital for care of the eye. In the United States, eye and ear hospitals were established during the 1800s in major cities of the east coast such as Boston, New York, and Philadelphia [1].

In the eastern United States the American Ophthalmological and Otological Society was established in 1864. The Western Ophthalmological and Otological Society was founded in Kansas City in 1896. This was later incorporated as the American Academy of Ophthalmology and Otolaryngology, the genesis of our current Academy of Otolaryngology. This combined society met together and published their Transactions together for many years until each became their own separate society in 1978 [2].

In the United States, physicians practicing Eye, Ear, Nose, and Throat were most common in the years between 1890 to 1930. Even in those years physicians tended to practice in one area or the other. At some sites the two specialities remained physically together such as the Massachusetts Eye and Ear Infirmary and in some private clinics. After the Flexner report in 1910, specialization began to develop more rapidly, with practitioners choosing either Ophthalmology or Otolaryngology. The American Board of Ophthalmology was established in 1916, and the American Board of Otolaryngology in 1924.

For many years the periorbital area has been a common ground shared by Ophthalmology, Otolaryngology, Plastic Surgery, Neurosurgery, and

E-mail address: thawlelys@wustl.edu

0030-6665/06/$ - see front matter © 2006 Elsevier Inc. All rights reserved.
doi:10.1016/j.otc.2006.06.004

Maxillofacial surgery. Trauma to the periobital areas sustained during World Wars I and II stimulated the advancement of care with resultant new techniques. Within ophthalmology training programs more subspeciality fellowships developed in the area of the periorbita. The journal of Ophthalmologic Plastic and Reconstructive Surgery was first published in 1985.

Otolaryngologists have developed and expanded their expertise in cosmetic facial plastic surgery incorporating some of the periorbital area. The most recent development has been the use of endoscopes and image guidance techniques by otolaryngologists within the nose and paranasal sinuses, allowing an expanding expertise and precision in applications of the periorbital area.

As both specialities race to keep pace with technologic advances, more applications continue to evolve. There continues to be a close working relationship between our specialities of Otolaryngology and Ophthalmology with mutual respect for our professional collegues.

The otolaryngologist–ophthalmologist relationship is frequently helpful in the areas of silent sinus syndrome, lacrimal duct problems, optic nerve decompression, orbital decompresson, drainage of subperiosteal abscesses, trauma of the orbit, tumor surgery, and complications of endoscopic sinus surgery.

Silent sinus syndrome

Spontaneous enophthalmos usually indicates orbital floor disruption secondary to malignancy, osteomyelitis, maxillary sinusitis, or systemic inflammatory disease. The silent sinus syndrome is thinning of the bony floor of the orbit, with resultant enophthalmos in otherwise asymptomatic maxillary sinus disease [3,4]. These cases are frequently associated with maxillary sinus hypoplasia, but normal sinuses demonstrated by normal sinus CT scans have been reported in patients years before development of enophthalmos [5]. The orbital floor is thinned and the other walls of the maxillary sinus may also be attentuated and pulled toward the lumen of the sinus, the medial wall being the next most common. In some cases there may be focal loss of bone. There have been reports of thickening of the other sinus walls. The sinus is not completely opacified in all cases. The disease is usually progressive, but in a few cases it may stabilize for long periods of time [6,7].

The etiology remains unknown but possibly is related to long-standing blockage of the ostium, defective aeration of the sinus, and resorption of air with resultant negative pressure. The presence of mucous in contact with the orbital floor and resultant thinning of bone may perhaps be similar to thinning of tympanic membranes secondary to long-standing serous otitis. Initially, it was thought that all of these cases were associated with long-standing hypoplasia of the maxillary sinus, but cases have occurred in normal appearing sinuses that later developed blockage of the maxillary sinus ostial area. The enophthalmos may develop over a relatively short period of time, not necessarily over many years [8].

Late enopthalmos following orbital decompression has been described with a postulated similar etiology to spontaneous enopthalmos. In cases of decompression where the inferior–medial orbital wall has been removed, the orbital fat may block the natural maxillary sinus ostia, leading to persistant mucous within the maxillary sinus with resultant enophthalmos at a latter time after the decompression [9].

In some cases, the eye needs to be supported with implants stabilized to bone [10]. These may be performed by the ophthalmologist or otolaryngologist. The ophthalmologist and otolaryngologist work together on these cases, with the sinus specialist opening the natural ostia of the maxillary sinus providing aeration and removal of any disease within the sinus. Some of these patients have intranasal structural abnormalities with deviation of the septum toward the ipsilateral side or narrowing of the middle meatus from a lateralized middle turbinate or concha bullosa. Adequate aeration of the maxillary sinus and opening of the natural ostia may include appropriate surgical modifications of the above-mentioned structural variations.

The disease usually stabilizes after adequate aeration of the maxillary sinus. In some cases, the enophthalmos improves after proper aeration with no orbital floor support. The decision to repair the orbital defect is dependent on each case and the surgeon. In these cases, it is ideal that ophthalmologist and otolaryngologist consult together, arriving at a combined agreed decision.

Dacryocystorhinostomy

Dacryocystorhinostomy is the standard surgery for blockage of the lacrimal outflow tract. The lacrimal sac is connected to the nose by removing the bone and mucosa between those structures. The traditional approach has been the external approach. In 1724, Woodhouse pierced the lacrimal bone, inserting a stent into the nose, and kept the connection to the nose patent with stents of gold, silver, or lead [11]. The external approach, the traditional ophthalmologic technique, involves a skin incision, removing the bone of the lacrimal sac fossa, opening the nasal mucosa, and suturing flaps to create a fistula into the nose. The external approach has been refined, and the current success rate is 80% to 90%.

The endonasal approach was described by Caldwell in 1893, but it did not become a popular technique because of lack of adequate instruments to visualize and work within the nose [12]. West described an intranasal approach in 1931. Compromised visualization could lead to increased bleeding and potential damage to the orbital and intracranial contents [13]. The endonasal approach was described again in 1950, but it has only been within the last 20 years that the intranasal approach has been popularized [14].

Endonasal visualization of the lacrimal sac area was accomplished by placing a light within the upper canalicula and into the lacrimal sac. This has been combined with using various lasers to remove mucosa and bone intranasally [14–17]. The anterior portion of the middle turbinate may be removed to more adequately visualize the lacrimal area. The anatomic landmark, the maxillary line, is an important surgical landmark for the cases that are performed endoscopically [18]. The endonasal technique has been used successfully with and without lasers with a success rate of 60% to 99%. It is also applicable for use in revision and pediatric cases [19,20].

Traditionally, ophthmalogists have performed most of the external approach cases but with the expertise of endoscopic nasal surgeons, otolaryngologists are increasingly performing these procedures endoscopically.

Optic nerve decompression

Traumatic injuries to the optic nerve is an area in which both ophthalmologists and otolaryngologists continue to work together to the benefit of the patient. The course of the optic nerve travels through anatomy in which the expertise of eye and sinus specialists as well as neurosurgeons is required. Depending on the area of damage, surgical approaches to the optic nerve include a craniotomy approach, extranasal transethmoidal approach, transorbital approach, transantral approach, intranasal microscopic approach, and an endoscopic nasal approach. These techniques may also be used to decompress the optic nerve in other disease entities such as psuedotumor cerebri, ischemic optic neuropathy, and endocrine orbitopathy.

Trauma producing edema, hematoma, or bony compression may respond to optic nerve decompression. The optic nerve is divided into three segments: the intraorbital segment, intracanalicular segment, and the intracranial segment. The intracanalicular segment is the area most frequently involved in indirect injuries [21].

In the endonasal endoscopic technique otolaryngologists approach the optic nerve medially through the sphenoid sinus. The optic nerve ususally resides just superior to the buldge produced by the carotid artery in the lateral sphenoid sinus wall. The bone overlying the optic nerve is thinned with a small bur and removed. The sheath and the annulus of Zinn may be incised depending on the opinion of the eye and sinus surgeons. The decompression is limited to the medial and inferior portions of the bony optic canal. A 180-degree decompression may be obtained by combining an external lateral transconjunctival approach with an endonasal sphenoidal approach [22,23]. Any orbital injury potentially involving the optic nerve should be evaluated by both an ophthalmologist and an endoscopic sinus surgeon to determine the most likely area of optic nerve damage and the appropriate approach [24].

There is still debate concerning treatment, as there may be spontaneous recovery with only medical treatment. These are cases where professional cooperation must exist closely between the eye specialist and the endoscopic sinus surgeon.

Orbital decompression

Historically, the expertise of ophthalmology and otolaryngology have blended together in the need for orbital decompression. Although indicated in other problems such as trauma, the exophthalmos of Graves' disease is the most common indication for orbit decompression. The four classic approaches have been superiorly into the cranial cavity by Naffziger [25], laterally into the temporal fossa by Kronlein, medially into the ethmoid sinuses by Sewall [26], inferiorly into the maxillary sinus by Hirsch [27], and the combined maxillary ethmoid approach through a Caldwell-Luc procedure by Walsh and Ogura [28,29] (Fig. 1). The removal of the floor of the orbit has the potential to produce the most diplopia.

Dr. Naffziger was born in California, and later studied under William Halstead and Harvey Cushing. He became the head of neurosurgery and Chairman of Surgery at the University of California. His major interest was the education and training of young surgeons. In 1931, he reported decompression of a right orbit for progressive exophthalmos through the anterior cranial fossa by removal of the orbital roof. He later reported 31 cases treated by this technique [30,31].

Dr. Rudolf Kronlein was born in Switzerland, and later succeeded Billroth and Rose as head of the surgery department at Zurich. He performed thoracic, abdominal, and intracranial surgeries. He was the first to deliberately remove a metastatic lesion from the lung. He collaborated with Joseph

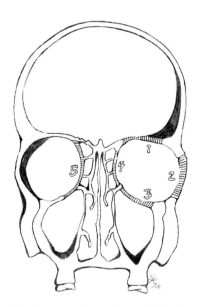

Fig. 1. Classic approaches for decompression of the orbit. 1. Naffziger, orbital roof; 2. Kronlein, lateral wall; 3. Hirsch, orbital floor; 4. Sewell, medial wall; 5. Walsh, Ogura, medial wall and orbital floor.

Lister, the father of aseptic surgery, and used carbolic acid to sterilize his instruments. He used the technique of the lateral approach to the orbit to remove a demoid cyst of the orbit. He did not operate for exophthalmos associated with Graves' disease, but was the first to design an operation that removed bone from the lateral orbit. In 1890, Julius Dollinger of Budapest used Kronlein's approach to successfully decompress the orbit in a patient with Graves'ophthalmopathy [30].

Dr. Oskar Hirsch was born in Moravia, Czechoslovakia. He trained in Vienna, becoming proficient in otolaryngology. He developed an endonasal technique for approaching the pituitary through the sphenoid sinus using a head light and reflection from a lamp. He reported a remarkable 400 cases of transsphenoidal pituitary cases with only a 5% mortality. Harvey Cushing visited him and learned his technique. In 1930, he published his technique for orbital decompression for Graves' ophthalmopathy by removing the orbital floor [30].

Dr. Walsh, chairman of Otolaryngology at Washington University in St. Louis, was primarily an otologist. He was followed as chairman by Dr. Joseph Ogura, who was famous as a leader in head and neck surgery and particularly conservation laryngeal surgery. They collaborated in their approach for orbital decompression through the medial and inferior wall of the orbit [28,29].

The development of techniques approaching the orbit for decompression has involved some illustrious and talented surgeons in the fields of ophthalmology, neurosurgery, and otolaryngology [31]. Our specialities are indebted to them for their creative and dedicated work in this singular area.

Recently, the development of intranasal endoscopic sinus surgery by otolaryngologists has allowed decompression of the orbit by removal of the medial wall of the orbit and portions of the orbital floor [32,33]. This has alleviated the need for external or conjunctival incisions. The success rate has been good with fewer complications. This technique also allows a more thorough decompression at the orbital apex area [33–35]. A combined transconjunctival and external approach for endoscopic orbital apex decompression in Graves Disease has been described as a procedure to enhance a safe apical decompression [23].

Irregardless of the technique, ophthalmologists frequently have to surgically address the diplopia by ocular muscle surgery. Orbital decompression is an ideal area for ophthalmogists and otolaryngologists to continue their historic association working together in decisions concerning the optimal combined treatment of the patient.

Subperiosteal orbital abscess drainage

This area involves the expertise of both ophthalmologist and endoscopic sinus surgeon. Subperiosteal abscesses arise on the medial wall of the orbit between the periosteum and lamina papyrcea. Traditionally, this area was drained by the ophthalmologists via an external approach from within the orbit. Otolaryngologist endoscopic sinus surgeons can now drain this area through an endonasal endoscopic approach by performing an intranasal ethmoidectomy and removing portions of the lamina papyrcea [36,37]. This allows the abscess to drain into the ethmoid sinus and nasal cavity. A combined external transcaruncular and transnasal endoscopic approach has also been suggested as perhaps providing better drainage of this area. Obviously, this area requires close cooperation and agreement on management between eye and sinus specialities.

Orbit trauma and tumor surgery

Orbital trauma has long been a field for cooperation between the ophthalmologist and otolaryngologist. The floor of the orbit may be approached through the conjunctiva of the inferior orbit or through the maxillary sinus via a Caldwell-Luc operation. As discussed previously, orbital decompression and apex decompression may be accomplished either externally or endonasally via an endoscope. In certain cases combined external and endonasal techniques may be appropriate depending on the particular circumstances and the experience and expertise of the surgeons [38].

Similar philosophy applies to tumor surgery involving the periorbital area. In general, endoscopic sinus surgery techniques are being increasingly used for tumor surgery, even in those which involve invasion of the orbit [39].

In trauma and tumor surgery of areas of the periobita close cooperation between eye and endoscopic sinus surgeons will frequently enhance the optimal result and prognosis for the patient.

Orbital complications of endoscopic sinus surgery

The orbit is frequently at risk in endoscopic sinus surgery, because it is the lateral margin of the ethmoid area. The lamina papyracea is thin bone and can be fractured with resultant hernation of fat, intraorbital bleading with orbital hematoma, and damage to the medial rectus. Anteriorly, the orbital fat and medial rectus are at risk. Posteriorly, the optic nerve is increasingly at risk as it is in a more medial plane and closer to the lateral wall of the posterior ethmoid cells. Superiorly, the ethmoid artery is at risk of transection with intra orbital bleeding. The lacrimal duct lies just anterior to the attachment of the uncinate process and is at risk for injury in that area.

The injuries may lead to loss of vision or diplopia, which may be temporary or permanent. The incidence of orbital complications is low because endoscopic sinus surgeons are increasingly well trained in residency and postgraduate courses. The advent of image guidance techniques is helpful, but does not alleviate the absolute requirement of detailed knowledge of anatomy and its variations and a cautious precise surgical technique along with a healthly respect for the inherent dangers in this surgery.

Intraorbital bleeding requires a quick response by the surgeon, and our ophthalmic collegues should be quickly consulted. Increasing vision loss and intraorbital pressure may require orbital decompression, lateral canthotomy and inferior cantholysis, and control of bleeding intranasally or by an external approach to the anterior ethmoid artery. Long-term diplopia secondary to damage to the medial rectus muscle should be followed by the ophthalmogist with possible surgical correction in the future.

Damage to the lacrimal duct system may repair itself by rerouting with only temporary epiphora. Long-term symptoms may require a dacryocystorhinostomy either by the ophthalmogist or endonasally by the endoscopic sinus surgeon.

The references for this survey highlight some of the important and interesting developments in selected areas of periorbital surgery. One can see various landmark techniques contributed by both otolaryngologists and ophthalmologists. As specialists in our seperate areas we continue our long mutually respected collaboration.

References

[1] Lederer FL. Address of the president, that they shall see, hear and speak. Trans Am Acad Ophthalmol Otolaryngol 1969;73:9–15.
[2] Straatsma BR. President's message. Trans Am Acad of Ophthalmol Otolaryngol 1977;84: 179–80.
[3] Soparkar CN, Patrinely JR, Cuaycong MJ, et al. The silent sinus syndrome, a cause of spontaneous enopthalmos. Opthalmology 1994;101:772–8.
[4] Gillman GS, Schaitkin BM. Asymptomatic enophthalmos: the silent sinus syndrome. Am J Rhinol 1999;13:459–62.
[5] Davidson JK, Soparkar CNS. Negative sinus pressure and normal predisease imaging in silent sinus syndrome. Arch Ophthalmol 1999;117:1653–4.
[6] Rose GE, Sandy C. Clinical and radiologic characteristics of the imploding antrum, or "silent sinus," syndrome. Ophthalmology 2003;110:811–8.
[7] Buono LM. The silent sinus syndrome: maxillary sinus atelectasis with enophthalmos and hypoglobus. Curr Opin Ophthalmol 2004;15:486–9.
[8] Soparkar CNS, Patrinely JR. Silent sinus syndrome—new perspectives? Ophthalmology 2004;111:414–5.
[9] Rose GE, Lund VJ. Clinical features and treatment of late enophthalmos after orbital decompression. Ophthalmology 2003;110:819–26.
[10] Thomas RD, Graham SM. Management of the orbital floor in silent sinus syndrom. Am J Rhinol 2003;17:97–100.
[11] Stallard AB. Eye surgery. 5th edition. Philadelphia (PA): Williams and Wilkins; 1973. p. 310.
[12] Caldwell GW. Two new operations for obstruction of the nasal duct, with preservation of the canaliculi and an incidental description of a new lacrymal probe. NY Med J 1893;57:581–2.
[13] West JW. The clinical results of the intranasal tear sac operation. Transaction of the Section of Ophthalmology. AMA; 1931. p. 169–72.
[14] Massaro BM. Endonasal laser dacryocystorhinostomy. A new approach to nasolacrimal duct obstruction. Arch Ophthalmol 1990;11:72–7.

[15] Gonnering RS, Lyon DB, Fisher JC. Endoscopic laser-assisted lacrimal surgery. Am J Oph-thalmol 1991;111:152–7.

[16] Seppa H, Grenman R, Hartikainen J. Endonasal CO2-Nd:YAG laser dacryocystorhinos-tomy. Acta Ophthalmol (Copenh) 1994;72:703–6.

[17] Tutton MK, O'Donnell NP. Endonasal laser dacryocystorhinostomy under direct vision. Eye 1995;9:485–7.

[18] Chastain JB, Cooper MH, Sindwani R. The maxillary line: anatomic characterization and clinical utility of an important surgical landmark. Laryngoscope 2005;115:990–2.

[19] Tsirbas A, Davis G, Wormald PJ. Revision dacryocystorhinostomy: a comparison of endo-scopic and external techniques. Am J Rhinol 2005;19:322–5.

[20] Kominek P, Cervenka S. Pediatric endonasal dacryocystorhinostomy: a report of 34 cases. Laryngoscope 2005;115:1800–3.

[21] Luxenberger W, Stammberger H. Endoscopic optic nerve decompression: the Graz experi-ence. Laryngoscope 1998;108:873–82.

[22] Kuppersmith RB, Alford EL. Combined transconjunctival/intranasal endoscopid approach to the optic canal in traumatic optic neuropthy. Laryngoscope 1997;107:311–5.

[23] Khan JA, Wagner DV. Combined transconjunctival and external apporoach for endoscopic orbital apex decompression in Gaves' disease. Laryngoscope 1995;105:203–6.

[24] Kountakis SE, Maillard AA. Endoscopic optic nerve decompression for traumatic blind-ness. Otolaryngol Head Neck Surg 2000;123:34–7.

[25] Naffziger. HC progressive exophthalmos following thyroidectomy: its pathology and treat-ment. Ann Surg 1931;94:582–4.

[26] Sewall EC. Operative control of progressive exophthalmos. Arch Otolaryngol 1936;24: 621–4.

[27] Hirsch O. Surgical decompression of malignant exophthalmos. Arch Otolaryngol 1950;51: 325–34.

[28] Walsh TE, Ogura JH. Transantral orbital decompression for malignant exophthalmos. Laryngoscope 1957;67:544–68.

[29] Ogura JH, Lucente FE. Surgical results of orbital decompression for malignant exophthalmos. Laryngoscope 1974;84:637–44.

[30] Alper MG. Pioneers in the history of orbital decompression for Graves' ophthalmopathy. Documenta Ophthalmologica 1995;89:163–71.

[31] Dallow RL, Netland PA. Management of thyroid-associated orbitopathy. In: Dallow RL, Netland PA, editors. Principles and practice of ophthalmology. 2000. p. 3082–9.

[32] Kennedy DW, Goodstein ML, Miller NR. Endoscopic transnasal orbital decompression. Arch Otolarynagol Head Neck Surg 1990;116:275–82.

[33] Metson R, Dallow RL, Shore JW. Endoscopic orbital decompression. Laryngoscope 1994; 104:950–7.

[34] Koay B, Bates G, Eliston J. Endoscopic orbital decompression for dysthyroid eye disease. J Laryngol Otol 1997;111:946–9.

[35] Michel O, Oberlander N, Neugebauer P. Follow-up of transnasal orbital decompression in severe Graves' ophthalmopathy. Ophthalmology 2001;108:400–4.

[36] Arjmand EM, Lusk RP, Muntz HR. Pediatric sinusitis and subperiosteal orbital abscess for-mation: diagnosis and treatment. Otolaryngol Head Neck Surg 1993;109:886–94.

[37] Pelton RW, Smith ME. Cosmetic consideration in surgery for orbital subperiosteal abscess in children. Arch Otolaryngol Head Neck Surg 2003;129:652–5.

[38] Chen C, Chen Y. Endoscopic assisted repair of orbital floor fractures. Plast Reconstr Surg 2001;108:2011–8.

[39] Huang H, Lie C, Lin K. Giant ethmoid osteoma with orbital extension, a nasoendoscopic appraoch using a intranasal drill. Laryngoscope 2001;111:430–2.

ELSEVIER
SAUNDERS

Otolaryngol Clin N Am
39 (2006) 855–864

OTOLARYNGOLOGIC
CLINICS
OF NORTH AMERICA

Anatomy of the Orbit, Lacrimal Apparatus, and Lateral Nasal Wall

John B. Chastain, MD, Raj Sindwani, MD, FACS, FRCS*

Department of Otolaryngology-Head and Neck Surgery, Saint Louis University School of Medicine, 3665 Vista Avenue, 6th Floor FDT, Saint Louis, MO 63110, USA

Endoscopic approaches to the orbit take advantage of key anatomic relationships that arise from the fact that the sinonasal tract and orbit are contiguous structures. Thus, a thorough understanding of both sinonasal and orbital anatomy is essential for safe and efficacious surgery in this complex region. Practical limits between the fields of otolaryngology and ophthalmology have produced to some extent a "no man's land" in which otolaryngologists feel as uneasy in the orbit as ophthalmologists do in the nose. For this reason, although we have chosen to highlight the structural features of the lateral nasal wall and medial orbit, we have also reviewed general aspects of the anatomy of the orbit, lacrimal apparatus, and the paranasal sinuses.

The Orbit

Osteology

The orbit is pyramidal in shape, with the posterior aspect open at the apex. The anterior orbit measures approximately 40 mm across horizontally and 32 mm vertically. The depth of the orbit is more variable, averaging 40 to 45 mm [1]. The orbit is comprised of seven bones. The frontal bone and the lesser wing of the sphenoid form the orbital roof. The floor of the orbit is formed by the orbital plates of the maxilla (medially), zygoma (laterally), and palatine bone (posteriorly). From anterior to posterior, the medial orbital wall consists of the frontal process of the maxilla, the lacrimal bone,

---

* Corresponding author.

E-mail address: Sindwani@slu.edu (R. Sindwani).

0030-6665/06/$ - see front matter © 2006 Elsevier Inc. All rights reserved.
doi:10.1016/j.otc.2006.07.003

the lamina papyracea of the ethmoid bone, and the sphenoid. The majority of the wall is comprised of the ethmoid bone, which is extremely thin except at its most posterior part [2]. The bony lacrimal fossa, bounded by anterior and posterior crests, is a prominent feature of the anterior medial orbital wall (Fig. 1). The average width of the lacrimal fossa, from the anterior crest to the posterior crest, is approximately 8 mm. The anterior lacrimal crest is formed by the frontal process of the maxilla, while the posterior crest is part of the thinner lacrimal bone. The vertical suture line between these bones is slightly closer to the posterior lacrimal crest but roughly bisects the fossa [3]. The lateral orbital wall is the thickest wall of the orbit, and is comprised of the zygoma and the greater wing of the sphenoid.

Foramina are present within the bony orbit through which numerous important structures pass. The largest of these is the superior orbital fissure, which averages 18 mm in length [4]. Its boundaries are formed by the lesser and greater wings of the sphenoid. The superior orbital fissure is divided into inferomedial and superotemporal aspects by the two tendons of the lateral rectus muscle. The inferomedial portion of the fissure contains structures that pass within the annulus of Zinn, including the inferior and superior divisions of the oculomotor nerve (cranial nerve III), the nasociliary branch of the ophthalmic division of the trigeminal nerve (CN V1), the abducens nerve (CN VI), and the sympathetic supply to the ciliary ganglion. The superotemporal aspect of the fissure transmits the frontal (CN V1), lacrimal (CN V1), and trochlear (CN IV) nerves. Vessels traversing the superior orbital fissure include the orbital branch of the middle meningeal artery, the recurrent branch of the lacrimal artery, the superior orbital vein, and the superior ophthalmic vein.

The inferior orbital fissure, bounded by the greater wing of the sphenoid, the maxilla, and the palatine bones, measures 20 mm in length. This fissure permits continuity among the orbit, the pterygopalatine fossa, and the infratemporal fossa. Through it traverse the infraorbital and zygomatic nerves

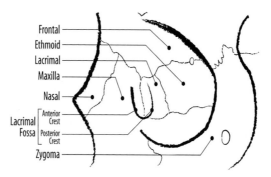

Fig. 1. Osteology of the orbit. The bones comprising the medial orbital wall include the frontal, ethmoid, and lacrimal bones, along with the frontal process of the maxilla. The anterior and posterior lacrimal crests are formed by the maxilla and the lacrimal bone, respectively.

(branches of the maxillary division (CN V2) of the trigeminal nerve), parasympathetic innervation to the lacrimal gland, the infraorbital artery, and the inferior ophthalmic veins. The infraorbital sulcus transmits the infraorbital neurovascular bundle along the orbital floor.

The optic canal transmits the optic nerve, its meningeal sheath, and the ophthalmic artery into the orbit through the lesser wing of the sphenoid. The optic canal is 5.5 to 11.5 mm long and 4.0 to 9.5 mm in diameter [5]. The intraorbital terminus of the canal is the optic foramen, located medial to the superior orbital fissure. Foramina along the medial wall of the orbit permit passage of branches of the ophthalmic artery into the ethmoid sinus. Deep to the anterior lacrimal crest, the anterior and posterior lacrimal arteries lie 20 mm and 35 mm, respectively, along the plane of the frontoethmoidal suture [6]. The nasociliary nerve accompanies the anterior ethmoid artery into the nasal cavity.

The lateral orbital wall transmits the lacrimal (CN V3) and zygomatic (CN V2) nerves and branches of the lacrimal artery via the zygomaticotemporal and zygomaticofacial canals. Posterolaterally within the orbit the meningeal foramen transmits the recurrent meningeal artery.

Whitnall's tubercle, located 3 to 4 mm posterior to the orbital rim and 11 mm inferior to the frontozygomatic suture, is an important landmark along the lateral orbital wall [7]. Several anatomic structures are normally attached to Whitnall's tubercle, including the check ligament of the lateral rectus, Lockwood's ligament, the pretarsal orbicularis, and the lateral canthal ligament.

The orbital roof is largely comprised of the orbital plate of the frontal bone, pneumatized anteriorly in approximately 65% to 85% of individuals by the frontal sinus air cells [8]. Two expanses located just below the anterior extent of the orbital roof house the lacrimal gland laterally and the trochlear fossa medially.

Extraocular muscles

All six extraocular muscles except the inferior oblique originate at the orbital apex. The medial, lateral, superior, and inferior recti originate from the annulus of Zinn, the ring of tendinous tissue at the orbital apex that encircles the optic foramen and the inferior portion of the superior orbital fissure. Intranasally, the region of the annulus of Zinn is located along the posterior lamina papyracea a few millimeters anterior to the face of the sphenoid sinus. The superior rectus and closely apposed levator palpebra superioris, as well as the superior oblique, originate from the apical aspect of the lesser wing of the sphenoid. The inferior oblique originates from the periosteum of the maxilla.

The rectus muscles insert in four quadrants on the globe, progressively farther away from the corneal limbus in a clockwise spiral, called the spiral of Tillaux, starting with the medial rectus [9]. As their names imply, the

858   CHASTAIN & SINDWANI

oblique muscles follow less direct routes than the rectus muscles. The inferior oblique courses posteriorly and laterally from its origin medially behind the lacrimal fossa, passes beneath the inferior rectus, and inserts on the inferior and lateral aspect of the globe. The superior oblique takes a circuitous route, beginning at the orbital apex above the annulus of Zinn, passing anterosuperiorly along the lesser wing of the sphenoid and into the trochlear fossa at the superomedial aspect of the anterior orbit. There it passes through the trochlea, a U-shaped cartilaginous structure at which point the superior oblique tendon turns at a 51- to 54-degree angle toward its insertion on the superolateral aspect of the globe.

Orbital connective tissue

The globe and its associated muscular and neurovascular structures are protected by a cushion of orbital fat and surrounding connective tissue. The periosteum of the bony orbit forms a continuous fibrous membrane, termed the periorbita, which lines the entire orbit. The periorbita serves as a significant barrier to regional infection, tumor spread, and surgical manipulation [10]. It is continuous posteriorly with dura mater through the superior orbital fissure and optic canal. Anteriorly, the periorbita is continuous with the periosteum. The orbital septum originates from a thickened portion of this periosteum anterior to the globe called the arcus marginalis. The orbital contents are also supported internally by a complex fascial framework principally comprised of the intermuscular septum and extraocular muscle sheaths, connective tissue joining the muscle sheaths to the periorbita and lids, and Tenon's capsule, a fibroelastic membrane surrounding the globe from the limbus to the dura. Orbital fat cushions and helps support the globe.

Vascular anatomy

The ophthalmic artery, a branch of the internal carotid system, is the major blood supply to the orbit [11]. It enters the orbit through the optic foramen, inferior to the optic nerve, and usually (in 85%) proceeds anteriorly beneath the superior oblique muscle. Ocular branches of the ophthalmic artery supply the globe and include the central retinal artery, ciliary arteries, and collateral branches to the optic nerve. Orbital branches include the lacrimal artery, muscular arteries, and periosteal branches. Extraorbital branches of the ophthalmic artery include the anterior and posterior ethmoid arteries, the supraorbital artery, the medial palpebral artery, the dorsal nasal artery, and the frontal (supratrochlear) artery. These vessels supply peripheral aspects of the orbit and the surrounding periorbital tissues including the forehead, brow, and nose.

The anterior and posterior ethmoid arteries traverse their respective foramina, which are located along the frontoethmoid suture along the medial orbit. These vessels supply parts of the extraocular muscle cone, ethmoid air cells, frontal sinus, lateral nasal wall, and nasal septum. Intranasally, the anterior ethmoid artery may be identified within or hanging below the roof of the ethmoid, and is susceptible to injury.

Anastomoses between the internal and external carotid systems provide redundancy in blood supply to the orbit. Venous drainage from the orbit is supplied by the superior and inferior ophthalmic veins which drain into the cavernous sinus.

Neurology

Innervation to the retina is provided by the optic nerve (CN II). The optic nerve is surrounded by a meningeal sheath in continuity with that of the central nervous system. The intraorbital portion of the nerve is approximately 6 mm longer than the distance from the globe to the optic foramen, permitting a full range of motion of the globe and preventing injury from proptosis and surgical traction [12].

The extraocular muscles are supplied by cranial nerves III, IV, and VI. Superior and inferior divisions of the oculomotor nerve (CN III) enter the superior orbital fissure to innervate the medial rectus, inferior rectus, inferior oblique, superior rectus, and levator palpebrae superioris. The trochlear nerve (CN IV) supplies the superior oblique muscle. The abducens nerve (CN VI) travels through the annulus of Zinn and then inserts on the inner surface of the lateral rectus muscle.

General sensory innervation to the orbit and face is supplied by the three divisions of the trigeminal nerve (CN V). The ophthalmic division (CN V1) enters the orbit through the superior orbital fissure. Its branches include the lacrimal, frontal, and nasociliary nerves. The lacrimal nerve supplies the lacrimal gland, conjunctiva, and upper eyelid. The frontal nerve travels superiorly and divides into the supraorbital and supratrochlear nerves, which innervate the tissues of the upper lid, brow, forehead, and frontoparietal scalp. The nasociliary nerve gives rise to the anterior and posterior ethmoidal nerves, long ciliary nerves to the globe, a sensory root to the ciliary ganglion, and its terminal branch, the infratrochlear nerve. These nerves supply sensation to the globe, conjunctiva, and ethmoid and sphenoid sinuses. The maxillary division (CN V2) of the trigeminal nerve enters the orbit via the inferior orbital fissure and courses within the infraorbital sulcus as the infraorbital nerve. Branches of this nerve supply the forehead, cheek, nose, upper lip, and inferior lid.

Sympathetic fibers to the orbit originate in the superior cervical ganglion and enter through the superior orbital fissure [13] to provide pupillary dilation, vasoconstriction, hidrosis, and constriction of eyelid smooth muscle. Parasympathetic fibers to the ciliary body and iris are supplied via short posterior ciliary nerves, while fibers to the lacrimal gland travel with the greater petrosal nerve (CN VII) [14].

The lacrimal apparatus

The lacrimal excretory system consists of the main lacrimal gland, 10 to 12 secretory ducts located within the superotemporal conjunctival fornix, and accessory glands (of Krause and Wolfring) located in the conjunctival fornices and in the palpebral conjunctiva, respectively. Whitnall's ligament provides structural support and prevents prolapse of the lacrimal gland [12]. The lacrimal apparatus provides for egress of tears via puncta located at the medial aspect of the eyelids. Each punctum opens into an avascular mound of fibrous tissue called the lacrimal papilla. The punctal opening, approximately 0.3 mm in diameter, leads to a canaliculus, which extends 2 mm vertically, turns 90 degrees toward the medial canthus, and travels through the orbicularis muscle for 8 mm before joining the lacrimal sac at an acute angle. The inferior and superior canaliculi coalesce to form a common canaliculus in 90% to 94% of individuals before joining the lacrimal sac [15]. The common canaliculus and lacrimal sac are located between the anterior and posterior limbs of the medial canthal ligament. The medial aspect of the common canaliculus contains the valve of Rosenmüller which prevents tear reflux.

The lacrimal sac averages 12 to 15 mm in height and usually extends 3 to 5 mm superior to the medial canthal ligament. It is immediately external to the orbit, within the lacrimal fossa, an indentation within the bony junction of the frontal process of the maxilla anteriorly and the thinner lacrimal bone posteriorly. Intranasally, the lacrimal sac lies an average of 8.8 mm above the insertion of the middle turbinate [16]. The rounded lower end of the lacrimal sac is continuous inferiorly with the nasolacrimal duct [2]. The duct travels within the bony nasolacrimal canal for approximately 11 mm [17] and continues 2 to 5 mm intranasally into the inferior meatus, usually emptying approximately 15 mm above the nasal floor and 4 to 6 mm posterior to the head of the inferior turbinate [18]. The duct's inferior course is also directed posteriorly and slightly laterally [19]. A mucosal fold, the valve of Hasner, is usually present at the nasal opening.

The paranasal sinuses

The paranasal sinuses, for the most part, surround the orbit on three of its four borders. Above and below the orbit are the frontal and maxillary sinuses. The maxillary sinus is the largest sinus air cell, and is located immediately beneath the orbit. Its natural ostium, located on the medial wall of the sinus, drains into the middle meatus and is hidden by the uncinate process. Occasionally, an accessory ostium may be seen along the medial wall of the sinus. The frontal sinuses may be quite large, asymmetric, or altogether absent [20]. Anterior ethmoid air cell development is closely related to frontal sinus development, and may cause pathologic obstruction of the frontal sinus outflow tract [21]. The frontal sinus ostium is located in the posteromedial aspect of the floor of the sinus and leads inferiorly to the frontal recess, which eventually drains into the middle meatus.

The ethmoid labyrinth is comprised of anterior and posterior groups of air cells separated by the basal (or ground) lamella of the middle turbinate. Anterior cells empty into the middle meatus via the ethmoid infundibulum and posterior cells drain into the superior meatus. The agger nasi is the anterior-most ethmoid cell(s), and appears as a swelling of the lateral nasal wall anterior to the superior origin of the middle turbinate [22]. The agger nasi cell forms the anterior boundary of the frontal recess and lies medial to the lacrimal bone. Anterior ethmoid cells commonly extend anteriorly to the level of the anterior lacrimal crest [23]. The ethmoid bulla is an anterior cell within the middle meatus that is seated laterally on the lamina papyracea itself. A well-pneumatized ethmoid bulla may extend to the skull base superiorly. Depending on the degree of pneumatization around the bulla, space above the bulla (suprabullar recess) or posterior to the bulla (retrobullar space) may be present [24]. The anterior face of the bulla appears as a bulbous curtain of bone oriented in the coronal plane, just posterior to the free edge of the uncinate process. Immediately posterior to the ethmoid bulla is the basal lamella, which also appears as a coronal curtain of bone attached to the lateral nasal wall. Its superior and medial aspects curve anteriorly to form the attachment of the entire length of the middle turbinate to the lateral nasal wall.

In addition, remarkable ethmoid cells include the infraorbital cell (Haller's cell), an ethmoid cell suspended from the orbital floor at the medial aspect of the maxillary sinus, the concha bullosa or pneumatized (usually middle) turbinate [25] and the sphenoethmoid (Onodi) cell, a posterior ethmoid cell that extends posterolaterally over the roof of the sphenoid sinus, and may contain the optic nerve [26].

The drainage pathway of the sphenoid sinus is into the sphenoethmoid recess through its 2 to 3 mm wide ostium, located approximately 10 mm superior to the floor of the sinus and 5 mm lateral to the septum [27]. Significantly, the sphenoid may partially pneumatize around the carotid artery and optic nerve, creating indentations within the sinus that may casually appear as additional sinus air cells [28,29]. Dehiscences over these areas (4% of optic nerves and 8% of carotid arteries) may exist increasing the risk of injury [30].

The lateral nasal wall

Several regions of the orbit and related structures may be accessed through the lateral nasal wall. The lacrimal system is housed within the anterior lateral wall, the orbit and orbital apex are separated from the nose by the lamina papyracea of the ethmoid, and exposure of the optic nerve is possible within the superolateral sphenoid.

The anatomy of the lateral nasal wall is dominated by the turbinates. Each turbinate is an oblong structure whose long axis is parallel to the floor of the nasal cavity. The turbinates are comprised of bone and are surrounded by a variable amount of fibrovascular erectile tissue covered by mucosa. Beneath each turbinate lies its corresponding meatus. Within the inferior meatus are the nasolacrimal duct opening and Woodruff's vascular plexus. The middle meatus contains the uncinate process, the ethmoid bulla, the frontal recess, and the maxillary sinus ostium. Pathology involving the sinuses may be impacted by common variations in middle turbinate configuration [25].

The uncinate process is a thin curtain of bone oriented in the parasagittal plane, whose anterior aspect curves slightly laterally to attach to the lateral nasal wall at the frontal process of the maxilla [31]. Inferiorly, the uncinate attaches to the ethmoidal process of the inferior turbinate. The uncinate process is lined by mucosa on both its medial and lateral aspects, with its posterior edge free within the middle meatus. The small two-dimensional cleft between the posterior edge of the uncinate process and the ethmoid bulla behind it is the hiatus semilunaris. Lateral to the uncinate process, the infundibulum is the three-dimensional space in which the maxillary sinus and anterior ethmoid air cells empty.

An important landmark for endoscopic sinus and orbital surgery is the maxillary line, a curvilinear eminence which projects from the anterior attachment of the middle turbinate superiorly and extends inferiorly along the lateral nasal wall to end at the root of the inferior turbinate (Fig. 2) [3]. The line is located near the head of the middle turbinate in the anteroposterior dimension. Extranasally, the maxillary line corresponds to the suture line between the lacrimal bone and the maxilla within the lacrimal fossa; intranasally, the maxillary line marks the attachment of the uncinate

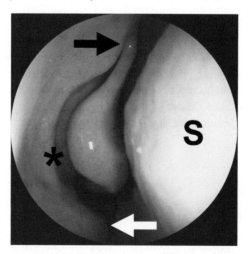

Fig. 2. Endoscopic view of the right lateral nasal wall in a live subject. The curvilinear maxillary line (*) begins superiorly at the middle turbinate attachment (*black arrow*) and then curves down along the lateral nasal wall to end at the root of the inferior turbinate (*white arrow*). S, septum. (*From* Chastain JB, Cooper MH, Sindwani R. The maxillary line: anatomical characterization and clinical utility of an important surgical landmark. Laryngoscope 2005;115(6): 990–2; with permission.)

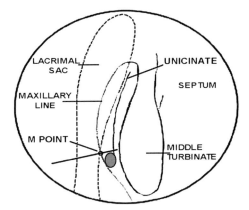

Fig. 3. An axial line through the midpoint (M point) of the C-shaped maxillary line is approximately at the level of the superior margin of the maxillary ostium posteriorly and just below the lacrimal sac-duct junction anteriorly. (*From* Chastain JB, Cooper MH, Sindwani R. The maxillary line: anatomical characterization and clinical utility of an important surgical landmark. Laryngoscope 2005;115(6):990–2; with permission.)

process to the maxilla. In the axial plane, the midpoint of the maxillary line marks the level of the superior aspect of the maxillary sinus ostium, which lies approximately 11 mm posteriorly, and the inferior aspect of the junction of the lacrimal sac and the nasolacrimal duct anteriorly (Fig. 3).

The lamina papyracea of the ethmoid bone separates the mid-orbit from the sinonasal cavity, and it courses posteriorly to end at the sphenoid face and the anterior skull base. The junction of the lamina papyracea with the skull base superiorly and the sphenoid face posteriorly forms an acute angle (termed the sphenoethmoid angle) in the posterosuperior ethmoid cavity.

Summary

A thorough understanding of the intricacies of orbital and paranasal sinus anatomy is critical to successful endoscopic surgery of the orbit and lacrimal apparatus.

References

[1] Lemke BN, Lucarelli MJ. Anatomy of the ocular adnexa, orbit, and related facial structures. In: Nesi FA, Lisman RD, Levine MR, editors. Smith's ophthalmic plastic and reconstructive surgery. St. Louis (MO): CV Mosby; 1998.
[2] Chow JM, Stankiewicz JA. Application of image-guidance to surgery of the orbit. Otolaryngol Clin North Am 2005;38(3):491–503.
[3] Chastain JB, Cooper MH, Sindwani R. The maxillary line: anatomic characterization and clinical utility of an important surgical landmark. Laryngoscope 2005;115(6):990–2.
[4] Natori Y, Rhoton A. Microsurgical anatomy of the superior orbital fissure. Neurosurgery 1995;36(4):762–75.

[5] Habal M, Maniscalco J, Rhoton A. Microsurgical anatomy of the optic canal: correlates to optic nerve exposure. J Surg Res 1977;22:527–33.

[6] Lemke B, Della Rocca R. Surgery of the eyelids and orbit: an anatomical approach. East Norwalk (CT): Appleton & Lange; 1990.

[7] Whitnall S. On a tubercle on the malar bone, and on the lateral attachments of the tarsal plates. J Anat Physiol 1911;45:426–32.

[8] Lee WT, Kuhn FA, Citardi MJ. 3D computed tomographic analysis of frontal recess anatomy in patients without frontal sinusitis. Otolaryngol Head Neck Surg 2004;131(3):164–73.

[9] Tillaux P. Traite d'anatomie topographique. Paris: Asselin et Houzeau; 1890.

[10] Curtin HD, Rabinov JD. Extension to the orbit from paraorbital disease. The sinuses. Radiol Clin North Am 1998;36(6):1201–13 [xi.].

[11] McNab A. Orbital vascular anatomy andvascular lesions. Orbit 2003;22(2):103–20.

[12] Whitnall S. Anatomy of the human orbit and accessory organs of vision. 2nd ed. London: Oxford University Press; 1932.

[13] Ruskell GL. Access of autonomic nerves through the optic canal, and their orbital distribution in man. Anat Rec A Discov Mol Cell Evol Biol 2003;275(1):937–8.

[14] Dutton J. The lacrimal systems. In: Dutton J, editor. Atlas of clinical and surgical orbital anatomy. Philadelphia (PA): WB Saunders; 1994.

[15] Yazici B, Yazici Z. Frequency of the common canaliculus: a radiologic study. Arch Ophthalmol 2000;118:1381–5.

[16] Wormald PJ, Kew J, Van Hasselt A. Intranasal anatomy of the nasolacrimal sac in endoscopic dacryocystorhinostomy. Otolaryngol Head Neck Surg 2000;123(3):307–10.

[17] Groell R, Schaffler G, Uggowitzer M, et al. Anatomy of the nasolacrimal sac and duct. Surg Radiol Anat 1997;19:189–91.

[18] Rose JG Jr, Lucarelli MJ, Lemke BN. Lacrimal, orbital, and sinus anatomy. In: Woog J, editor. Manual of endoscopic lacrimal and orbital surgery. New York: Elsevier; 2003.

[19] Warwick R, Williams PL, editors. Gray's anatomy. 35th edition. Philadelphia (PA): WB Saunders; 1973.

[20] Daniels DL, Mafee MF, Smith MM, et al. The frontal sinus drainage pathway and related structures. AJNR Am J Neuroradiol 2003;24(8):1618–27.

[21] Bent JP, Cuilty-Siller C, Kuhn FA. The frontal cell as a cause of frontal sinus obstruction. Am J Rhinol 1994;8:185–91.

[22] Yanagisawa E, Mirante JP, Christmas DA. Vertical insertion of the middle turbinate: a sign of the presence of a well-developed agger nasi cell. Ear Nose Throat J 2002;81(12):818–9.

[23] Whitnall SE. The relation of the lacrimal fossa to the ethmoidal cells. Ophthal Rev 1911;30: 321–5.

[24] Bolger WE, Mawn CB. Analysis of the suprabullar and retrobullar recesses for endoscopic sinus surgery. Ann Otol Rhinol Laryngol Suppl 2001;186:3–14.

[25] Joe JK, Ho SY, Yanagisawa E. Documentation of variations in sinonasal anatomy by intraoperative nasal endoscopy. Laryngoscope 2000;110(2, Part 1):229–35.

[26] Kantarci M, Karasen RM, Alper F, et al. Remarkable anatomic variations in paranasal sinus region and their clinical importance. Eur J Radiol 2004;50(3):296–302.

[27] Kim HU, Kim SS, Kang SS, et al. Surgical anatomy of the natural ostium of the sphenoid sinus. Laryngoscope 2001;111(9):1599–602.

[28] Rosenberger HC. The clinical availability of the ostium maxillae: a clinical and cadaver study. Ann Otol Rhinol Laryngol 1938;47:177–82.

[29] Dixon FW. A comparative study of the sphenoid. Ann Otol Rhinol Laryngol 1937;46: 687–98.

[30] Fujii K, Chambers S, Rhoton A. Neurovascular relationships of the sphenoid sinus. A microsurgical study. J Neurosurg 1979;50:31–9.

[31] Isobe M, Murakami G, Kataura A. Variations of the uncinate process of the lateral nasal wall with clinical implications. Clin Anat 1998;11:295–303.

ELSEVIER
SAUNDERS

Otolaryngol Clin N Am
39 (2006) 865–893

OTOLARYNGOLOGIC
CLINICS
OF NORTH AMERICA

Radiologic Evaluation of Lacrimal and Orbital Disease

Philip D. Kousoubris, MD*, David A. Rosman, MD, MBA

Neuroradiology Division, Department of Diagnostic Radiology, Lahey Medical Center, 41 Mall Road, Burlington, MA 01805, USA

Dysfunction or disease of the nasolacrimal ductal system (NLDS) is a common ophthalmologic problem, with the patient presenting with epiphora, lacrimal sac mass, or inflammation. The spectrum of disease varies from congenital absence or aberrancy of ductal structures to the more common acquired stenoses and obstructions of adulthood. Primary lacrimal sac and duct tumors are exceedingly rare. Infection is a much more common disease entity, especially in children and occasionally in adults. The radiologic lacrimal evaluation has evolved during the past 4 decades from x-ray dacryocystograms (DCG) to nuclear medicine isotope examination to CT and MRI evaluation. Some new techniques also have emerged from this past decade's increasing computer processor power, which, when applied to older CT methods, results in three-dimensional (3D) views of the NLDS. Orbital processes of particular interest to the oculoplastic surgeon are evaluation of Graves' dysthyroid orbitopathy and orbital wall trauma, which rely primarily on CT diagnostic techniques.

Plain-film radiographic evaluation relies on the Caldwell (posteroanterior) projection, the lateral view, and a Waters view of the orbits and paranasal sinus region. The Caldwell view details ethmoid and frontal anatomy, whereas the Waters view best demonstrates the maxillary sinuses. Conventional radiographs are still obtained as preliminary films for a DCG but are considered obsolete for the trauma patient [1,2]. DCG was first described by Ewing in 1909 [3]. Since the first use of the oil-based contrast agent lipiodol, the examination has evolved to use either water-soluble

Portions of this article are reprinted from: Kousoubris PD. Radiologic Evaluation of Lacrimal and Orbital Disease. In: John J. Woog, Ed. Manual of Endoscopic Lacrimal and Orbital Surgery. Philadelphia: Butterworth/Heineman, 2004; with permission.

* Corresponding author.
E-mail address: drphilxr@yahoo.com (P.D. Kousoubris).

Sinografin iodinated contrast or newer non-ionic contrast media. The indications for DCG are numerous. This type of study generally is used to evaluate obstruction, tumor, trauma, or congenital abnormality. Acute dacryocystitis is a relative contraindication to DCG because of patient discomfort and the potential risk of infection associated with instrumentation of the infected lacrimal outflow system. In patients who have epiphora, DCG may be performed to determine the nature, degree, and level of obstruction or other pathology. A sialogram (Rabinov-type) blunt-tip catheter of appropriate caliber (21–30 gauge in diameter) is selected to infuse a small amount (1–2 cm^3 per duct) of non-ionic 61% iopamidol contrast (Isovue 300, Bracco Diagnostics, Princeton, NJ). Nonionic aqueous contrasts come in a variety of iodine concentrations, from 200 g/L to 370 g/L, and can be tailored to exposure technique and patient comfort level. Higher iodine concentrations may be more irritating to the patient, but water-soluble agents are preferred to oil-based compounds such as Ethiodol.

Macrodacryocystography using magnification fluoroscopy with bilateral injections should be considered as a routine study, because the asymptomatic side may be considered the patient's control normal, and the radiation exposure is not significantly greater than with a unilateral study. The quality of the DCG depends to a great degree on operator technique, because adequate contrast volume and flow, which rely on cannula position and size and contrast selection and use, are needed to define obstructions.

The advantage of digital radiography is the reduced radiation exposure to the patient when compared with conventional film-screen technique, at the cost of reduced resolution [4]. Other digital advantages are the ability to manipulate image contrast and brightness settings infinitely (manipulation that often is necessary with contrast DCG) and the ability to subtract the background structures from the image. The latter technique is referred to as digital-subtraction dacryocystography (DS-DCG) (Fig. 1) [5]. Complete filling of the normal nasolacrimal system generally occurs within 10 seconds and has one tenth the radiation dose per exposure as compared with routine radiographs [4]. Finally, both oblique frontal projections and slightly off-lateral views are obtained while injecting contrast through the ductal systems.

CT examination after contrast DCG study provides bony detail of the orbits and sinuses adjacent to the nasolacrimal system while allowing soft tissue density characterization of lesions within the duct, sac, or the eyelid and surrounding tissues. Three-millimeter cuts in the coronal and axial planes should be considered a minimal requirement, and newer multidetector techniques facilitate cuts as thin as 0.625 mm or less. Although the radiation dose can be as high as 5 cGY (1 cGy = 1 rad) for thin cuts of 1 mm or less, these slices offer superb anatomic detail necessary for the small size of the NLDS. A reduced electrical current (80 mA/s) technique is desirable to decrease patient radiation exposure, because it requires only one scan after contrast injection through bilaterally cannulated lacrimal systems, eliminating additional radiation for the coronal images. This technique is

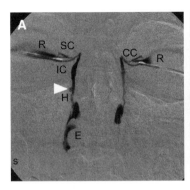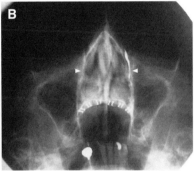

Fig. 1. (*A*) Normal DS-DCG frontal view. A possible small diverticulum (*arrowhead*) on the right above the valve of Hasner (H) region is an incidental finding. Superior (SC), inferior (IC), and common canaliculi (CC) opacify simultaneously with bilateral globe reflux (R). Nasal cavity contrast efflux (E) indicates NLDS patency bilaterally. (*B*) Modified Waters view, unsubtracted normal DCG, best depicts the posteriorly coursing nasolacrimal ducts (*arrowheads*).

patterned after that of Ashenhurst and colleagues [6]. Zeinrich and colleagues [7] have performed topical contrast administration before CT, as a more physiologic evaluation with increased patient comfort over punctal cannulation. The lens can be shielded with lead or bismuth during fluoroscopic DCG and subsequent CT [8]. The CT image will be degraded severely by star artifact from the high-density lead shields, obscuring vital structures. The authors have found that the extended-range processing algorithm used by one vendor's multidetector scanner (Siemens, Erlangen, Germany) produces extremely sharp contrast CT-DCG images because of the ability of the scanner software to register the higher density of contrast and bone more accurately by extending the upper Hounsfield unit (HU) range. The same type of algorithm is available on General Electric multidetector units (General Electric, Milwaukee, WI).

3D reconstruction of thin-slice, overlapping CT data can yield striking depiction of the anatomy by using both volume-rendered and maximum-intensity-projection techniques widely available on most scanners and their workstations. In essence, the lacrimal system contrast column will be shown in 3D form with lighted and shaded surfaces. The two techniques often are complementary. The one disadvantage to CT-DCG, even with 3D reconstruction, is that it does not offer any dynamic insight into lacrimal flow. Like plain-film DCG, the study is subject to variable interpretation [9].

Radionuclide evaluation of the lacrimal system was first described in 1972 by Rassomondo and colleagues [10]. The DSG method can both quantitate tear flow dynamics (in radioactive counts/second) and qualitate the dynamics (in terms of relative physiologic flow). The test is well tolerated and can easily be done bilaterally, because the radionuclide tag is introduced by micropipette into the inferior fornix of the lid. During acquisition, the traveling radiolabeled tears are visualized in real time on a video monitor.

The actual time for half of the activity to decline (T1/2) varies institutionally. Generally, it takes 2 to 6 minutes for tracer activity to leave the conjunctival sac [9]. If there is a partial or completely obstructed system, the time–activity slope will remain relatively flat or show abnormal decline (transit of labeled-tears). The study end point is reached when tracer reaches the nasal cavity. The dacryoscintigram is not universally performed but is clinically useful in the evaluation of pediatric epiphora [11], in unclear cases of partial or complete obstruction, and in patients whose puncta cannot be cannulated because of size or trauma. The normal dacryoscintigram has been found to be always associated with a normal radiographic DCG and is more sensitive than radiography in the detection of obstruction [9,12]. The clinically asymptomatic side in a bilateral DSG study has been shown to have abnormal flow in up to 40% of cases [13].

Unfortunately, transit times are variable throughout the ductal system, as first described by Chavis and colleagues [14] in a study of 100 patients. The main limit of scintigraphy is its low resolution compared with other imaging modalities [15]. Although some authors have advocated using the DSG as a screening test in patients who have epiphora, its role at present remains complementary to other imaging modalities.

The prime advantage of MRI over CT is its superior tissue contrast ability, including the separation of fluid signal from surrounding soft tissue. The technique involves no ionizing radiation and a noninvasive contrast application but has the drawback of increased scan time and cost compared with CT. Diluted gadolinium has been applied as a MR contrast agent in a dilute 1:100 solution (0.5% gadolinium meglumine) with sterile saline, both in drop form and by direct canalicular injection [16]. Imaging is performed within 5 to 10 minutes of contrast administration, because the contrast persists in the nasolacrimal system for approximately 20 minutes. Cannulation of the puncta can be performed before the MR study to assess an obstructing lesion more fully but negates the functional aspect of topically applied contrast. Axial T1-weighted images are obtained with or without the use of fat suppression. The multiplanar ability of MRI allows imaging in any obliquity, so coronal and sagittal views are easily obtained. No adverse local reaction or pain associated with gadolinium drops has been reported; the drops, apparently, are well tolerated.

MR-DCG is not widely used in the routine evaluation of epiphora or mass lesions; however, some authors use it as a first-line test because it delivers no ionizing radiation to the lens. MR-DCG was shown to have a comparable accuracy when compared with CT-DCG by surgical correlation of stenosis in a study of 25 patients [17]. MR-DCG can be performed with or without administration of lacrimal ductal contrast. Congenital intranasal dacryocystoceles are exceptionally well seen as cystic structures, including characterization of cyst contents, by noncontrast MRI [18]. MR-DCG has been shown to depict lacrimal ductal anatomy adequately, but the results do not always correlate with conventional DSG results [19].

Some researchers have compared eyedrop-contrast MR-DSG with DS-DSG; they have found MR to be more accurate than DS-DCG in detecting the level of obstruction and in three cases were able to trace contrast further in the duct than with DS-DCG [20]. Use of both intravenous and conjunctival gadolinium contrast has been reported, but this combination is rarely used [21]. A very fast acquisition pulse sequence that is heavily T2-weighted, relying on half-Fourier single-shot technique (HASTE, Siemens Medical Systems, and SSFSE, GE Medical Systems) can image the ductal system functionally after irrigation with topical saline as a contrast agent, but this technique is not widely used [22]. In summary, occasionally MR-DCG is clinically useful in diagnosing pediatric lacrimal obstruction and in complicated cases involving soft tissue tumors and is the subject of ongoing investigation of a wider diagnostic role.

Lacrimal ultrasound was first described by Oksala [23] in 1959 in the setting of diagnosing acute dacryocystitis. Usually B-scale (or "grayscale") images are produced of the lacrimal sac and duct, with the lacrimal crests also seen. Gross anatomic abnormalities related to lacrimal sac size and contents, such as dacryoliths, abscesses, and diverticula, can be defined quickly. Lacrimal sac contents can be assessed in disease states as a dark fluid- or debris-filled sac (ie, in obstruction and infection) or as solidly replaced by echogenic stone or tumor [24]. Normal lacrimal sac and duct should appear as an echo-free tubular structure. Although ultrasound lacks anatomic detail and is unable to define sites of lacrimal obstruction accurately, it is performed easily in the outpatient setting and lacks ionizing radiation.

The generalization can be made that there is no single standard in the current diagnostic battery of imaging tests for lacrimal drainage disorders. Instead, each modality contributes unique information to the final diagnosis.

Specific lacrimal disorders

Congenital dacryostenosis

Congenital dacryostenosis is included in a spectrum of dysgenesis of the lacrimal system. The lacrimal puncta may be atretic. If only an upper or lower lid is involved, conventional and DS-DCG can be performed through the apposing canaliculus to outline the level and extent of hypoplasia by contrast refluxing into the affected limb. Atresia of the entire canaliculus is usually detectable by DCG. Punctal and canalicular atresia also may be associated with fistula formation [25–27]. Punctal atresia with absence of the salivary glands is a rare autosomal dominant disorder that may be diagnosed by CT examination of the neck [28]. Duplication of a canaliculus, which often is asymptomatic, will appear on DCG as a separate linear contrast channel in the upper or lower lid [29–32]. A fistula can appear on ultrasound as an echolucent (dark) track from the skin connecting to the lacrimal sac [33]. The thin membrane that may be present at the level of the valve of Hasner at birth usually ruptures with inspiratory effort at birth or becomes perforated within 1 month postnatally, but it can persist for 9 to 12 months [34–36]. Obstruction may be associated with a bluish medial canthal mass or nasal cavity cyst [9,37]. Such cysts can enlarge into the nasal cavity through expansion of the posterior lacrimal crest or can extend through and expand the duct to present as a mass in the lower nasal cavity. The classic triad detectable by CT scanning includes ductal expansion and rounded medial and nasal cavity cystic masses of water-like low density [38,39]. MRI further differentiates the cystic lesions from meningoceles, encephaloceles, and nasal gliomas, which must be entertained in the differential list [9,40]. Cross-sectional imaging is the preferred modality for the primary investigation of medial canthal masses, without the need for contrast injection into the lacrimal system.

Diverticula of the lacrimal system are not common. They usually arise from the duct–sac junction but can arise from any portion of the lacrimal drainage system. Diverticula may be congenital, or they may be acquired in the setting of chronic inflammation, obstruction, or manipulation of the ductal system. They almost always are saccular in configuration and may have a wide or narrow neck as seen by DCG [41]. Canalicular diverticula are similar in appearance [42]. CT-DCG may be valuable in some cases, because small stones or debris that may form in the diverticular lumen are more easily visualized than on plain-film DCG (Fig. 2) [43].

Fistulas of the lacrimal system were first described in 1675 by Rasor [44] and can be congenital or acquired from many causes. The fistulas may be internal, external, or even blind-ending, but most arise from the region of the common canaliculus [45]. Fistulas are well demonstrated as a track of contrast by DS-DCG and CT-DCG.

Dysgenesis of the lacrimal sac and duct can occur at any level. Total atresia of the nasolacrimal duct is rare [46,47]. Abrupt termination of the contrast column in a small blind pouch would be expected in ductal atresia

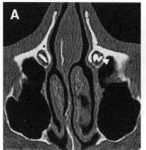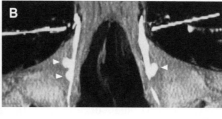

Fig. 2. Diverticula. (*A*) Axial CT-DCG reveals a left ductal "double-barrel" contrast configuration, the lateral contrast lobe being the diverticulum (*arrowhead*). (*B*) Three-dimensional CT-DCG of the same patient elegantly depicts diverticula (*arrowheads*) from surrounding anatomy.

by DCG. CT-DCG axial sections may demonstrate hypoplasia or atresia of the lacrimal crests and duct, with luminal replacement by the ethmoid bone. Nasoseptal deformity also may contribute to nasolacrimal duct obstruction. In Gray's [48] series of 100 patients who had nasolacrimal ductal obstruction, all were found to have septal deformity or deviation correlating to the blockage.

Acquired dacryostenosis

Acquired dacryostenosis can be primary, associated with a fibroinflammatory obstruction of the ductal system of unknown cause, or secondary, attributable to a definable cause such as tumor, trauma, inflammation, infection, or radiation therapy [49,50]. The most commonly encountered entity is so-called "primary acquired nasolacrimal duct obstruction" (PANDO), which presents as epiphora or a medial canthal mass [51]. A number of radiologic findings have been made regarding PANDO. First, the width of the canal is narrower in women than in men, perhaps explaining the greater incidence of nasolacrimal duct obstruction in women [43,52]. Studies have demonstrated a high prevalence of sinus disease associated with nasolacrimal ductal obstruction [53]. Other, less common causes of acquired obstruction that may be imaged include lacrimal primary neoplasm, dacryolithiasis, sarcoid, Wegener's granulomatosis, foreign bodies, and melanin casts [54,55]. Canalicular obstruction or stenosis may occur from traumatic laceration, punctual plug placement, infection, chronic use of topical medication, or, rarely, papilloma formation [56]. The location of the obstruction may be defined by DS-DCG. CT scans may offer additional information if the obstruction is associated with a mass. Canaliculitis usually results in ectasia of the canaliculus, with associated contour beading, diverticula, or other luminal irregularity [57]. Canalicular ectasia without stenosis suggests chronic inflammation. Small filling defects within the canaliculi may reflect stones, which, although nonspecific, commonly occur with the sulfur granules of *Actinomyces* infection [58,59].

In common canalicular obstruction, prompt reflux is seen into the superior canaliculus from inferior punctal injection without passage into the sac. Common canalicular stenosis should be suspected if any of these DCG findings are seen: caliber is less than 1 mm, diameter is less than the ipsilateral canaliculus, and canalicular dilatation occurs with increased injection pressure [43].

On conventional and DS-DCG, stenosis and complete obstructions are commonly seen in the adult patient at the sac–duct junction or, less frequently, within the nasolacrimal duct. Normally the lacrimal sac and duct are smooth in caliber, with the duct measuring 1 to 4 mm in size [60]. The ductal contrast column in patients who have PANDO may terminate abruptly or taper over a long segment on DCG. Frequently, concentric soft tissue density reflecting the fibroinflammatory mucosal changes can be seen on CT-DCG at the affected segment, ultimately filling in the lumen with soft tissue density at the obstructing point or narrowing the central contrast column [61]. Lacrimal sac dilatation above the stenosis can assume a globular, pear-shaped, or cylindrical configuration (Fig. 3) [43]. The normal diameter of the sac is approximately 4 mm, and the upper limit of normal is 7 to 8 mm [60]. Sac dilatation can be assumed if there is significant size asymmetry (>1–2 mm) to the contralateral side, as well as an enlarged diameter, depending on any associated pathologic conditions. If the sac retains a smooth outline, there usually is no associated inflammatory change of the mucosa; an irregular contour suggests inflammation. Observation of the ductal column in at least two planes is helpful for accurate delineation of a true stenosis. CT-DCG is considered technically superior to MR-DCG for the evaluation of the canaliculi, but sac and duct pathology are equally well seen by both techniques [62].

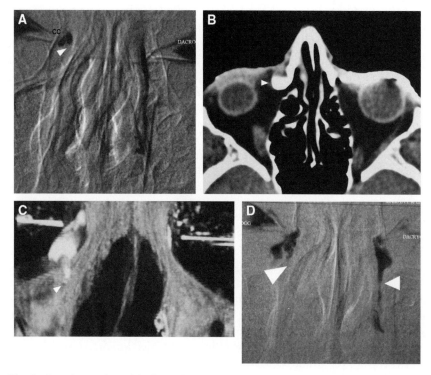

Fig. 3. Complete and partial obstruction. (*A*) Subtracted DCG depicts right sac complete obstruction (*arrowhead*), common canaliculus dilated (CC). The left nasolacrimal system is of normal appearance. (*B*) Axial CT-DCG in the same patient shows a contrast–tear fluid level (*arrowhead*) in the dilated, obstructed right sac. The left sac shows air and contrast density from normal washout. (*C*) 3D-DCG view of the same patient better depicts the level of obstruction than *A*, with a trace amount of contrast in the normal left system. (*D*) Subtracted DCG in a different patient with complete obstruction at the right sac–duct junction (*arrowhead*) and partial obstruction from stricture at the left sac–duct junction (*arrowhead*).

Partial obstructions may present the clinician without a clear diagnosis as to cause or level of obstruction. Partial blockage of the common canaliculus may be detected with greater sensitivity by DCG than by clinical syringing and probing [31]. Conversely, DCG findings may be normal findings in patients who have functional or partial obstruction [15].

DCG is heavily technique dependant, and functionally significant stenoses may be demonstrated only if the rate of contrast flow overcomes the total capacitance of the ductal system; this rate of flow can be difficult to achieve, even with cannulated technique. Partial obstruction commonly appears on DCG as a relative stenosis, with passage of contrast delayed as compared with the contralateral side. MR-DCG, using topical gadolinium or saline contrast, has been touted as more physiologic than CT-DCG and DCG, and can differentiate between stenosis and obstruction, as evidenced in a series of 18 patients [63]. In another study, topical gadolinium contrast medium was used along with dynamically acquired rapid T1 MR pulse sequences to depict the time course of contrast flow in a cinematic fashion. This study characterized the amount of time needed for contrast passage in partial obstructions as "intermediary" between complete obstruction and normal [64]. Most recently, in a series of 12 patients, fast dynamic MR-DCG pulses characterized the actual passage of gadolinium and saline drops through the nasolacrimal system, showing a bolus passing after several eyeblinks (Jones's theory of the orbicularis oculi nasolacrimal pump) [65].

Partial obstructions commonly are shown as areas of concentric soft tissue that narrow but preserve the contrast column (see Fig. 3). A report by Janssen and colleagues [66] described a mean minimum bony ductal dimension of 3.5 mm in normal controls and 3.0 mm in patients who had ductal obstruction, with significant overlap in diameter between the groups. The study did not address ductal morphology in partial obstructions. A similar morphologic study quantitated the anteroposterior diameter of 71 normal patients' bony nasolacrimal ducts, confirming that the bony diameter of the duct is smaller in women than in men and suggesting a relationship between PANDO and ductal size. The study did not address cases of obstruction [67]. There has been no quantitative study of ductal bony canal morphology in partial nasolacrimal obstructions in the literature, although partial obstructions frequently are documented by DCG during balloon dacryoplasty or by endoscopy of the lacrimal system [68,69]. Also, because of the great variability in thickness of the lacrimal ductal epithelium, no study to date has evaluated this soft tissue contribution to obstructed versus normal ducts [61].

Dacryolithiasis

Dacryoliths have been found during surgery with a frequency of 10% to 30% in patients who have chronic inflammation of the lacrimal system, and they may be associated with fungal elements [70]. In a series reported by Berlin and colleagues [71], 11 of 70 patients who underwent dacryocystorhinostomy were found to have lacrimal sac stones. Six of these patients demonstrated septate hyphae consistent with the presence of fungus. On pathologic examination, the dacryoliths also may represent aggregates of cellular debris, fibrinous material, and leukocytes, with or without microbial pathogens [72]. As documented in a report by von Graefe, canalicular dacryoliths were known to be associated with *Actinomyces* infection as early as 1854 [73]. *Candida* species also have been cultured from lacrimal calculi [74]. Topical epinephrine breakdown products also have been reported as black dacryoliths associated with nasolacrimal obstruction [55,75]. A variety of foreign bodies, such as eyelashes, have been reported in the literature to cause filling defects in the lacrimal sac [76,77].

Filling defects of the duct or lacrimal sac appear on DCG as dark objects in bright contrast. Pathologic filling defects should not change in size and shape, as would artifact such as introduced air bubble. Thick secretions or debris could mimic dacryolith-like filling defects. Occasionally dacryoliths show increased calcific density best appreciated by CT scan (≥ 90 HU). CT-DCG offers the benefit of demonstrating a DCG filling defect while providing CT information on the density of the lesion and surrounding bony architecture (Fig. 4). Calculi have been reported in diverticula of the nasolacrimal system as well, and diverticula may be well demonstrated on DCG. MRI scans may depict a dacryolith if water or gadolinium contrast material is used. Neoplasms represent the other major category in the differential diagnosis of filling defects examined by DCG.

Nasolacrimal neoplasms

Lacrimal sac tumors are considered rare, with the largest series reported in the literature numbering 115 in an Armed Forces Institute of Pathology

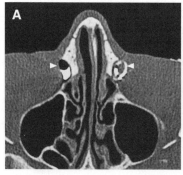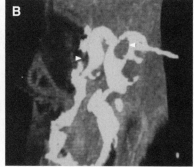

Fig. 4. Dacryoliths. (*A*) Axial CT-DCG at the sac level reveals bilateral sac-filling defects (*arrowheads*). The defect on the right is air density (*black*). The density on the left is of soft tissue quality (*gray*). (*B*) 3D CT-DCG rendering of the patient in *A*, obliquely rotated to show essentially no difference in quality of multiple sac and duct filling defects. These defects have a limited, nonspecific appearance when compared with *A*. The patient had multiple dacryoliths.

review by Stefanyszyn and colleagues [78]. The rate of malignancy of lacrimal sac tumors varies from 50% to 70% to as high as 90% in the series by Ni [79]. Generally, epithelial tumors comprise the majority of sac tumors, followed by sarcomas, melanomas, neural tumors, lymphoma, and other rare lesions. Patients may present with intermittent epiphora and dacryocystitis [80].

The most common benign epithelial tumor is the papilloma. Papillomas may develop foci of squamous cell carcinoma in situ, with up to a 10% to 15% transformation rate [81,82]. Papillomas may have a characteristic lacy interstitial contrast pattern and appear as irregular-contour filling defects on DCG [83]. Inverting papillomas may expand through bone into adjacent sinonasal structures, such as the ethmoid air cells or nasal cavity [84]. Recurrent conjunctival papillomas may erode into the lacrimal sac and obstruct the upper nasolacrimal system [85]. CT scans may reveal a homogeneous soft tissue density, similar to that of muscle. Osseous lacrimal bone lesions include hemangiomas, osteomas, and fibro-osseous lesions, among others (Fig. 5).

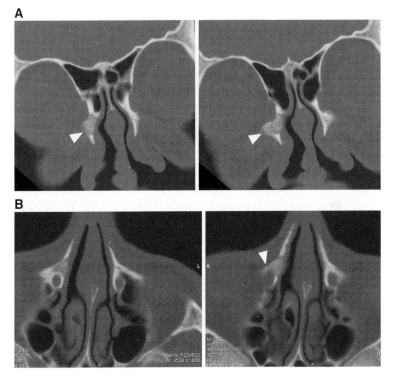

Fig. 5. Primary lacrimal bone lesion. (A) Coronal noncontrast CT orbits reveals ground-glass lucency affecting the right anterior lacrimal crest, sac level. (B) Axial CT orbits do not show any bony expansion by focal fibrous dysplasia into the sac. The finding was incidental and was completely inconspicuous on plain-film examination.

Other benign epithelial lesions include oncocytomas, polyps, fibromas, and benign mixed neoplasms. If small, these tumors may not be visible by DCG or may present as sharply defined filling defects.

Of malignant epithelial tumors, squamous cell carcinoma predominates, followed by transitional cell carcinoma [86]. A sharply defined filling defect on DCG is typical of smaller carcinomas, whereas larger, invasive tumors tend to be more irregular in contour. Invasive neoplasms may cause extra-luminal tracking of contrast into adjacent structures. Dilatation or irregu-larity of the sac and bone destruction may be additional findings with malignant disease. A well-circumscribed mass that is isointense to brain on T1 studies and dark and nonhomogeneously enhancing on T2 studies has been described by Rahangdale and colleagues [87] in a single case report of MRI findings in a patient who had squamous cell neoplasia of the lacri-mal sac. Other T2-dark nasolacrimal lesions may include pseudotumor, melanoma, lymphoma, fibrosis, and dacryolithiasis. MRI findings are non-specific in differentiating squamous cell neoplasms from other nasolacrimal abnormalities. Other malignant epithelial tumors include adenocarcinoma, mucoepidermoid, adenoid cystic carcinoma, and poorly differentiated carcinomas [88].

Of the nonepithelial malignant nasolacrimal tumors, sac melanoma de-serves mention as a rare entity [89–92]. Central nervous system and intraoc-ular melanomas can be characteristically T1-bright and T2-dark because of melanin's intrinsic signal and paramagnetic properties. Billing and colleagues [93], however, reported a case of malignant melanoma of the lac-rimal sac that was intermediate on both T1 and T2 with some enhancement with gadolinium. Because the T1 hyperintensity depends on the paramagnetic properties, amelanotic lesions can be isointense on T1. Gliezal and colleagues [94] advocated CT scan; they noted the insidious onset of this lesion and suggested that any persistent dacryocystitis should raise concern for malignant melanoma. Other nonepithelial malignant tumors include tumors of mesenchymal origin, of which benign fibrous histiocytoma is the most common, followed in frequency by malignant fibrous histiocytoma and hemangiopericytoma. Lymphomas and neural sheath tumors constitute the remainder of the nonepithelial neoplasms. Lymphomas occur more commonly than neural sheath tumors in the sinonasal passages, secondarily invading the nasolacrimal system. Frank bone destruction is atypical in lym-phoma but has been reported [95].

The MRI characteristics of lacrimal sac tumors are nonspecific in general. Indeed, Rubin and colleagues [96] have reported that the ability of MRI to dif-ferentiate between lacrimal sac diverticulum and regional neoplasm is limited. MRI may be useful, however, in distinguishing solid from cystic masses, and gadolinium infusion aids in this determination. Secondary invasion of the lac-rimal system can occur from benign and malignant neoplasms arising in sur-rounding structures. Sinus osteomas, fibro-osseous lesions, Wegener's granulomatosis, dermoids, and other orbital and paranasal sinus diseases may involve the lacrimal system. The most common extrinsic lesions affecting the nasolacrimal system are ethmoid sinus mucoceles. The bone expansion associated with these lesions is depicted best by CT [97].

Thyroid orbitopathy in Graves' disease

The early stage of Graves' ophthalmopathy is marked by congestive orbital inflammation that is directed toward the connective tissue of the muscle sheath endomysium but spreads outward with disease progression. Fibrosis occurs in the later stages. The muscle bellies that are enlarged, in the order of greatest frequency, are the inferior, medial, and superior rectus-levator palpebrae complex. The tendons of the extraocular muscles are classically spared, except in some severe cases. The lateral rectus is involved least frequently and is almost never affected in isolation.

In contrast to orbital pseudotumor, thyroid orbitopathy is bilateral in approximately 90% of patients. In unusual cases of isolated muscular enlargement, the inferior and the medial rectus are the most commonly involved. Koornneef [98] elegantly described a possible reason for this distribution. The orbital connective tissue support system is best developed around the inferior oblique and inferior rectus muscles; these muscles, therefore, are most prone to becoming enlarged as a result of mucopolysaccharide deposition. Not infrequently, the author finds central hypodensity by CT and signal hyperintensity on T1-weighted MRI images that diminishes markedly in signal with fat-suppression sequences within the affected muscle (Fig. 6). In patients who have thyroid-associated orbitopathy, lipogenesis, along with mast cell infiltration and fibrosis, has been observed histopathologically in 16 of 23 Mueller's muscle specimens [99]. Because of edema, increased signal in the bellies can be found on T2-weighted images, and this signal can decrease with favorable response to steroid therapy [100,101]. Short tau inversion recovery imaging also has been found useful in such instances and offers intrinsic fat suppression, highlighting edema as bright against a dark background of fat [102]. This particular sequence should be considered an important sequence in routine orbital imaging protocols.

The lipogenic form of the disorder, usually seen in young women, is found in approximately 10% of patients, with increased fat apparent in the lids and orbit on CT scan [103]. Cushingoid and obese patients may also present with excessive orbital fat bilaterally [104]. Globe subluxation, defined as protrusion of the equator of the globe beyond the orbital rim with lid retraction, and optic nerve tethering are seen in the lipogenic form of the disease, as well as in numerous other conditions [105]. Prolapse of fat through the superior orbital fissure, correlating with compressive optic neuropathy, has been reported as a more sensitive and specific sign than dilatation of the optic nerve sheath and distention of the superior ophthalmic vein [106]. This finding, however, is also seen in many normal patients, so it should not be interpreted as a definitive indicator of thyroid orbitopathy.

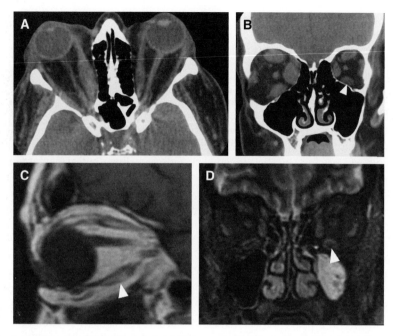

Fig. 6. Dysthyroid orbitopathy. (*A*) Axial CT scan reveals bilateral proptosis and right greater than left myositic enlargement of the cone. (*B*) Coronal mid orbital CT scan shows minimal lucent fatty density in the enlarged muscles (*arrowhead*). (*C*) MRI sagittal T1 pulse in *C* shows T1 bright intramuscular fatty signal (*arrowheads*). (*D*) Signal decreases appropriately in intensity on short tau inversion recovery coronal pulse. The same patient was imaged after orbital decompression 2 months later than *A,* emphasizing MRI's greater sensitivity in depicting minimal soft tissue changes as compared with CT.

Anterior protrusion and enlargement of the lacrimal glands has also been described with Graves' disease.

Pentetreotide (Octreoscan, a synthetic derivative of somatostatin) that has been labeled with 111-Indium is used to localize tumors having surface or membrane receptors for somatostatin. It is thought that retro-orbital lymphocytes express somatostatin receptors on the cellular surface in patients who have active Graves' ophthalmopathy. Pentetreotide has been found to accumulate avidly in the muscles of dysthyroid orbitopathic patients and can be used to assess response to immunotherapy, because decreased uptake is expected [107,108]. This radionuclide scan is helpful in assessing treatment response in patients who have normal scans (Lanreotide, Somatuline).

Orbital trauma

Orbital trauma can result in bony fracture or soft tissue injury to the globe, optic nerve, and orbital soft tissues. Imaging with CT should be done with 3-mm axial cuts; and with coronal imaging, whether by direct scanning or by reformatting the axial data, as an essential addition. The primary reason for coronal images is that inferior orbital fractures, the most common type, can be missed easily on axial-only sections. In the special case of orbital foreign body evaluation, 1.5-mm axial cuts are advised, because objects significantly smaller than a slice thickness of 3 mm may be missed. MRI may be helpful when optic nerve injury or other subtle soft tissue abnormalities need to be evaluated. There is no primary role for plain films in the evaluation of orbital trauma, because they will miss 5% to 10% of fractures and in general are inferior to CT scanning.

Blowout fractures

The most common type of orbital fracture is the "blowout" fracture, in which blunt trauma compresses the orbital contents, raising intraorbital pressure which is relieved through one of the orbital walls. Controversy exists whether the disruptive force is transmitted by the orbital rim or the globe [109]. The typical blowout fracture involves the inferior orbital floor; less commonly, the medial orbital wall (lamina papyracea) is involved. It is postulated from cadaveric studies that less force is required to fracture the inferior wall than the medial wall [110]. The fracture may be comminuted, and small fragments may impale the inferior rectus muscle. The muscle usually herniates with fat through the fracture defect. Entrapment of a muscle can be caused secondarily by fat herniating through the fracture defect, without the muscle, carrying with it supporting connective tissue elements around the inferior rectus and inferior oblique muscles [111]. Although the muscle does not lie within the defect, gaze impairment is apparent clinically. The entrapped muscle may show a distorted shape, such as a "vertical" (asymmetric) inferior rectus on coronal scans (Fig. 7). The force of transmitted sinus air pressure into the orbit is exemplified by a case report of a

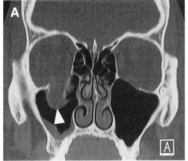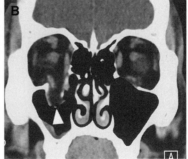

Fig. 7. Inferior orbital wall fracture. (*A*) Coronal CT scan outlines the trapdoor fragment (*arrowhead*) entering the maxillary sinus using bone detail algorithm. (*B*) Soft tissue windowed coronal view reveals fat density in the blowout and a vertical orientation to the inferior rectus contour (*arrowhead*).

70-year-old woman inciting a floor fracture from excessive nose blowing [112]. Damage to the infraorbital nerve is quite common, with the fracture traversing the canal, yielding hypoesthesia. The optic canal must be inspected radiographically in severe injuries, typically high-speed motor vehicle impacts or falls from a height, because the optic strut can fracture and impinge the nerve. The surgeon will be interested in the fracture extent anteroposteriorly for surgical planning purposes; sagittal reformatted views created parallel to the optic nerve are extremely helpful in this regard [113]. Surgery is recommended within 2 weeks of injury in cases of clinically symptomatic diplopia and evidence of orbital soft tissue entrapment on CT examination or large orbital floor fractures that may cause the potential for enophthalmos or hypo-ophthalmos [114]. In about one third of inferior blowout fractures, there is an associated medial wall fracture, the medial blowout fracture, which usually is not surgically significant. When isolated, orbital emphysema is more common in medial blowouts than in floor fractures and usually is found near the site of fracture. Sinus mucosal tearing is a prerequisite for orbital emphysema, and medial wall fractures also are commonly associated with intrasinus acute hemorrhage, which is hyperdense on CT [115]. Medial rectus muscle entrapment rarely occurs in medial blowouts. The medial rectus muscle can be enlarged from edema or hematoma, however [116]. CT will resolve cases of congenital lamina papyracea dehiscence that are not associated with hemorrhage and have well-defined cortical margins at the defect. MRI has been used to assess a small series of adults who had complex strabismus and demonstrated unknown medial orbital wall fractures in three of the six patients [117]. MRI can demonstrate orbital floor fractures as sensitively as CT, but CT remains superior to MRI in depicting small and associated fractures [118]. An unusual orbital fracture variant is the "blow-in" fracture, in which the fracture fragments are driven upward to impinge on the inferior rectus muscle. This fracture has been reported as a relatively rare fracture of the greater sphenoid wing-lateral orbital wall, with pan-muscular impingement [119]. Surgical repair of orbital wall fracture relies on synthetic allograft meshes, such as Teflon, Silastic, or polypropylene (Marlex) mesh, and porous polyethylene (Medpor). Titanium plates and mesh as thin as 0.4 mm can be used to reconstruct large bony gaps. CT will visualize various types of grafts, usually in the setting of suspected graft migration, extrusion, or infection. Titanium produces less artifact than stainless steel on MRI scan, does not deflect or cause a change in temperature while in the magnet, and can be scanned safely in a standard 1.5T MRI unit [120]. On CT, the thinner the titanium mesh size, the less streak or star artifact will occur from computer reconstruction. Medpor polyethylene implants are porous, appearing as a hypodense, linear strip on CT, in contrast to adjacent soft tissue, bone, or mucosa. The mean density of this implant varies between −30 and −50 HU, midway between the mean densities of water and fat [121]. Fibrovascular ingrowth of the Medpor implants can be assessed serially by contrast MRI. Gadolinium enhancement occurs as early as 1.5 months after implantation and in globe implants can enhance centripetally over the first 6 months' time [122]. If a nonmetallic graft is not well seen by CT, MRI imaging in the coronal plane, using T1-weighted sequences with and without fat-suppression, is most helpful. Autografts of cartilage (ie, nasal septum) have been described for fracture repair and promoted as less prone to complication. Autografts appear as soft tissue density against the dark orbital fat by CT [123].

Silent sinus syndrome

The silent sinus syndrome was first reported in 1994 by Soparkar and colleagues [124] in a series of 19 patients. Also known as imploding antrum and chronic maxillary sinus atelectasis, silent sinus syndrome consists of the defined criteria of maxillary sinus volume loss, painless enophthalmos or hypoglobus, and subclinical maxillary sinusitis [125]. The inciting anatomic event seems to be obstruction of the anterior ostiomeatal unit (OMU) at the infundibulum, with the uncinate process commonly deviated laterally toward the inferior orbital wall, which it may oppose (Fig. 8). Manometric studies have confirmed negative maxillary intrasinus pressure of the affected side as a result of OMU obstruction, compared with the contralateral isobaric maxillary antrum [126]. All four maxillary sinus walls typically are retracted, but the inferior orbital wall always is affected and usually is thinned [127]. The radiologic finding of maxillary sinus volume loss can be misinterpreted easily as hypoplasia of the antrum, which should not be associated with hypoglobus and OMU obstruction [128]. The disease process is treated by functional endoscopic sinus surgery by creating a nasal antral window or maxillary antrostomy [129,130]. In some cases, there is resolution of the enophthalmos from the aeration created by the antrostomy. If, after several months, radiographic evidence of resolution is not

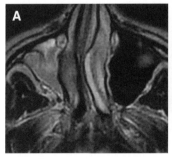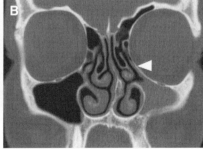

Fig. 8. Silent sinus syndrome. (*A*) Axial T2-weighted MRI image of the first patient shows a much smaller right maxillary antral volume, occupied by central T2 faintly bright inspissated secretion. (*B*) A different patient, coronal CT bone windowed image, clearly depicting a laterally deviated uncinate process opposing the inferior orbital wall (*arowhead*). (Images courtesy of Dr. Peter Hildenbrand.)

demonstrated, a second stage of reconstruction of the orbital floor can be undertaken [131].

Orbital hematomas

Orbital hematomas may be significant, because they can cause increased orbital pressure leading to optic neuropathy. Proptosis of the globe and lengthening of the optic nerve are clues to increased orbital pressure. Subperiosteal orbital hematomas are rare, affecting younger individuals who have a weaker attachment of the periorbita to bone. The subperiosteal hematomas are formed, ellipsoid, hyperdense masses that abut bone in the extraconal orbit (Fig. 9). They can present anywhere in the orbit,

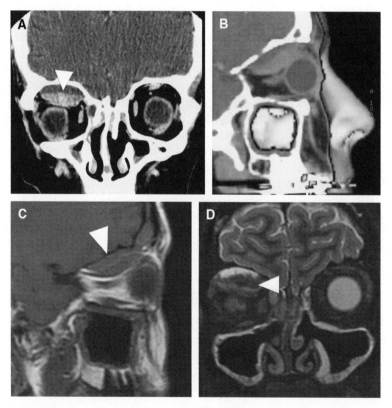

Fig. 9. Hematic cyst. (*A*) Coronal CT shows a fluid–fluid level hematocrit effect (*arrowhead*) in a sharply circumscribed right orbital mass inseparable from the bony roof, subperiosteal. (*B*) Sagittal reformat best depicts the true anterior-posterior extent of hemorrhage, with hypoglobus. (*C*) T1 sagittal plane image showing the lesion (*arrowhead*) to be mildly hyperintense to muscle, deflecting the superior rectus-levator complex inferiorly. (*D*) The short tau inversion recovery coronal plane image again shows the hematocrit effect, dark aggregated red blood cells and cellular debris (*arrowhead*); plasma above is of fluid signal, T2 bright. This cyst resolved slowly over the next 3 months.

including the muscles. The orbital roof is the most common site for hematic cysts [132]. A persistent hematoma, particularly one that is adjacent to the frontal bone, may evolve into a hematic cyst analogous to the pathologic temporal bone cholesterol cyst (or "granuloma"). Blood breakdown products may exert an osmotic effect, resulting in progressive cyst enlargement. Because of their proteinaceous content, hematic cysts are hyperdense on CT and hyperintense on all MR pulse sequences, without significant enhancement unless infected or inflamed [133].

Zygomaticomaxillary complex fracture

A tripod fracture is diagnosed when there is diastasis of the zygomatico-frontal in association with fractures involving the zygomatic arch fractures and the inferior orbital rim. The rim fracture usually extends posteriorly along the floor. The resulting maxillary fragment rotates inferomedially, yielding a flattened cheek (Fig. 10). Currently, the fracture is commonly referred to as a fracture of the zygomaticomaxillary complex. It is usually tetrapod in configuration, involving the four bony support points of the zygoma, maxilla, orbit, and frontal bone. The zygomaticomaxillary complex fracture can be considered a fracture of the "lateral orbital buttress," one of three proposed facial buttresses [134]. CT scanning is the preferred diagnostic method. 3D, surface-shading, reformatted views of the bony anatomy in several projections are helpful in the surgical planning process.

LeFort fractures

Fractures of the midface may affect the orbits. These fractures originally were described by René LeFort in the 1800s, based on his experiments his experiments on cadavers. The LeFort I fracture results from a blow to the upper lip, resulting in a "floating palate" but no orbital injury. LeFort II fractures result in a pyramid-shaped central fracture fragment extending

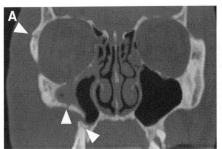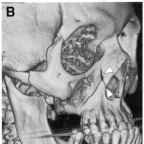

Fig. 10. Zygomaticomaxillary fracture. (*A*) A coronal CT image depicts some of the right zygomaticomaxillary fracture lines (*arrowheads*). (*B*) The extent of injury is shown more fully by volume-rendered 3D views. This patient also had a right nasal cavity pyriform aperture fracture (*arrowheads*).

outward from the nasofrontal sutures to the medial orbits bilaterally and inferolaterally to the zygomaticomaxillary sutures. The pterygoid plates are fractured. The central pyramidal fragment is displaced posteriorly, creating a "dishface" deformity. The LeFort III fractures result in a "floating face" deformity, so called because the fracture radiates from the nasal bridge outwards and posteriorly along the orbital floors, with separation of the upper zygomata from the cranium. The fracture lines in a LeFort III injury can be likened to the outline of wire-rimmed glasses (Fig. 11). The lateral orbital walls are included in the fracture arc, as are the pterygoid plates. The ethmoid plate, sphenoid sinus, and optic canals may be involved, and cerebrospinal fluid rhinorrhea indicates a breach of the dura.

Nasoethmoidal complex fractures

Fractures of the nasoethmoidal complex result when the nasal bones impact the anterior cribriform plate and frontal sinuses (Fig. 12). With increasing severity of injury, the ethmoid orbital plates can be fractured. The medial canthal tendon overlying the lacrimal sac is injured and impairs the lacrimal pump system. Damage to the nasolacrimal system, with chronic fibrosis leading to epiphora, is a frequent concern, as with other midface

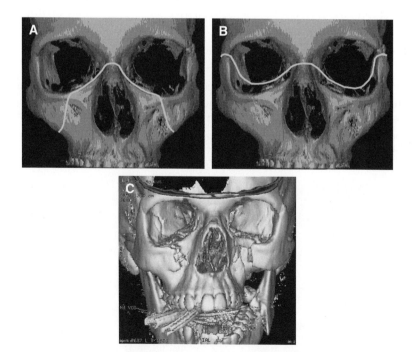

Fig. 11. Lefort fracture. (*A*) Fracture line pattern of LeFort II injury. (*B*) LeFort III type fracture line pattern. (*C*) Volume-rendered anterior projection CT scan of patient suffering LeFort II fracture "dishface" deformity from high-speed motor vehicle accident.

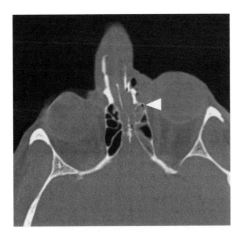

Fig. 12. Nasoethmoidal complex fracture. Mild impaction of the left lacrimal and nasal bones into the anterior ethmoid labyrinth (*arrowhead*). Dark air lucency at the medial canthal region is from trauma and is not within the lacrimal sac.

injuries (ie, LeFort fractures). Leakage of cerebral spinal fluid also is a frequent complication because of the thin dural covering of the cribriform plate. Infection and pneumocephalus may result.

Optic canal fracture

Fractures of the optic canal are rare, occurring most commonly in association with midface injuries of the LeFort type or, more unusually, in isolation. Orbital apex fracture is commonly seen with optic canal injury, as extension of lines of force. Sphenoid fractures are almost always present, and sinus blood levels should be sought out (Fig. 13). Nerve edema, perineural hematoma, and frank transection of the optic nerve at the apex or canal can occur. The optic canal itself can be imaged in an oblique sagittal plane by CT or by MRI to assess injury fully but is imaged adequately on thin-cut coronal CT. MRI demonstrates the status of the optic nerve more fully than CT in clinically ambiguous cases, with optic nerve swelling and edema usual findings. Actual transection of the optic nerve is rare but may be seen on CT as discontinuity of the nerve or on MRI as a better-defined gap associated with traumatic findings.

Injury to the globe

Globe injury can manifest as penetrating or blunt injury. The blunt trauma mechanism more commonly results in blowout fracture, whereas penetrating injuries spark a search for foreign body and signs of ocular hypotonia. The globe may appear completely normal in the presence of clinical globe rupture, but the classic ''flat-tire'' appearance of a shrunken and irregular contoured globe is quite characteristic for rupture radiographically

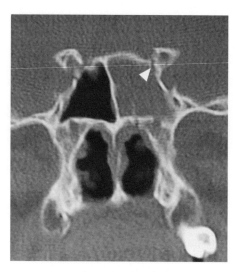

Fig. 13. Optic canal fracture. Bilateral sphenoid bone fractures track vertically into both optic canals, particularly the left (*arrowhead*). There is no bone fragment impinging the canals.

by CT. Subtler cases may show mildly decreased volume in the anterior chamber unilaterally as the only CT finding.

The lens can also sublux or dislocate from the anterior chamber. If the lens shows decreased density compared with the contralateral side, there may be acute edema resulting in traumatic cataract formation, which will be obvious clinically.

Ocular hypotonia can result in a serous choroidal detachment, seen as a subretinal semilunar or crescentic water-density collection bulging into the vitreous with wide sparing of the area around the nerve disc, in contrast to retinal detachment. In many cases, however, it is difficult to distinguish retinal from choroidal detachment. Hemorrhagic choroidal detachments usually cannot be differentiated from the serous type by shape, because both are in the same compartment. Hemorrhage is usually hyperdense by CT and follows hemorrhagic MR signal. Hemorrhage has complex signal patterns on MRI [135], but commonly is imaged in the early and late sub-acute phase as T1-bright signal. Acute hemorrhage is high density on CT. In contrast to detachment, choroidal effusion appears as a crescentic or fully concentric thickening of the uvea central to the sclera with increased signal on T1- and T2-weighted MR sequences [136].

Unenhanced thin-slice CT is the preferred modality for evaluating ocular trauma and the presence of a foreign body. MRI can offer even more information on vitreous abnormalities if the clinical examination is not clear.

Orbital foreign bodies

Orbital foreign bodies such as metal, wood, vegetable matter, and plastic can enter the globe or orbit. Intraocular air seen on CT should cause suspicion of penetrating injury with a potential foreign body (Fig. 14). Air under the lid can be mistaken for a foreign body or injury. Detection of wood foreign bodies is difficult, because dry wood can mimic air lucency, both being black. With proper windowing and level settings, however, dry and fresh wood can be distinguished from fat and air on CT. On MRI, dry wood is hypointense on all sequences because of the lack of mobile protons [137]. T1-weighted imaging has been preferred because of its speed and intrinsic orbital contrast. CT is preferred over MRI for the detection of wooden foreign body, despite case reports of false-negative findings by CT [138,139].

There have been reports of contact lenses migrating into the lid, subconjunctiva, and even into the postseptal orbit. A contact lens "reappearing" over the cornea 12 years after its disappearance has been reported [140]. Other unusual foreign bodies reported in the literature include pens, pencils, teeth, and spearlike metallic objects [141].

Plastic compounds can have low CT densities, in the −100 HU range [142]. Depending on their composition, plastics may not be seen by CT [143]. The HU can considerably vary with plastic and glass compounds. Glass also may not be visualized by conventional radiography [144]. Experimentally, glass has been readily detected by CT [145]. Metal is visualized easily by CT; MRI obviously is contraindicated in these cases. Metallic star artifact from CT reconstruction algorithm can easily blur out the true margins of the object, making precise localization more difficult. Newer algorithms by some manufacturers, such as the Siemens CT units that employ "extended scale," can compensate for the star artifact by increasing the upper HU range.

As an overall generalization, CT may miss nonmetallic foreign bodies, so clinical information is paramount in the work-up. CT should be performed in at least 1.5-mm thin axial cuts to detect small foreign bodies reliably. Both 1-mm and 3-mm cuts will reliably detect all metallic foreign bodies larger than 0.06 mm^3; the difference in detection sensitivity between helical and conventional technique is not significant [146]. Additional planes of imaging are also helpful, particularly oblique sagittal views oriented along the optic nerve.

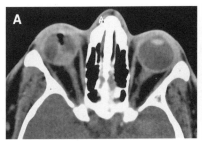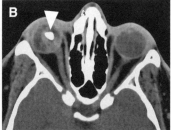

Fig. 14. Metallic foreign body. (*A*) Air lucency in the vitreous associated with more posterior hyperdense hemorrhage, right globe. (*B*) Very high-density metallic foreign body (*arrowhead*) accounts for the air and hemorrhage, a penetrating injury with clinical globe rupture.

References

[1] Schuknecht B, Graetz K. Radiologic assessment of maxillofacial, mandibular, and skull base trauma. Eur Radiol 2005;15:560–8.

[2] Lweandowski RJ, Rhodes CA, McCarroll K, et al. Role of routine nonenhanced head computed tomography scan in excluding orbital, maxillary, or zygomatic fractures secondary to blunt head trauma. Emerg Radiol 2004;10:173–5.

[3] Ewing AE. Roentgen ray demonstration of the lacrimal abscess cavity. Am J Ophthalmol 1909;24:1.

[4] Galloway JE, Kavic TA, Raflo GT. Digital subtraction macrodacryocystography. A new method of lacrimal system imaging. Ophthalmology 1984;91:956–62.

[5] Lloyd GA, Welham RAN. Subtraction macrodacryocystography. Br J Radiol 1974;47: 379–82.

[6] Ashenhurst M, Jaffer N, Hurwitz JJ, et al. Combined computed tomography and dacryocystography for complex lacrimal problems. Can J Ophthal 1991;26:27–31.

[7] Zinreich SJ, Miller NR, Freeman LE, et al. Computed tomographic dacryocystography using topical contrast media for lacrimal system visualization. Orbit 1990;9:79–87.

[8] Perisinakis K, Raissaki M, Theocharopoulos N, et al. Reduction of eye lens radiation dose by orbital bismuth shielding in pediatric patients undergoing CT of the head: a Monte Carlo study. Med Phys 2005;32:1024–30.

[9] Hurwitz JJ, Kassel EE. Dacryocystography. In: Hurwitz JJ, editor. The lacrimal system. Philadelphia: Lippincott-Raven; 1996. p. 63–72.

[10] Rossomondo RM, Carlton WH, Trueblood JH, et al. A new method of evaluating lacrimal drainage. Arch Ophthalmol 1972;88:523–5.

[11] Heyman S, Katowitz JA, Smoger B. Dacryoscintography in children. Ophthalmic Surg 1985;16:703–9.

[12] Rose JDG, Clayton CB. Scintigraphy and contrast radiography for epiphora. Br J Radiol 1985;58:1183–6.

[13] Amanat LA, Hilditch TE, Kwok CS. Lacrimal scintigraphy II: its role in the diagnosis of epiphora. Br J Ophthalmol 1983;67:720–8.

[14] Chavis RM, Welham RAN, Maisley MN. Quantitative lacrimal scintillography. Arch Ophthalmol 1978;96:2066–8.

[15] Guzek JP, Ching AS, Hoang T, et al. Clinical and radiologic lacrimal testing in patients with epiphora. Ophthalmology 1997;104:1875–81.

[16] Goldberg RA, Heinz GW, Chiu L. Gadolinium magnetic resonance imaging dacryocystography. Am J Ophthalmol 1993;115:738–41.

[17] Manfre L, de Maria M, Todaro E, et al. MR dacryocystography: comparison with dacryocystography and CT dacryocystography. AJNR Am J Neuroradiol 2000;21:1145–50.

[18] Menestrina LE, Osborne RE. Congenital dacryocystocele with intranasal extension: correlation of computed tomography and magnetic resonance imaging. J Am Osteopath Assoc 1990;90:264–9.

[19] Yoshikawa T, Hirota S, Sugimora K. Topical contrast-enhanced magnetic resonance dacryocystography. Radiat Med 2000;18:355–63.

[20] Kirchhof K, Hahnel S, Jansen O, et al. Gadolinium-enhanced magnetic resonance dacryocystography in patients with epiphora. J Comput Assist Tomogr 2000;24:327–31.

[21] Hoffman KT, Anders N, Hosten N, et al. High resolution functional magnetic resonance tomography with Gd-DTPA eyedrops in diagnosis of lacrimal apparatus diseases. Opthalmologe 1998;95:542–8.

[22] Takehara Y, Kurihashi K, Isoda H, et al. [Dynamic magnetic resonance dacryocystography using half Fourier single shot fast spin echo sequence]. Nippon Igaku Hoshasen Gakkai Zasshi 1998;58:524–6 [in Japanese].

[23] Oksala A. Diagnosis by ultrasound in acute dacryocystitis. Acta Ophthalmol (Copenh) 1959;37:176.

[24] Jedrzynski MS, Bullock JD. Lacrimal ultrasonography. Ophthalmic Plast Reconst Surg 1994;10:114–20.

[25] Howard R, Caldwell J. Congenital fistula of the lacrimal sac. Am J Ophthalmol 1969;67: 931–4.

[26] Welham RAN, Bergin DJ. Congenital lacrimal fistulas. Arch Opthalmol 1985;103: 545–8.

[27] Tsibidas P, Roussos J. Supernumerary lacrimal canaliculi. Ann Ophthalmol 1979;11:265–7.

[28] Ferreira AP, Gomez RS, Castro WH, et al. Congenital absence of lacrimal puncta and salivary glands: report of a Brazilian family and review. Am J Med Genet 2000;1994: 32–4.

[29] Velhagen K. Der Augenarzt. 3rd edition. Leipzig (Germany): Thieme; 1975.

[30] Irfan A, Cassels-Brown MN. Comparison between syringing/probing, macrodacryocys-tography, and surgical findings in the management of epiphora. Eye 1998;12:197–202.

[31] Irfan S, Cassels-Brown A, Nelson M. Comparison between nasolacrimal syringing/prob-ing, macrodacryocystography and surgical findings in the management of epiphora. Eye 1998;12:197–202.

[32] Williams A, Pizzuto M, Brodsky L, et al. Supernumerary nostril: a rare congenital defor-mity. Int J Pediatr Otorhinolaryngol 1998;44:161–7.

[33] Rochels R, Lieb W, Nover A. Echographische diagnostik bei erkrankungen der ableitenden tranenwege. Klin Monatsbl Augenheilkd 1984;185:243.

[34] Freitag SK, Woog JJ. Congenital nasolacrimal obstruction. Ophthalmol Clin North Am 2000;13:705–18.

[35] Paoli C, Francois M, Polonovski JM, et al. [Cysts of the lacrimal tracts in the newborn infant]. Ann Otolaryngol Chir Cervicofac 1993;110:266–70 [in French].

[36] Guerry D III, Kendig EL Jr. Congenital impatency of the nasolacrimal duct. Arch Ophthal-mol 1948;19:193–202.

[37] Meyer JR, Quint DJ, Holmes JM, et al. Infected congenital mucoceles of the nasolacrimal duct. AJNR Am J Neuroradiol 1993;14:1008–10.

[38] Castillo M, Merten DF, Weissler MC. Bilateral nasolacrimal duct mucocele, a rare cause of respiratory distress: CT findings in two newborns. AJNR Am J Neuroradiol 1993;14: 1011–3.

[39] Raflo GT, Horton JA, Sprinkle PM. An unusual intranasal anomaly of the lacrimal drain-age system. Ophthalmic Surg 1982;13:741–4.

[40] Friedman DP, Rao VM, Flanders AE. Lesions causing a mass in the medial canthus of the orbit: CT and MR features. AJR Am J Roentgenol 1993;160:1095–9.

[41] Sinnreich Z. Lacrimal diverticula. Orbit 1998;17:195–200.

[42] Adjemian A, Burnstine MA. Lacrimal canalicular diverticulum: a cause of epiphora and discharge. Ophthal Plast Reconstr Surg 2000;16:471–2.

[43] Weber AL, Rodriquez-DeVelasquez A, Lucarelli MJ, et al. Normal anatomy and lesions of the lacrimal sac and duct. Neuroimaging Clin N Am 1996;6:199–217.

[44] Freitag SK, Woog JJ, Kousoubris PD, et al. Helical computed tomographic dacryocystog-raphy with three-dimensional reconstruction: a new view of the lacrimal drainage system. Ophthal Plast Reconstr Surg 2002;18(2):121–32.

[45] Sullivan TJ, Clarke MP, Morin JD, et al. The surgical management of congenital lacrimal fistulae. Aust N Z J Ophthalmol 1992;20:109–14.

[46] McNab AA. Congenital absence of the nasolacrimal duct. J Pediatr Ophthal Strabismus 1998;35:294–5.

[47] Pereira L, Dammann F, Duda SH, et al. [Value of dacryocystography in localization diag-nosis of lacrimal ductstenosis]. Rofo 1997;166:498–501 [in German].

[48] Gray LP. Relationship of septal deformity to snuffly noses, poor feeding, sticky eyes and blocked nasolacrimal ducts. Int J Pediatr Otorhinolaryngol 1980;2:201–15.

[49] Yeatts RP. Acquired nasolacrimal duct obstruction. Oculoplastic Surgery Update 1996; 13(4):719–29.

[50] Lindberg JV, McCormick SA. Primary acquired nasolacrimal duct obstruction. A clinico-pathologic report and biopsy technique. Ophthalmology 1986;93:1055–63.

[51] Bartley GB. Acquired lacrimal drainage obstruction: an etiologic classification system, case reports and a review of the literature: part 1. Ophthalmic Plast Reconstr Surg 1992;8: 237–42.

[52] Groessl SA, Bryan SS, Lemke BN. An anatomic basis for primary acquired nasolacrimal duct obstruction. Arch Ophthalmol 1997;115:71–4.

[53] Kallman JE, Foster JA, Wulc AE, et al. Computed tomography in lacrimal outflow obstruction. Ophthalmology 1997;104:676–82.

[54] Dryden RM, Wulc AE. Pseudoepiphora from cerebrospinal fluid leak: case report. Br J Ophthalmol 1986;70(8):570–4.

[55] Spaeth GL. Nasolacrimal duct obstruction caused by topical epinephrine. Arch Ophthalmol 1967;77:355–7.

[56] Migliori ME, Putterman AM. Recurrent conjunctival papilloma causing nasolacrimal duct obstruction. Am J Ophthalmol 1990;110:17–22.

[57] Kassel EE, Schatz CJ. Lacrimal apparatus. In: Som PM, Curtin HD, editors. Head and neck imaging. St. Louis (MO): CV Mosby; 1996. p. 1154.

[58] Berlin AJ, Rath R, Rich L. Lacrimal system dacryoliths. Ophthalmic Surg 1980;11: 435–6.

[59] Sathananthan N, Sullivan TJ, Rose GE, et al. Intubation dacryocystography in patients with a clinical diagnosis of chronic canaliculitis. Br J Radiol 1993;66:389–93.

[60] Malik SR, Gupta AK, Chaterjee S, et al. Dacryocystography of normal and pathological lacrimal passages. Br J Ophthal 1969;53:174–9.

[61] Francis IC, Kappagoda MB, Cole IE, et al. Computed tomography of the lacrimal drainage system: retrospective study of 107 cases of dacryostenosis. Ophthal Plast Reconstr Surg 1999;15:217–26.

[62] Caldemeyer KS, Stockberger SM, Broderick LS. Topical contrast-enhanced CT and MR dacryocystography: imaging the lacrimal drainage apparatus of healthy volunteers. AJR Am J Radiol 1998;171:1501–4.

[63] Hoffmann KT, Hosten N, Anders N. High-resolution conjunctival contrast-enhanced MRI dacryocystography. Neuroradiology 1999;41:208–13.

[64] Pariselle J, Froussart F, Sarrazin JL, et al. Contribution of MRI in the dynamic study of the lacrimal outflow system. J Fr Ophtalmol 1999;22:628–34.

[65] Amrith S, Goh PS, Wang SC. Tear flow dynamics in the human nasolacrimal ducts-a pilot study using dynamic magnetic resonance imaging. Graefes Arch Clin Exp Ophthalmol 2005;243:127–31.

[66] Janssen AG, Mansour K, Bos JJ, et al. Diameter of the bony lacrimal canal: normal values and values related to nasolacrimal duct obstruction: assessment with CT. AJNR Am J Neuroradiol 2001;22:845–50.

[67] Groessl SA, Bryan SS, Lemke BN. An anatomic basis for primary acquired nasolacrimal duct obstruction. Arch Ophthalmol 1997;115:71–4.

[68] Mullner K, Bodner E, Mannor GE. Endoscopy of the lacrimal system. Br J Ophthalmol 1999;83:949–52.

[69] Lee JM, Song HY, Han YM, et al. Balloon dacryocystoplasty: results in the treatment of complete and partial obstructions of the nasolacrimal system. Radiology 1994;192: 503–8.

[70] Wilkins RB, Pressly JP. Diagnosis and incidence of lacrimal canaliculi. Ophthalmic Surg 1980;11:787–9.

[71] Berlin AJ, Rath R, Rich L. Lacrimal system dacryoliths. Ophthalmic Surg 1980;11(7): 435–6.

[72] Jones LT. Tear-sac foreign bodies. Am J Ophthalmol 1965;60:111.

[73] Veirs EW. Lacrimal disorders, diagnosis, and treatment. St. Louis (MO): CV Mosby; 1976. p. 54–9, 74–6.

[74] Bacin F, Kantelip B. [One case of dacryolithiasis of the lacrimal sac]. J Fr Ophtalmol 1981; 4(2):113–6 [in French].

[75] Bradbury JA, Rennie IG, Parsons MA. Adrenaline dacryolith: detection by ultrasound examination of the nasolacrimal duct. Br J Ophthalmol 1998;72(12):935–7.

[76] Jay JL, Lee WR. Dacryolith formation around an eyelash retained in the lacrimal sac. Br J Ophthalmol 1976;60:772.

[77] Epley KD, Karesh JW. Lacrimal sac diverticula associated with a patent lacrimal system. Ophthalmic Plast Reconstr Surg 1999;15(2):111–5.

[78] Stefanyszyn MA, Hidayat AA, Pe'er JJ, et al. Lacrimal sac tumors. Ophthalmic Plast Reconstr Surg 1994;10(3):169–84.

[79] Ni C, Cheng SC, Dryja TP, et al. Lacrimal gland tumors: a clinicopathological analysis of 160 cases. Int Ophthalmol Clin 1982;22(1):99–120.

[80] Sutula FC. Tumors of the lacrimal gland and sac. In: Albert DM, Jakobiec FA, editors. Principles and practice of ophthalmology. Philadelphia: WB Saunders; 1994. p. 1952–67.

[81] Vrabec DP. The inverted Schneidarian papilloma: a clinical and pathological study. Laryngoscope 1975;85:186–220.

[82] Karcioglu ZA, Caldwell DR, Reed HT. Papillomas of the lacrimal drainage system: a clinicopathologic study. Ophthalmic Surg 1984;15:670.

[83] Williams R, Ilsar M, Welham RAN. Lacrimal canalicular papillomatosis. Br J Ophthalmol 1985;69:464–7.

[84] Bosley CE, Pruet CW. Inverted sinonasal papillomas. Ear Nose Throat J 1984;63:509–13.

[85] Migliori ME, Putterman AM. Recurrent conjunctival papilloma causing nasolacrimal duct obstruction. Am J Ophthalmol 1990;110(1):17–22.

[86] Bonder D, Fischer MJ, Levine MR. Squamous cell carcinoma of the lacrimal sac. Ophthalmology 1983;90:1133–5.

[87] Rahangdale SRN, Castillo M, Shockley W. MR in squamous cell carcinoma of the lacrimal sac. AJNR Am J Neuroradiol 1995;16:1262–4.

[88] Stefanyszyn MA, Parnell JR, Mamalis N, et al. Primary adenoid cystic carcinoma of the lacrimal sac: report of a case. Ophthalmic Plast Reconstr Surg 1994;10(2):124–9.

[89] Levine MR, Dinar Y, Davies R. Malignant melanoma of the lacrimal sac. Ophthalmic Surg Lasers 1996;27(4):318–20.

[90] Malik TY, Sanders R, Young JD. Malignant melanoma of the lacrimal sac. Eye 1997;11 (Pt 6):935–7.

[91] McNab AA, McKelvie P. Malignant melanoma of the lacrimal sac complicating primary acquired melanosis of the conjunctiva. Opthalmic Surg Lasers 1997;28(6):501–4.

[92] Kuwabara H, Takeda J. Malignant melanoma of the lacrimal sac with surrounding melanosis. Arch Pathol Lab Med 1997;121(5):517–9.

[93] Billing K, Malhotra R, Selva D, et al. Magnetic resonance imaging findings in malignant melanoma of the lacrimal sac. Br J Ophthalmol 2003;87:1187–8.

[94] Gleizal A, Kodjikian L, Lebreton F, et al. Early CT-scan for chronic lacrimal duct symptoms—case report of a malignant melanoma of the lacrimal sac and review of the literature. J Craniomaxillofac Surg 2005;33:201–4.

[95] Spielmann AC, Debelle L, Lederlin P, et al. [Massive bone destruction: an atypical sign of orbital lymphoma]. J Fr Ophtalmol 1998;21(10):769–72 [in French].

[96] Rubin PA, Bilyk JR, Shore JW, et al. Magnetic resonance imaging of the lacrimal drainage system. Ophthalmology 1994;101:235–43.

[97] Weber AL. Tumors of the paranasal sinuses. Otolaryngol Clin North Am 1988;21:439–54.

[98] Koornneef L. Eyelid and orbital fascial attachments and their clinical significance. Eye 1988;2(Pt 2):130–4.

[99] Cockerham KP, Hidayat AA, Brown HG, et al. Clinicopathologic evaluation of the Mueller muscle in thyroid-associated orbitopathy. Ophthal Plast Reconstr Surg 2002;18(1):11–7.

[100] Ohnishi T, Noguchi S, Murakami N. Extraocular muscles in Graves ophthalmopathy: usefulness of T2 relaxation time measurements. Radiology 1994;190(3):857–62.

[101] Utech CI, Khatibnia U, Winter PFMR. T2 relaxation time for the assessment of retrobulbar inflammation in Graves' ophthalmopathy. Thyroid 1995;5(3):185–93.

[102] Laitt RD, Hoh B, Wakeley C. The value of the short tau inversion recovery sequence in magnetic resonance imaging of thyroid eye disease. Br J Radiol 1994;67(795):244–7.

[103] Forbes G, Gorman CA, Brennan MD. Ophthalmopathy of Graves' disease: computerized volume measurements of the orbital fat and muscle. AJNR Am J Neuroradiol 1986;7(4): 651–6.

[104] Peyster RG, Ginsberg F, Silber JH. Exophthalmos caused by excessive fat: CT volumetric analysis and differential diagnosis. AJR Am J Roentgenol 1986;146(3):459–64.

[105] Rubin PA, Watkins LM, Rumelt S. Orbital computed tomographic characteristics of globe subluxation in thyroid orbitopathy. Ophthalmology 1998;105(11):2061–4.

[106] Birchall D, Goodall KL, Noble JL. Graves ophthalmopathy: intracranial fat prolapse on CT images as an indicator of optic nerve compression. Radiology 1996;200(1):123–7.

[107] Kahaly GJ, Förster GJ. Somatostatin receptor scintigraphy in thyroid eye disease. Thyroid 1998;8(6):549–52.

[108] Krassas GE, Kahaly GJ. The role of OctreoScan in thyroid eye disease. Eur J Endocrinol 1999;140(5):373–5.

[109] Waterhouse N, Lyne J, Urdang M, et al. An investigation into the mechanism of orbital blowout fractures. Br J Plast Surg 1999;52:607–12.

[110] Rhee JS, Kilde J, Yoganadan N, et al. Orbital blowout fractures: experimental evidence for the pure hydraulic theory. Arch Facial Plast Surg 2002;4:98–101.

[111] Harris GJ, Garcia GH, Logani SC, et al. Orbital blow-out fractures: correlation of preoperative computed tomography and postoperative ocular motility. Trans Am Ophthalmol Soc 1998;96:329–47 [discussion: 347–5].

[112] Oluwole M, White P. Orbital floor fracture following nose blowing. Ear Nose Throat J 1996;75:169–70.

[113] Rake PA, Rake SA, Swift JQ, et al. A single reformatted oblique sagittal view as an adjunct to coronal computed tomography for the evaluation of orbital floor fractures. J Oral Maxillofac Surg 2004;62:456–9.

[114] Burnstine MA. Clinical recommendations for repair of isolated orbital floor fractures: an evidence-based analysis. Ophthalmology 2002;109:1207–10.

[115] Shinohara H, Shirota Y, Fujita K. Implication of differences in the incidence of orbital emphysema in ethmoidal and maxillary sinus fractures. Ann Plast Surg 2004; 53:565–9.

[116] Merle H, Gerard M, Raynaud M. Isolated medial orbital blow-out fracture with medial rectus entrapment. Acta Ophthalmol Scand 1998;76:378–9.

[117] Ortube MC, Rosenbaum AL, Goldberg RA, et al. Orbital imaging demonstrates occult blow out fracture in complex strabismus. J AAPOS 2004;8:264–73.

[118] Freund M, Hahnel S, Sartor K. The value of magnetic resonance imaging in the diagnosis of orbital floor fractures. Eur Radiol 2002;12:1127–33.

[119] Yoshioka N, Tominaga Y, Motomura H, et al. Surgical treatment for greater sphenoid wing fracture (orbital blow-in fracture). Ann Plast Surgt 1999;42:87–91.

[120] Sullivan PK, Smith JF, Rozzelle AA. Cranio-orbital reconstruction: safety and image quality of metallic implants on CT and MRI scanning. Plast Reconstr Surg 1994;94:589–96.

[121] Wladis EJ, Wolansky LJ, Turbin RE, et al. Computed tomographic characteristics of porous polyethylene orbital implants. Presented at the 2003 ASOPRS Scientific Symposium. Anaheim, California, November 15, 2003.

[122] De Potter P, Duprez T, Cosnard G. Postcontrast magnetic resonance imaging assessment of porous polyethylene orbital implant (Medpor). Ophthalmology 2000;107:1656–60.

[123] Lai A, Gliklich RE, Rubin PA. Repair of orbital blow-out fractures with nasoseptal cartilage. Laryngoscope 1998;108:645–50.

[124] Soparkar CN, Patrinely JR, Cuaycong MJ, et al. The silent sinus syndrome. A cause of spontaneous enophthalmos. Ophthalmology 1994;101:1763–4.

[125] Numa WA, Desai U, Gold DR, et al. Silent sinus syndrome: a case presentation and comprehensive review of all 84 reported cases. Ann Otol Rhinol Laryngol 2005;114:688–94.

[126] Kass ES, Salman S, Montgomery WW. Manometric study of complete ostial occlusion in chronic maxillary atelectasis. Laryngoscope 1996;106:1255–8.

[127] Hourany R, Aygun N, Della Santina CC, et al. Silent sinus syndrome: an acquired condition. AJNR Am J Neuroradiol 2005;26:2390–2.

[128] Erdem T, Aktas D, Erdem G, et al. Maxillary sinus hypoplasia. Rhinology 2002;40:150–3.

[129] Illner A, Davidson HC, Harnsberger HR, et al. The silent sinus syndrome: clinical and radiographic findings. AJR Am J Roentgenol 2002;178:503–6.

[130] Nkenke E, Alexiou C, Iro H. Management of spontaneous enophthalmos due to silent sinus syndrome: a case report. Int J Oral Maxillofac Surg 2005;34:809–11.

[131] Thomas RD, Graham SM, Carter KD, et al. Management of the orbital floor in silent sinus syndrome. AJR Am J Roentgenol 2003;17:97–100.

[132] Gunalp I, Gunduz K. Cystic lesions of the orbit. Int Ophthalmol 1996;20:273–7.

[133] Privat C, Bellamy J, Courthaliac C, et al. [Chronic hematic cyst of the orbit (orbital subperiosteal hematoma)]. J Radiol 2000;81:811–4 [in French].

[134] Strong EB, Sykes JM. Zygoma complex fractures. Facial Plast Surg 1998;14(1):105–15.

[135] Gomori JM, Grossman RI. Mechanisms responsible for the MR appearance and evolution of intracranial hemorrhage. Radiographics 1988;8:427–40.

[136] Mafee MF. Eye and orbit. In: Som PM, Curtin HD, editors. Head and neck imaging. St. Louis (MO): CV Mosby; 1996. p. 1022–3.

[137] McGuckin JF Jr, Akhtar N, Ho VT, et al. CT and MR evaluation of a wooden foreign body in an in vitro model of the orbit. AJNR Am J Neuroradiol 1996;17(1):129–33.

[138] Specht CS, Varga JH, Jalali MM, et al. Orbitocranial wooden foreign body diagnosed by magnetic resonance imaging. Dry wood can be isodense with air and orbital fat by computed tomography. Surv Ophthalmol 1992;36(5):341–4.

[139] Wesley RE, Wahl JW, Loden JP, et al. Management of wooden foreign bodies in the orbit. South Med J 1982;75(8):924–6, 932.

[140] Roberts-Harry TJ, Davey CC, Jagger JD. Periocular migration of hard contact lenses. Br J Ophthalmol 1992;76(2):95–7.

[141] Bullock JD, Warwar RE, Bartley GB, et al. Unusual orbital foreign bodies. Ophthalmic Plast Reconstr Surg 1999;15(1):44–51.

[142] Duker JS, Fischer DH. Occult plastic intraocular foreign body. Ophthalmic Surg 1989; 20(3):169–70.

[143] Myllylä V, Pyhtinen J, Päivänsalo M, et al. CT detection and location of intraorbital foreign bodies. Experiments with wood and glass 1987;146(6):639–43.

[144] Lindahl S. Computed tomography of intraorbital foreign bodies. Acta Radiol 1987;28: 235–40.

[145] Lakits A, Steiner E, Scholda C, et al. Evaluation of intraocular foreign bodies by spiral computed tomography and multiplanar reconstruction. Ophthalmology 1998;105(2): 307–12.

[146] Chacko JG, Figueroa RE, Johnson MH, et al. Detection and localization of steel intraocular foreign bodies using computed tomography. A comparison of helical and conventional axial scanning. Ophthalmology 1997;104(2):319–23.

ELSEVIER
SAUNDERS

Otolaryngol Clin N Am
39 (2006) 895–909

OTOLARYNGOLOGIC
CLINICS
OF NORTH AMERICA

Traditional Approaches to the Orbit

Aayesha M. Khan, MD, Mark A. Varvares, MD*

*Department of Otolaryngology-Head and Neck Surgery, Saint Louis University School
of Medicine, 3635 Vista Avenue at Grand Boulevard, 6 FDT, Saint Louis, MO 63104, USA*

The orbit is a complex anatomic region that houses, protects, and supports the globe and its intricate network of nerves, vessels, muscles, and glandular and connective tissue structures. It occupies an important functional and aesthetic location, being in close proximity to the cranium, nasal passageways, sinuses, oral cavity, and the bone and soft tissues of the midface. The management of patients with orbital processes can be challenging due to the wide variety of diseases that can develop as an intrinsic problem, as direct extension from cranial, bony, sinonasal, and cutaneous origins, as well as from distant sources (eg, hematogenous spread of infection or metastatic disease from lung, prostate, or breast). Clinical history and physical examination is crucial, and imaging is helpful in localizing the disease process; however, definitive diagnosis and management often requires surgical intervention. A thorough knowledge of orbital anatomy and its adjacent structures is essential to perform any surgical procedure involving the orbit. This article briefly discusses the orbital anatomy, focuses on the principles of orbital surgery, and details the traditional, that is, external, surgical techniques.

Surgical anatomy

The orbit begins to develop in the sixth week of gestation, and ossification is completed shortly after birth. It consists of seven bones that form a four-sided pyramid that becomes three-sided near the apex and has a volume of approximately 30 cm^3. Anteriorly it forms a wide rim that Whitnall [1] described as a spiral with its two ends overlapping medially on the either side of the lacrimal fossa. The superior orbital rim is formed by the frontal bone, the lateral rim by the zygomatic bone, the medial rim by the frontal

* Corresponding author.
E-mail address: mark.varvares@tenethealth.com (M.A. Varvares).

0030-6665/06/$ - see front matter © 2006 Elsevier Inc. All rights reserved.
doi:10.1016/j.otc.2006.08.008
oto.theclinics.com

process of the maxillary bone joined by the maxillary process of the frontal bone, and the inferior orbital rim by the maxillary bone medially and the zygomatic bone laterally. The orbital roof consists of the thin orbital plate of the frontal bone that separates the orbit from the frontal sinuses anteriorly and the anterior cranial fossa posteriorly. Prominent frontal sinuses that extend posteriorly can limit the exposure gained by the superior approach to the orbit [2]. The posterior 1.5 cm of the orbital roof is formed by the lesser wing of the sphenoid bone as the roof tapers backwards and downwards toward the orbital apex into the anterior clinoid process. The optic nerve enters the orbit through the optic foramen located in the posterior orbital roof. The lacrimal gland fossa is located in the lateral orbital roof and the trochlear fossa in the anteromedial orbital roof.

The lateral orbital wall is formed by the zygomatic bone anteriorly and the greater wing of the sphenoid bone posteriorly. It is extremely thick anteriorly, thin in the middle where it forms the medial wall of the temporalis fossa, and becomes thick again posterior to the sphenozygomatic suture. This varying thickness of the lateral orbital wall is important to recognize in the lateral approaches to the orbit [3]. The Whitnall's tubercle is 1.2 to 1.5 cm posterior to the lateral orbital rim, and marks the attachment of the lateral canthal tendon, which should be reattached if injured during surgery. The posterior extent of the lateral wall is defined by the superior orbital fissure created by the gap between the greater and lesser wings of the sphenoid bone, and the inferior orbital fissure created by the gap between the maxillary bone and the greater wing of the sphenoid bone.

The medial orbital walls are approximately parallel to each other and to the mid-sagittal plane. From anterior to posterior, the medial orbital wall is formed by the frontal process of the maxillary bone, which is a thick bone that forms the medial orbital rim; the lacrimal bone, a thin plate that contains the posterior lacrimal crest and forms the posterior half of the lacrimal sac fossa; the lamina papyracea of the ethmoid bone, which is a thin plate (0.2–0.4 mm) that separates the orbit from the ethmoid air cells; and the body of the sphenoid bone, which completes the medial wall to the apex. The frontoethmoid suture line marks the superior limit of the medial orbital wall. It contains the anterior and posterior ethmoidal foramina approximately 20 to 25 mm and 32 to 35 mm posterior to the anterior lacrimal crest, respectively [4,5]. These foramina transmit corresponding arteries, and should be identified to prevent hemorrhage and also because they mark the approximate level of the cribriform plate that separates the floor of the anterior cranial fossa and the roof of the ethmoid sinus. A cerebrospinal fluid leak can occur if the medial orbital wall is penetrated superior to these foramina.

The orbital floor is the shortest orbital wall, formed primarily by the orbital plate of the maxillary bone overlying the maxillary sinus. The anterolateral segment is formed by the zygomatic bone and the posterior segment by the palatine bone. The floor forms a triangular wedge from the maxillary-ethmoid buttress to the inferior orbital fissure horizontally, and the orbital rim to the posterior wall of the maxillary sinus, that is, it does not reach the orbital apex. The infraorbital groove transmitting the infraorbital nerve and artery begins at the inferior orbital fissure and runs forward in the maxillary bone, becoming the infraorbital canal anteriorly ending as the infraorbital foramen 6 to 10 mm inferior to the inferior orbital rim. The floor is thin medial to the infraorbital canal, and surgery on the orbital floor requires special attention to prevent injury.

The four rectus muscles define the muscle cone dividing the orbit into extraconal and intraconal compartments. Surgical spaces have been described (Fig. 1) and include (1) subperiosteal space, which is a potential space between the periorbita and bony walls; (2) peripheral space between the periorbita and extraocular muscle cone; (3) central space encompassed by extraocular muscles; and (4) Episcleral or Tenon's space between the Tenon's capsule and the sclera [6]. The site of involvement determine the selection of the surgical approach.

Principles of orbital surgery

The first procedure for removal of the globe for ocular cancer was performed by a barber surgeon, George Bartisch, in the sixteenth century [7]. There are many indications for orbital surgery that may require biopsy, resection, or reconstruction. The surgical approaches to the orbit are designed to enable the most direct access to the lesion/area of interest, and depend on the location of the lesion within the orbit. Surgical intervention on the anterior half of the orbit is approached via an anterior orbitotomy and that in the posterior half by lateral or more extensive transcranial approaches.

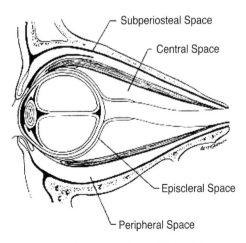

Subperiosteal Space

Central Space

Episcleral Space

Peripheral Space

Fig. 1. Surgical spaces of the orbit. (*From* Osguthorpe JD, Saubders RA, Adkins WY. Evaluation of and access to posterior orbital tumors. Laryngoscope 1983;93:766–71; with permission.)

The optimum surgical approach should provide wide exposure, which is the key to adequate resection with minimal risk of morbidity and mortality. Achieving meticulous hemostasis is imperative to prevent increase in intraocular pressure and risk to optic nerve. In the case of orbital lesions, size of the lesion and involvement of adjacent structures are additional important determinants of the surgical approach. A multidisciplinary approach with collaboration with the neurosurgeon or the ophthalmologist may be required. The use of endoscopes has made significant advances in the surgical techniques involving the orbit; the focus of this article, however, is to detail the various external, or so-called traditional approaches.

Anterior orbitotomy

This approach is used to gain access to the anterior half of the orbit and in some cases also to the posterior orbit. Anterior orbitotomy is defined as a transcutaneous or transconjunctival approach to the orbital or periorbital space that does not involve removal of the lateral orbital wall [8]. Removal of the inferior rim to access the floor or enter the maxillary sinus, and removal of the superior orbital margin to improve exposure to the superoanterior orbital space are included in this technique. The location of the incision used in the anterior approach is further determined by the quadrant (medial, lateral, superior, or inferior) and the surgical space involved. Cosmesis is an important consideration when planning a cutaneous incision, which should be placed along the relaxed skin tension lines. The transcutaneous approaches (Fig. 2) are categorized as extraperiosteal (orbital rim) or trans-septal (eyelid) [9]. The transconjunctival approach was first described

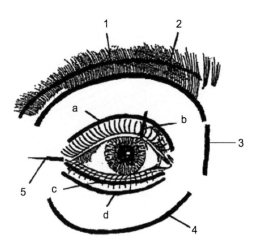

Fig. 2. Cutaneous incisions for anterior orbitotomy. Extraperiosteal incisions 1–5: (1) brow; (2) subbrow; (3) Lynch; (4) inferior rim; (5) lateral canthal. Trans-septal incisions a–d: (a) upper eyelid; (b) vertical lid-split; (c) subciliary; (d) mid-tarsal.

in 1924 [10], and started to be used for repairing facial trauma in the 1971 [11]. It provides quick and easy access via a cosmetically ideal incision, and is categorized as presepatal when the orbital septum is not violated, or retroseptal, which is more direct but violates the orbital septum, resulting in extrusion of orbital fat into the surgical field [12]. Both the extraconal and intraconal spaces can be accesed. Studies have shown a lower incidence of ectropion or lid position complications with the transconjuctival approach [13,14].

Anterior medial approaches (superomedial orbitotomy)

The medial orbit including the roof and floor, the nasolacrimal sac and duct, the anterior and posterior ethmoid foramina, the ethmoid sinus for external ethmoidectomy, the sphenoid sinus via the posterior ethmoid air cells, and the optic nerve via the sphenoid sinus is easily accessed via this approach.

The transcutaneous approach uses the Lynch incision, which is a slightly curved vertical incision beginning along the inferior aspect of the medial brow, approximately midway between the inner canthus and the dorsum of the nose and extending 2 to 3 cm inferiorly. Dissection is carried down to the periosteum, which is incised and elevated. The anterior and posterior ethmoidal arteries should be identified and cauterized. The medial canthal ligament may be elevated, and should be reapproximated. Care should be taken to prevent detachment of the trochlea and injury to the lacrimal sac. For extensive lacrimal sac and duct lesions, the Lynch incision can be extended inferiorly to include a lateral rhinotomy. The subperiosteal space can be easily approached to drain a subperiosteal abscess. Disadvantages include limited access to the orbital floor and the residual scar, which can be unacceptable. Many modifications have been described, inclusion of the Z-plasty being the most commonly used to prevent webbing and scarring (Fig. 3).

The transconjunctival approach can be used to access the medial orbital wall and both the medial extraconal space via the transcaruncular and medial intraconal space via the medial inferior fornix approach. The trans-caruncular approach requires an incision through the medial conjunctiva, between the plica and the caruncle, posterior to the lacrimal puncta and canaliculi, and extending into the superior and inferior fornices [9]. Cotton-tip applicators are used for careful blunt dissection, which is carried behind the lacrimal sac, along the posterior limb of the medial canthal tendon known as Horner's muscle. The medial wall and inferomedial floor (for orbital decompression), trochlea, retrotrochlear space, medial rectus, as well as the superior oblique muscle can be accessed.

The medial inferior fornix approach gives access to the anterior intraco-nal space and is primarily used for optic nerve sheath fenestration. A medial 180° conjunctival incision near the corneal limbus is made using scissors,

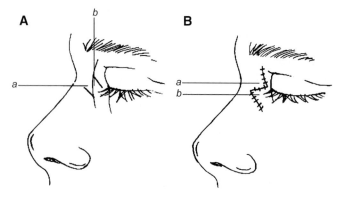

Fig. 3. Z-plasty modification of Lynch incision. (*A*) Preoperative; (B) postoperative. a,b positions of two skin flaps (*From* Patel BCK, Eisa MS, Flaharty P, et al. Orbital decompression for thyroid eye disease. In: Toth BA, Keating RF, Stewart WB, Eds. Atlas of Orbitocranial Surgery, 2nd edition. London: Martin Dunitz Ltd; 1999; with permission).

and if needed, relaxing incisions in the superior and inferior fornices can be made. This approach requires resection and medial retraction of the medial rectus muscle. The Tenon's capsule is then entered, which exposes the orbital fat, and care should taken at this point not to damage the vortex veins. Careful blunt dissection along the globe exposes the anterior nerve sheath, which is frequently covered with posterior ciliary vessels. These are end-arteries, and injury should be avoided. The central retinal artery enters the ventral surface of the optic nerve 8 to 15 mm posterior to the globe, and its disruption can result in rapid and irreversible blindness. After hemostasis is achieved, the medial rectus muscle is reattached and the conjunctiva closed.

Anterior lateral approaches

Lacrimal gland tumors, lesions involving the intra- or extraconal spaces inferior to the lacrimal gland and the lateral canthal ligament, can be accessed using the anterior lateral approach. Deeper lesions of the lateral orbit require a lateral osteotomy which, by definition, is not included in the anterior lateral approaches and will be discussed later.

The lateral rim approach uses a transcutaneous incision to expose the anterior lateral extraconal space [9]. A transverse incision from the lateral canthus toward the temporal fossa is made, and a lateral canthotomy followed by cantholysis of the superior and inferior crura is performed. The limbs are tagged with 4.0 sutures and reflected, the periosteum at the lateral rim is incised, and the periorbita is then elevated off the lateral orbital wall and incised to enter the desired space. Care should be taken not to injure the zygomaticotemporal and zygomaticfacial vessels. After the completion of the procedure the lateral canthal tendons are sewn together and to the periosteum and the incision closed. Eyelid retraction and lateral canthal rounding are risks involved with this incision.

Both the anterior lateral extraconal and intraconal spaces as well as the inferolateral orbit can be accessed via the transconjunctival approach. The incision begins in the lateral inferior fornix followed by canthotomy and cantholysis. The extraconal space can be accessed by the same technique described above. The intraconal space is accessed through the lateral conjunctiva.

Anterior superior approaches

The extra- and intraconal anterosuperior and superonasal spaces can only be accessed transcutaneously using the extraperiosteal (brow and sub-brow) or the trans-septal (upper eyelid crease and vertical lid-split) approaches (Fig. 2). A transconjunctival approach for the anterior superior spaces has not been described.

The brow and subbrow incisions provide direct access to the anterosuperior orbit all the way to the apex. The incision is carried down to the periosteum, which is then incised and elevated at the superior orbital rim to the area of interest, at which point the periosteum is opened and orbital fat encountered. Cotton-tip applicators and malleable retractors are used to keep the orbital fat out of the surgical field. Care should be taken to preserve the supraorbital and supratrochlear neurovascular bundles. Ten to 12 mm of the lateral superior orbital rim can be safely removed without the risk of entering the intracranial cavity, and provides access for deeper and more infiltrative lesions. The superomedial rim is often aerated by the frontal sinus and can be entered, resulting in injury to the nasofrontal duct or the sinus mucosa if the rim is excised in the medial region. Obliteration of the frontal sinus is necessary in that situation. A preoperative CT scan identifies the sinuses and can guide the extent of resection. At the completion of the procedure it is not important to close the periosteum at the rim before closing the soft tissue and skin.

The upper eyelid crease incision is cosmetically more appealing than the brow and subbrow incisions, and can be used to access both the intra- and extraconal spaces. After making the skin incision, orbicularis is divided and the orbital septum is opened, resulting in extrusion of orbital fat, which is then retracted superiorly. Careful dissection is carried posteriorly, separating adhesions between the fat and the levator muscle until adequate exposure of the extraconal space is achieved. The intraconal space can be entered by dividing and disinserting the levator aponeurosis and Mueller's muscle, traditionally achieved by making a transverse incision that can result in alteration of lid height and contour leading to ptosis or lid retraction. A vertical incision prevents this problem. The frontal branch of the facial nerve should be identified and preserved. At the completion of the procedure, the orbicularis may or may not be closed depending on the degree of edema and the laxity of the skin; however, the septum should not be closed because suturing the orbital septum can lead to lagophthalmos.

The vertical lid-split incision was first described by Byron Smith in 1966, as providing improved exposure for removal of anterior superonasal orbital tumors [15]. It has also been shown to provide improved exposure for accessing the deeper intraconal superonasal space without resulting in ptosis or lid retraction [16]. An iris scissors is used to make a vertical, full-thickness incision through the eyelid skin, orbicularis, and the tarsal plate, perpendicular to the lid margin at the junction of its medial and central one third. The incision is extended to the conjunctival fornix and then directed inferiorly through the bulbar conjunctiva to the superonasal limbus. The medial orbit is accessed by performing posterior dissection and the intraconal space by incising the muscular septum between the superior and medial rectus muscles. It is important to identify the tendon of the superior oblique muscle, which traverses the surgical field and is at risk of getting injured. The operating microscope can be used to aid biopsy or removal of the lesion. At completion, the bulbar fornix and palpebral conjunctiva are reapproximated with absorbable sutures, the tarsal plate carefully realigned at the lid margin, and the orbicularis and skin closed.

Anterior inferior approaches

The inferior orbital rim, orbital floor, inferior intra- or extraconal space, the lacrimal duct, and orbital apex can be accessed. The transcutaneous approach is mostly used in cases of severe conjunctival disease when a transconjunctival approach is unsuitable or in cases of extensive orbital floor or nasoethmoid fractues. The transcutaneous approaches include the extraperiosteal (infraorbital) and the trans-septal (lower eyelid) approaches. The infraorbital incision also known as the inferior rim incision, provides the most direct access to the orbital rim and floor but results in a cosmetically objectionable scar. The skin, orbicularis, and periosteum are incised simultaneously and dissection is carried in the subperiosteal plane to expose the area of interest. The lower eyelid approach uses two incisions: (1) the subciliary or lower blepharoplasty, and (2) the subtarsal or mid-lid incision. The subciliary incision is made 2 mm inferior and parallel to the superior free margin of the lower lid, and extends from the medial canthal region to the lateral orbit, ending in one of the relaxed skin tension lines. Dissection is in either the subcutaneous plane between the orbicularis and the skin to the level of the infraorbital rim, or via the skin–muscle technique, which requires dissecting through the orbicularis muscle to raise a flap [17]. Both techniques preserve the position of the pretarsal orbicularis; however, in the first technique the orbicularis muscle is detached from the inferior tarsus. In both techniques the periosteum is incised at the inferior orbital rim and subperiosteal dissection is performed. The subtarsal or mid-lid incision was popularized by John Converse in 1944 [18]. The incision is made 5 to

7 mm inferior to the lower lid margin through the skin and orbicularis, and dissection is carried in the preseptal plane to the level of the orbital rim. The periosteum is incised below the inferior rim, leaving a band of pretarsal orbicularis muscle and its innervation to the tarsal plate.

The transconjunctival approach, also known as the inferior fornix approach, has the advantage of a cosmetically hidden scar [19]. The inferior fornix is exposed by retraction of the lower lid with a Desmarres' retractor, and a malleable retractor placed inside the orbital rim. The incision is made along the entire length and dissection is performed in the preseptal or retroseptal plane. Care should be taken not to injure the lacrimal system when dissecting medially. Exposure may be limited using the transconjunctival approach alone. A lateral canthotomy/cantholysis or combining a transcaruncular incision can improve exposure.

Approaches to the posterior orbit

Access to the posterior half of the orbit and orbital apex generally requires removal of one or more orbital walls or a more extensive procedure requiring a transcranial approach when there is intracranial extension. The transcranial approaches require neurosurgical collaboration, and are not discussed in this article. The next section details the more traditional, external approaches to the posterior orbit.

Lateral orbitotomy with osteotomy

Removal of the lateral orbital wall (to excise a large dermoid) was first described by Kronlein, in 1888 [20]. The Kronlein operation, also called the Swift operation, is now only of historic significance. It required an incision over the lateral orbital rim and removal of the lateral orbital wall. The bony defect was covered with orbital periosteum and temporalis muscle. The scar and the absence of the lateral orbital wall, which exposes the orbit to injury, are the main disadvantages of this technique. In 1954, Berke [21] described a modification of Kronlein's operation in which a horizontal incision beginning at the lateral canthus and extending 3 to 4 cm into one of the crow's feet was made through skin and orbicularis. This approach also required cantholysis of the superior and inferior crura of the lateral canthal tendon before raising the skin muscle flap. Various incisions have since been described. The Stallard-Wright is an S-shaped incision beginning above the frontozygomatic suture and extending inferiorly to the level of the lateral canthus and then posteriorly for 25 mm [22]. A hockey-stick incision begins inferior to the lateral one third of the brow and follows the superior orbital rim to approximately 3.5 cm posterior to the lateral canthus and then continues posteriorly along the superior border of the zygomatic arch [23]. An upper eyelid crease incision or for the more inferior lesions, the subciliary incision extending into one of the crow's feet have also been described.

The more extensive bicoronal incision has been used when additional exposure or adjunctive procedures are required or rarely to avoid a facial scar
[24].

Once adequate exposure of periosteum of the frontal and zygomatic
bones at the lateral orbital rim has been obtained, skin–muscle flaps are
retracted with 4-0 silk sutures. The periosteum is incised approximately
2 mm posterior and parallel to the orbital margin and extended superiorly
above the zygomaticofrontal suture and inferiorly on the zygomatic arch.
The periosteum and the temporalis muscle are elevated and reflected posteriorly. The periorbita is then meticulously elevated off the lateral orbital rim
and wall and a malleable retractor is placed between the globe and the lateral orbital wall. Drill holes are made above and below the planned osteotomies, and a saw is used to make the cuts while continuing to protect the
contents of the orbit with a broad malleable retractor. Irrigating and suc-
tioning while making the osteotomies improves exposure and prevents
heat necrosis of the bone. If additional removal of bone from the temporalis
fossa is required, a rongeur or a cutting burr on the drill can be used. Bleeding can be controlled using bone wax. Once adequate exposure is achieved,
the periorbita is incised in an anterior–posterior direction, the lateral rectus
muscle identified and retracted, and the lesion identified and biopsied or
excised as indicated. At completion of the procedure, the periorbita is
loosely closed using absorbable sutures, the bone segment replaced, and
secured using wires or mini- or microplates. A drain is placed in the temporalis fossa and brought out through the skin posterior to the incision. The
periosteum, temporalis muscle subcutaneous tissue, and skin are closed.
This approach can be combined with anterior medial or inferior approaches
to achieve improved exposure. Complications are rare, and include lateral
rectus dysfunction, diplopia, injury to the ciliary ganglion leading to persistent mydriasis, or injury to the lacrimal gland. Serious injuries include
orbital infections, hematoma, optic nerve injury, and loss of vision.

LeFort I orbitotomy

This relatively recent technique was described by Dailey and colleagues
[25] to remove a 10 × 20 mm cavernous hemangioma of the inferomedial
orbital apex. The incision is made in the maxillary gingivobuccal sulcus between the first molars. The anterior and lateral maxilla is exposed using
a periosteal elevator and a LeFort I osteotomy is made, which separates
the maxilla from the nose and the zygoma on each side, slightly above the
floor of the maxillary sinuses. A straight osteotome is used to section the
medial, lateral, and posterior walls of the maxillary sinus and a curved
osteotome to separate the ptyregoid plates from the posterior maxilla, which
is then down-fractured. It is important to preserve a vascular pedicle in the
posterolateral buccal mucosa and soft palate. The patients head is tilted
backward and toward the operative side and held in place using a Mayfield

head holder. The maxilla is retracted inferiorly and a transanatral ethmoidectomy is performed skeletonizing the orbital apex. The inferomedial orbital wall is removed using rongeurs (Fig. 4), the periorbita opened sharply, and infraorbital dissection carried. At the completion of the procedure, the periorbita is left open, the maxilla rigidly fixed in position, and buccal mucosa closed. This technique is thought to cause less morbidity than a transcranial approach required to access the inferomedial apex. The disadvantages include temporary hypoesthesia of the infraorbital nerve distribution and alteration in sensation of the maxillary teeth.

Orbital decompression—The traditional way

The indications for orbital decompression include compressive optic neuropathy, and more commonly, complications of severe proptosis from thyroid ophthalmopathy. Early orbital decompression surgery involved removal of one orbital wall. As techniques evolved, all four orbital walls were used. The more advanced approaches use the transnasal endoscopic techniques. The next section describes the more traditional approaches (Fig. 5).

Lateral decompression

The first report of orbital decompression for Grave's disease was published by Dollinger in 1911, when he used Kronlein's lateral orbitotomy technique of removing the lateral orbital wall [26]. Any of the lateral orbitotomy techniques described above may be used for removal of the lateral

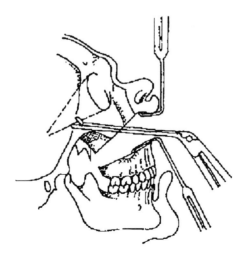

Fig. 4. Sagittal section representation for removal of inferomedial orbital bone through LeFort I orbitotomy. (*From* Dailey RA, Dierks E, Wilkins J, et al. LeFort I orbitotomy: a new approach to the inferonasal orbital apex. Opthal Plast Reconstr Surg 1998;14(1):27–31; with permission.)

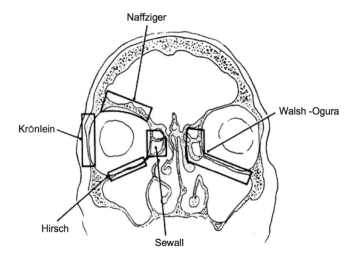

Fig. 5. Traditional approaches for orbital decompression. (*From* Girod DA. Management of Thyroid Eye Disease (Graves' Ophthalmopathy). In: Cummings C, Haughey B, Thomas JR, et al, Eds. Otolaryngology Head and Neck Surgery, 4th edition. St. Louis: Mosby, 2005; with permission.)

orbital wall. The periorbita is incised and the orbital fat is allowed to prolapse in the temporalis fossa. The orbital rim is usually replaced. Complete removal without replacement of the lateral orbital rim requires repositioning the upper and lower canthal tendons to the anterior edge of a periosteal bridge. This technique has also been described [27,28], but may result in cosmetic deformities. For more aggressive lateral decompression, the posterior surface of the lateral wall can be thinned and the residual orbital rim advanced and rotated outward and rigidly fixed [29]. Isolated lateral decompression is not suitable for compressive optic neuropathy. The potential complications of lateral decompression include an obvious scar, injury to the frontal branch of the facial nerve, cosmetic deformities, and injury to the lacrimal gland.

Inferior decompression

Removal of the orbital floor for decompression was first described by Hirsch in 1930 [30]. The Caldwell-Luc approach was used to enter the maxillary sinus, and its roof was removed from either side of the infraorbital nerve canal. The periorbita was excised, which allowed the fat to prolapse into the maxillary sinus. A transantral window was created in the nasoantral wall of the inferior meatus. This technique was considered safe, simple, and did not result in an external scar. A transantral approach, or any of the anterior inferior approaches described to perform the inferior decompression, may be used. Once the orbital rim in exposed and the periosteum elevated, the orbital floor is fractured medial to the infraorbital nerve and the bone removed using rongeurs or Takahashi forceps laterally up to the base of the lateral wall and posteriorly to the posterior wall of the maxillary sinus, which is identified by the thick bone formed by the fusion of the orbital floor, the superomedial wall of the maxillary sinus, and the inferolateral wall of the ethmoid sinus. The posterior removal is essential when treating compressive optic neuropathy.

Superior decompression

A transcranial approach for removal of the orbital roof as far posterior as the optic foramen was described by Naffziger in 1931 [31]. A frontal bone flap is created for unilateral or bilateral decompression, after which the dura is peeled back from the orbital plate, which is removed widely, limited only by the frontal sinus anteriorly and the ethmoids medially. The posterolateral wall is removed and the pterion and sphenoidal ridge are rongeured. The superior orbital rim is preserved to maintain contour. The periorbita is opened widely and the orbital contents allowed to decompress superiorly being in contact with the dura. Achieving meticulous hemostasis is essential. The bone flaps are replaced and soft tissue closed. Disadvantages include prolonged postoperative healing time, higher morbidity, and transmission of cerebral pulsations to the eye.

Medial decompression

In 1936, Sewall [32] described orbital decompression by removing the ethmoid plate via an external approach. The transcutaneous or transconjunctival approaches for anterior medial orbitotomy may be used. The periosteum should be elevated in its entire length including the anterior and posterior lacrimal crests and the lacrimal fossa. The lacrimal sac is carefully dissected laterally. Elevating the periosteum superior to the lacrimal fossa detaches the medial canthal ligament. The anterior and posterior ethmoid arteries are identified and cauterized, the suture line between the lacrimal bone, lamina papyracea, and orbital process of the frontal bone identified. This indicates the level and direction of the roof of the ethmoid and cribriform plate, which is important to know to prevent entering the intracranial cavity. The lacrimal plate or fossa is penetrated to enter the anterior ethmoid cells. Total ethmoidectomy is then completed. The periosteum may be left unapproximated, but the caruncle and conjunctiva need to be closed with interrupted absorbable sutures.

Combined approaches

Transantral orbital decompression using a combination of the Hirsch and Sewell techniques was reported by Walsh and Ogura [33] in 1957. A sublabial incision is used to gain access to the inferior and medial walls. A three-wall decompression was described by Tessier [34] in 1969, and McCord and Moses [35] in 1979. Kennerdell and Maroon [36] used the lateral orbitotomy combined with a transconjunctival incision to achieve four-wall decompression. The inferomedial two-wall technique is the most commonly used technique. The amount of reduction is highly variable; however, on average, single-wall decompression results in approximately 4 mm, two-wall decompression in 6 mm, three-wall decompression in 10 mm, and four-wall decompression in 16 mm of reduction in proptosis [37].

Summary

The selection of the surgical approach to the orbit depends on the indication for surgery and the location, size, and extent of the lesion. For the anterior half of the orbit, anterior orbitotomy provides adequate exposure. For the posterior half, more extensive procedures with osteotomy are necessary. This article details the external approaches to the orbit. The traditional approaches for orbital decompression for Grave's ophthalmopathy are also described.

References

[1] Whitnall SE. The anatomy of the human orbit and accessory organs of vision. New York: Oxford University Press; 1932. p. 1–252.
[2] Doxanas MT. Orbital osteology and anatomy. In: Toth BA, Keating RF, Stewart WB, editors. An atlas of orbitocranial surgery. London: Martin Dunitz, Ltd. 1999. p. 1–10.
[3] Dutton JJ. Clinical and surgical orbital anatomy. Ophthalmol Clin North Am 1996;9(4): 527–39.
[4] Ducasae A, Delattre JF, Segal A, et al. Anatomical basis of the surgical approach to the medial wall of the orbit. Anat Clin 1985;7:15.
[5] Kirchner JA, Yanagisawa E, Crelin ES. Surgical anatomy of the ethmoidal arteries: a laboratory study of 150 orbits. Arch Otolaryngol 1961;74:382.
[6] Osguthorpe JD, Saubders RA, Adkins WY. Evaluation of and access to posterior orbital tumors. Laryngoscope 1983;93:766–71.
[7] Albert DM. In: Albert DM, Jakobiec FA, Azar DT, et al, editors. Principles and practice of ophthalmology. 2nd edition. Vol. 1. Philadelphia: W.B. Saunders; 2000.
[8] Goldberg RA. Anterior orbitotomy. In: Toth BA, Keating RF, Stewart WB, editors. An atlas of orbitocranial surgery. London: Martin Dunitz Ltd. 1999. p. 45–55.
[9] Wojno TH. Surgical approaches to orbital disease. Ophthalmol Clin North Am 1996;9(4): 581–9.
[10] Bourquet J. Les hernies graisseuse de l'orbite: notre traitment chirurgical. Bull Acad Med (Paris) 1924;92:1270.
[11] Tenzel RR, Miller GR. Orbital blowout fracture repair, conjunctival approach. Am J Ophthalmol 1971;7:1141.
[12] Kushner GM. Surgical approaches to the infraorbital rim and orbital floor: the case for the transconjunctival approach. J Oral Maxillofac Surg 2006;64:108–10.
[13] Jacono AA, Moskowitz B. Transconjunctival versus transcutaneous approach in upper and lower belpharoplasty. Facial Plast Surg 2001;17:21.

[14] Patel PC, Soboto BT, Patel NM, et al. Comparison of transconjunctival versus subciliary approaches for orbital fractures. A review of 60 cases. J Craniomaxillofac Trauma 1998;4: 17–21.

[15] Smith B. The anterior surgical approach to orbital tumors. Trans Am Acad Ophthalmol Otolaryngol 1966;70:607–11.

[16] Kersten RC, Kulwin DR. Vertical lid split orbitotomy revisited. Ophthal Plast Reconstr Surg 1999;15(6):425–8.

[17] Wilson S, Ellis E. Surgical approaches to the infraorbital rim and orbital floor. The case for the subtarsal approach. J Oral Maxillofac Surg 2006;64:104–7.

[18] Converse JM. Two plastic operations for repair of orbit following severe trauma and extensive comminuted fracture. Arch Ophthalmol 1944;31:323.

[19] Kushner GM. Surgical approaches to the infraorbital rim and orbital floor: the case for the transconjunctival approach. J Oral Maxillofac Surg 2006;64:108–10.

[20] Kronlein RU. Zur Pathologie und Behandlung der Dermoidcysten der Orbita. Beitr Klin Chirl 1889;4:149–63.

[21] Berke RN. A modified Kronlein operation. Arch Ophtalmol (Paris) 1954;51:609–32.

[22] Stallard HB. A plea for lateral orbitotomy with certain modifications. Br J Ophthalmol 1960; 44:718.

[23] Kennerdell JS, Maroon JC, Malton ML. Surgical approaches to orbital tumors. Clin Plast Surg 1988;15(2):273–82.

[24] Stewart WB, Levin PS, Toth BA. The technique of coronal flap approach to the lateral orbitotomy. Arch Ophthalmol 1988;106:1724–6.

[25] Dailey RA, Dierks E, Wilkins J, et al. Lefort I orbitotomy: a new approach to the infer nasal orbital apex. Ophthal Plast Reconstr Surg 14(1):27–31.

[26] Dollinger J. Die Drukentlastung der Augenhohl durch Entfernung der auBeren Orbitalwand bei hochgradigen exophthalmos (Morbus Basedow) und konsekutiver Hornhuaterkrangkung. Dtsch Med Wochenschr 1911;37:1888–90.

[27] Leone CR, Priest KL, Newman RJ. Medial and lateral wall decompression for thyroid ophthalmopathy. Am J Ophthalmol 1989;108:160–6.

[28] McCord CD. Orbital decompression for Graves' disease: exposure through lateral canthal and inferior fornix incision. Ophthalmology 1981;88:533–41.

[29] Walk AE, Popp JC, Bartlett SP. Lateral wall advancement in orbital decompression. Ophthalmology 1990;97:1358–69.

[30] Hirsch VO, Urbanek GR. Behandlung eines excessiven exophthalmos (Basedow) durch Entfernung von orbital fett von der Kieferhohle aus. Monatsschr F Ohrenh 1930;64:212–3.

[31] Naffziger HC. Progressive exophthalmoses following thyroidectomy: its pathology and treatment. Ann Surg 1931;94:582–6.

[32] Sewell EC. Operative control of progressive exophthalmos. Arch Otolaryngol 1936;24: 621–4.

[33] Walsh TE, Ogura JH. Transantral orbital decompression for malignant exopthalmos. Laryngoscope 1957;67:544–68.

[34] Tessier P. Expansion chirurgicale de l'orbite. Ann Chir Plast 1969;14(2):7–14.

[35] McCord CD, Moses JL. Exposure of the inferior orbit with fornix incision and lateral canthotomy. Ophthalm Surg 1979;10:53–63.

[36] Kennerdell JS, Maroon JC. AN orbital decompression for severe dysthyroid exophthalmos. Ophthalmology 1982;89:467–72.

[37] Patel BCK, Eisa MS, Flaharty P, et al. Orbital decompression for thyroid eye disease. In: Toth BA, Keating RF, Stewart WB, editors. An atlas of orbitocranial surgery. London: Martin Dunitz, Ltd. 1999. p. 119–51.

ELSEVIER
SAUNDERS

Otolaryngol Clin N Am
39 (2006) 911–922

OTOLARYNGOLOGIC
CLINICS
OF NORTH AMERICA

Office Evaluation of Lacrimal and Orbital Disease

Renzo A. Zaldívar, MD[a],*, Daniel E. Buerger, MD[b],
David G. Buerger, MD[b], John J. Woog, MD, FACS[a]

[a]Department of Ophthalmology, Mayo Clinic, 200 First Street SW,
Rochester, MN 55905, USA
[b]Pittsburgh Oculoplastic Associates, 3471 Fifth Avenue #1115, Pittsburgh, PA 15213, USA

Evaluation of the lacrimal system

The anatomy of the lacrimal system is reviewed elsewhere in this issue. Tears are produced by the main and accessory lacrimal glands and are drained by the lacrimal excretory system. Disorders of the lacrimal system most frequently cause a complaint of tearing. Tearing may be a result of hypersecretion from the glands or insufficient drainage of tears through the nasolacrimal system. A thorough office evaluation will identify the cause of abnormal tearing in most patients.

History

A thorough evaluation of the lacrimal system begins with a complete history of the patient's symptoms to determine if the tearing secondary to overproduction or insufficient drainage. The overproduction of tears frequently produces bilateral, intermittent tearing with minimal discharge or crusting. Tearing secondary to insufficient drainage, or epiphora, often occurs constantly and is, by contrast, often unilateral. This condition may be accompanied by complaints of ocular discharge or eyelid crusting, particularly upon awakening. With complete obstruction of the outflow system, infection may develop in the lacrimal system, causing swelling, redness, and tenderness in the medial canthal region. Episodes of lacrimal sac

Portions of this article are reprinted from: Buerger DE, Buerger DG, Woog JJ. Office Evaluation of Lacrimal and Orbital Disease. In: John J. Woog, Ed. Manual of Endoscopic Lacrimal and Orbital Surgery. Philadelphia: Butterworth/Heineman, 2004; with permission.
* Corresponding author.
E-mail address: zaldivar.renzo@mayo.edu (R.A. Zaldívar).

doi:10.1016/j.otc.2006.07.006

infection (dacryocystitis) are usually associated with significant pain around the eye and may progress to periorbital, facial, or, in the case of pediatric patients in particular, orbital cellulitis.

Examination

Physical examination is used to confirm information from the history and to determine the cause of tearing. It is helpful to evaluate each segment of the outflow pathway in an orderly manner following the normal course of tear drainage. The external examination includes an inspection of eyelid position, contour, and function in relation to operation of the lacrimal pump. Eyelid malpositions such as ectropion, in which the punctum is not apposed to the globe, can be associated with epiphora. Facial nerve paresis may be associated with tearing secondary to paralytic ectropion or weakness of the orbicularis muscle required for normal lacrimal pump function. Maceration of the eyelid skin is frequently seen in cases of constant or long-standing tearing.

Punctal abnormalities, in addition to punctal ectropion, may be associated with epiphora. Each punctum is evaluated for patency. The punctum normally is 0.3 mm in diameter; congenital or acquired stenosis or occlusion may interfere with tear discharge. Swelling and erythema surrounding the punctum or canaliculus may signify canaliculitis. In such cases, pressure over the canaliculus, not the lacrimal sac, often results in reflux of mucopurulent discharge or stones.

Palpation of the medial canthus may reveal a mass in the area of the lacrimal sac. Distention or inflammation of the sac can be seen in the medial canthus with outflow obstruction, typically below the level of the medial canthal tendon. Lacrimal sac tumors may extend above the medial canthal tendon. Other masses that may extend above the tendon include paranasal sinus tumors or mucoceles, orbital or nasal epidermoid/dermoid cysts, and meningoencephaloceles. Applying pressure over the sac often results in tenderness and reflux through the puncta. In cases of dacryocystitis, the reflux may be purulent or mucopurulent in nature. Acute dacryocystitis produces a red, swollen, and painful mass in the medial canthus, which may rupture spontaneously (Fig. 1). Nasal examination is performed to allow evaluation of the inferior and middle meatus and to facilitate identification of sinonasal disorders that may contribute to lacrimal outflow obstruction.

Biomicroscopic (slit-lamp) examination, performed by an ophthalmologist, may reveal elevation of the precorneal tear film in the setting of lacrimal obstruction. In addition, slit-lamp examination may demonstrate subtle lacrimal sac reflux as well as evidence of eyelid, conjunctival, corneal, or intraocular inflammation that may be associated with lacrimal hypersecretion.

Several diagnostic tests may be helpful in localizing an obstruction in the lacrimal outflow system. A combination of these tests may be most effective in diagnosing outflow obstruction. The basic Schirmer secretion test is

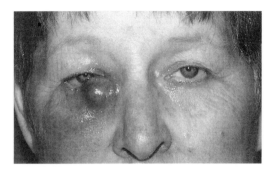

Fig. 1. Acute dacryocystitis.

performed to quantitate tear production. Strips of white filter paper (41 Whatman) are placed at the junction of the middle and lateral thirds of the lower eyelids after administration of a topical anesthetic. With the eyes closed, tear production is measured along the length of the filter paper over a period of 5 minutes. A normal test result yields more than 10 mm but less than 30 mm of tears. In cases of lacrimal outflow obstruction, the measurement may be greater than 30 mm. A normal or low measurement does not rule out the possibility of lacrimal system obstruction because of the possibility of concurrent hyposecretion.

The fluorescein dye disappearance test is performed easily in the office. A topical anesthetic and fluorescein dye (Fig. 2) are placed in the inferior fornix of each eye. The tear film in each eye is observed and compared over a period of 5 to 10 minutes. The fluorescein dye should drain rapidly through a patent outflow system. Persistent dye in the tear film after 10 minutes indicates an abnormality of lacrimal outflow, which may be

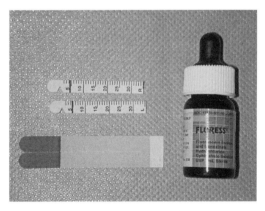

Fig. 2. Filter paper strips (*top*) are placed in the inferior fornix to assess tear secretion. Fluorescein in strip form (*bottom left*) or in solution form (*bottom right*), combined with local anesthetic, may be used to assess the tear film.

functional or anatomic. An abnormal result from a dye disappearance test should prompt additional ancillary testing.

Punctal dilation and canalicular probing are used to evaluate the patency of the proximal lacrimal system. Difficulty with dilation may indicate clinically significant punctal stenosis. Likewise, difficulty with probing through the canaliculus may indicate canalicular strictures and stenosis. Tearing may improve once the areas of stenosis are opened with the lacrimal probe. Easy probing to the lacrimal sac usually is a good indication of patency through the puncta and canaliculi.

Lacrimal irrigation is a simple test that may be used to diagnose the location and extent (complete or partial) of an obstruction. A 23- to 27-gauge cannula attached to a syringe containing sterile saline solution (Fig. 3) is introduced into the proximal canaliculus (usually the lower one) following punctal dilation. Irrigation is generally performed bilaterally, even in patients who have unilateral epiphora, because the normal eye serves as a basis for comparison during this study. With a patent or partially patent lacrimal system the irrigant should pass into the nose. Reflux through the same punctum indicates canalicular obstruction. Reflux through the opposite punctum indicates obstruction distal to the common canaliculus (Fig. 4). Distention of the lacrimal sac or reflux of mucopurulent material may occur with nasolacrimal duct obstruction. Reflux of a bloody solution can indicate lacrimal system inflammation, a lacrimal sac tumor, or trauma to the tissues during insertion of the cannula.

Jones dye tests may be used to differentiate further between functional and anatomic outflow problems. As with the dye disappearance test, the primary dye test is performed by placing topical anesthetic and fluorescein dye in the conjunctival sac. Topical 4% lidocaine and oxymetazoline nasal sprays may be used to anesthetize and vasoconstrict the inferior meatus and

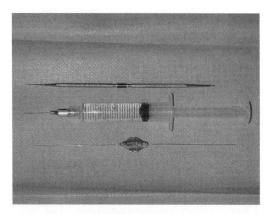

Fig. 3. A punctum dilator (*top*), a lacrimal cannula attached to a syringe containing saline irrigant (*middle*), and a lacrimal probe (*bottom*) are used to assess canalicular patency.

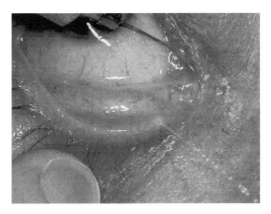

Fig. 4. Reflux of fluorescein-containing saline solution from the superior canaliculus following irrigation through the inferior canaliculus in a patient who has complete nasolacrimal duct obstruction.

turbinate within the nasal cavity. A cotton-tipped applicator is placed beneath the inferior turbinate near the opening of the nasolacrimal duct. Recovery of fluorescein dye in the nose (positive result) indicates a functionally and anatomically patent system. No recovery of dye (negative result) suggests a functional or anatomic blockage. The secondary dye test is performed if no dye is recovered during the primary test. After removal of residual fluorescein from the conjunctival sac, a clear saline solution is placed into the inferior canaliculus using a syringe and cannula. The irrigant is retrieved from the nose by tilting the patient's head forward over a basin. Fluorescein dye within the irrigant (positive result) indicates that dye traveled to the lacrimal sac through a functional upper system and that the lower system is at least partially open but is not functional. Recovery of a clear irrigant (negative result) indicates a functional problem with the upper system.

Further testing outside the office may include a dacryocystogram to evaluate the anatomy of the lacrimal outflow system. This test involves injection of contrast material into the lower canaliculus during serial radiography. The lacrimal outflow system, as well as any anatomic abnormalities, can be visualized as the dye flows down through the sac and nasolacrimal duct. Radiologic evaluation of the lacrimal outflow system is discussed elsewhere in this issue.

In summary, evaluation of the lacrimal system is best performed in a logical sequence to determine whether any functional or anatomic block may be causing abnormal tearing. A thorough office evaluation must include a complete history from the patient and a physical examination supplemented with the appropriate ancillary tests. This strategy will allow determination of the specific cause of abnormal tearing, which is critical in providing appropriate treatment.

Evaluation of the orbit

The office evaluation of a potential orbital disorder should, first and foremost, distinguish orbital from periorbital, intraocular, and sinonasal disorders. A complete evaluation, beginning with a detailed history, is essential in establishing a probable diagnosis and in guiding further work-up and management.

Two of the most common encountered orbital disorders in clinical practice are Graves' disease or thyroid eye disease (TED) and orbital fractures. The endoscope is a useful surgical tool in the management of each of these entities. The remainder of this article focuses on the office evaluation of these disorders.

Thyroid eye disease

Graves' orbitopathy is discussed in detail elsewhere in this issue. By way of brief summary, however, TED is usually diagnosed in the presence of hyperthyroidism, but it may be present in euthyroid or hypothyroid patients. The signs and symptoms may be unilateral or bilateral and often are asymmetric (Fig. 5). Certain criteria have been established to facilitate the diagnosis of TED (Fig. 6). One of the major criteria is the presence of eyelid retraction on clinical examination. In the presence of eyelid retraction, the diagnosis can be made with the presence of one of the following: thyroid dysfunction, exophthalmos, optic nerve dysfunction, or extraocular muscle involvement. In the absence of eyelid retraction, the diagnosis can be made with the presence of thyroid dysfunction and one of the following: exophthalmos, optic nerve dysfunction, or extraocular muscle involvement. Endocrinologic consultation may be helpful in documenting subtle thyroid dysfunction or evidence of autoimmune disease that may support a diagnosis of TED.

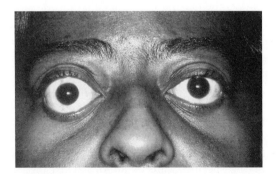

Fig. 5. Eyelid retraction and proptosis in a patient who has thyroid eye disease.

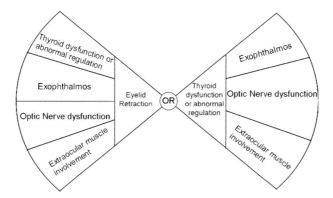

Fig. 6. Diagnostic criteria for thyroid eye disease. (*Reprinted from:* Bartley GB, Gorman CA. Diagnostic criteria for Graves' ophthalmopathy. Am J Ophthalmol 1995;119:792–5; with permission.)

History

Presenting ophthalmic symptoms of TED are often nonspecific and variable. Some degree of ocular irritation and discomfort is present in most patients, but unless it is severe, it usually is not the main reason patients seek evaluation and treatment. Conjunctival injection and tearing are also present in a large percentage of patients. Symptoms that may prompt patients to seek attention are diplopia, proptosis, eyelid retraction, and pain or pressure around the eye. Patients usually note proptosis as a bulging of one eye. When the proptosis is symmetric, it is usually not noticed by the patients until it is at least moderate in degree. Review of old photographs (eg, an old driver's license) may assist in detecting subtle change. Eyelid retraction is usually noticed as an asymmetry in the upper eyelid position. Patients sometimes believe the normal eyelid is actually ptotic. Patients may also complain of diplopia at presentation. Less commonly, they may notice decreased visual acuity and, less often, are aware of visual field impairment. Additional points of interest in terms of a patient's health history include symptoms referable to hyperthyroidism or hypothyroidism as well as a family history of thyroid dysfunction. It also is helpful to inquire about cigarette smoking, because smoking may be associated with dysthyroid orbitopathy.

Examination

After obtaining a complete history, the examination begins with tests of visual function. Best-corrected visual acuity is checked first, both at a distance and near. If necessary, a refraction should be performed to ensure that a refractive error is not responsible for visual loss. Because compressive optic neuropathy affects peripheral vision and color vision first, it is important to test these parameters routinely to help monitor disease progression. Color vision is checked with each eye individually using standard color-vision testing books. Confrontation visual fields may be performed, but a formal screening visual field should be performed if there is any question of compressive optic neuropathy. A careful pupillary examination with the swinging flashlight test can help in the diagnosis of an afferent pupillary defect, which is another useful sign of early compressive optic neuropathy.

Extraocular muscle inflammation and enlargement in Graves' disease may result in limitation of eye movement and double vision. Eye muscle function is evaluated by determining the alignment of the globes in primary position and then assessing extraocular motility. If the globes are normally aligned or orthophoric in primary gaze and reading position (downgaze), the patient will not experience diplopia. To assess ocular alignment, a cover-uncover test is performed in which each eye in turn is occluded and uncovered while the patient fixates on a distant target. Corrective movements of the uncovered eye are assessed. If the eye is deviated downward, for example, a rapid upward movement of the eye will be evident when it is uncovered. Hypotropia is seen with unilateral restriction of an inferior rectus muscle, whereas an esotropia is seen with restriction of the medial rectus muscle. The inferior and medial recti are more commonly involved than the superior and lateral recti. The physician can then assess extraocular motility as the patients' eyes follow a flashlight, checking each field of gaze and documenting how far each eye can move in each cardinal direction. Limitation of upward and lateral gaze with associated diplopia is encountered most commonly.

External examination of the periorbital area entails determination of the position of the globes relative to the bony orbit and of the eyelids relative to the globe. Eyelid retraction is the most common clinical finding in TED, and TED is the most common cause of eyelid retraction. There are several measurements that may help quantitate the degree of retraction and facilitate monitoring of disease progression. The upper eyelid normally rests just below the superior limbus, whereas the lower eyelid rests just at the inferior limbus. Scleral show between the upper and lower eyelid margins and the limbus, measured in millimeters, is a good indication of eyelid retraction. The vertical interpalpebral height is measured centrally, with the patient looking in primary gaze. Measurement of the temporal palpebral fissure height may be useful as well in patients who have TED because of the tendency for eyelid retraction to be more pronounced temporally in patients who have this disorder. The margin reflex distance is the distance between the corneal light reflex and the upper eyelid margin with the patient in primary gaze (Fig. 7).

Observation of upper eyelid movement also may be helpful in the evaluation of TED. Normally, the upper eyelid descends smoothly and completely with downward rotation of the globe in downgaze. Lid lag (Fig. 8), characterized by delayed or incomplete downward movement of the lid in downgaze, is observed in many patients who have upper eyelid

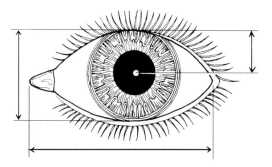

Fig. 7. The margin-reflex distance (MRD) is the distance between the papillary light reflex and the upper eyelid margin.

retraction. Lid lag is encountered most frequently in the setting of TED but also may occur after eyelid surgery or trauma or in patients who have congenital ptosis. Lagophthalmos, defined as incomplete eyelid closure, also may be observed in patients who have TED, as well as in those who have other disorders, including facial nerve paresis.

Proptosis is defined as forward movement of the eye. Most commonly it is measured by using an exophthalmometer (Fig. 9) to determine the amount of protrusion of the corneal surface of the globe in front of the lateral orbital rim. TED is the most common cause of unilateral and bilateral proptosis in adulthood.

Slit-lamp examination findings in TED include conjunctival injection or chemosis and superficial punctate keratopathy, a signs of corneal exposure. Initially, the conjunctival injection may be localized over the inflamed rectus muscles. Injection of the interpalpebral conjunctiva may be noted in the setting of lagophthalmos and exposure keratopathy. Exposure keratopathy can be exacerbated by dry eye causing localized or generalized punctate staining of the cornea. Another conjunctival/corneal finding is superior

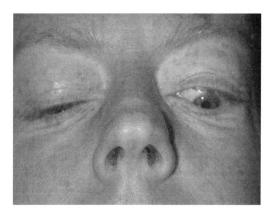

Fig. 8. Lid lag in a patient who has thyroid eye disease.

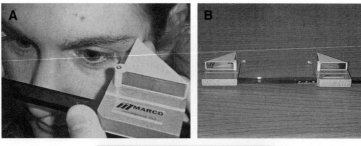

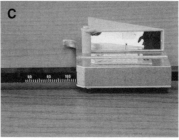

Fig. 9. Globe prominence relative to the lateral orbital rim is assessed using the exophthalmometer. (*A*) The exophthalmometer is placed against the lateral orbital rim. (*B*) The position of the corneal image is located in the prism following alignment of the lines within the prism to avoid parallax error. (*C*) The numeric scale on the central bar of the instrument is used to measure the intercanthal distance.

limbic keratoconjunctivitis, a focal inflammation of the superior bulbar conjunctiva and superior limbus of the cornea. Fine filaments also may be present on the superior corneal surface. Intraocular pressure may be normal or elevated in primary position. In upgaze, the intraocular pressure may increase secondary to restriction of globe rotation associated with inferior rectus enlargement. The fundus usually is not affected until severe orbital congestion occurs. If compressive optic neuropathy develops, the optic nerve head may become swollen, and the vessels on the nerve head may dilate. Later, pallor may occur.

Orbital fractures

Orbital trauma may damage the facial bones and adjacent soft tissues. Although fractures involving any of the orbital rims or walls, either singly or in combination, may occur, in the authors' experience, indirect or "blowout" fractures involving the orbital floor and medial wall are most commonly encountered. With orbital trauma, there is a high incidence of associated ocular trauma, including subconjunctival hemorrhage, hyphema or iritis, corneoscleral rupture, vitreous hemorrhage, and retinal trauma. A complete ocular examination, including a visual acuity test, must be performed initially to assess the integrity of the globe.

History

The patient's clinical history will reveal the nature of the trauma and will guide the examiner in the search for associated injuries and possible foreign bodies. Symptoms may include pain, especially with extraocular movements, diplopia, facial numbness, and trismus. Pain usually is not extreme unless there is true entrapment of a muscle in a trapdoor fracture. In such cases, surgery should proceed urgently to free the muscle and decrease the risk of vascular compromise and the associated risk of muscle necrosis or fibrosis secondary to persistent incarceration. Diplopia, commonly seen with blowout fractures, may be noted on vertical gaze with orbital floor fractures and on horizontal gaze with medial wall fractures. Midfacial or dental numbness is fairly common with orbital floor fractures because of injury to the infraorbital nerve. Trismus is encountered with injury to the lateral rim and zygomatic arch, as occurs in tripod fractures.

Examination begins by assessing the integrity of the globe. Ocular injuries are frequently associated with orbital fractures and may require specific treatment before management of orbital trauma. After globe injuries have been excluded, a more focused periorbital examination may commence. External inspection often reveals periorbital edema and ecchymosis. The orbital rim is palpated for deformities and tenderness. Crepitus of the eyelids, from orbital emphysema, is seen often with medial wall fractures and much less commonly with orbital floor fractures. Patients who are diagnosed as having orbital fractures or who are thought to have an orbital fracture should be instructed not to blow their noses to avoid forcing air into the orbit. Hypoesthesia of the cheek and upper lip may be associated with fractures of the orbital floor.

The position of the globe is assessed as described for TED. With orbital floor fractures, the globe may be proptotic in the acute phase because of periorbital edema. As the edema resolves, enophthalmos may develop in patients who have large floor fractures, especially when associated with medial wall fractures. The superior sulcus may appear deeper, and the vertical

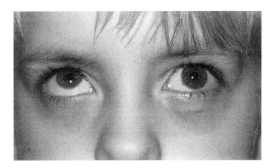

Fig. 10. Restriction of upgaze in the left eye secondary to inferior rectus muscle entrapment in a patient with an orbital floor fracture.

palpebral fissure may appear smaller in association with enophthalmos. Even without enophthalmos, vertical globe displacement (globe ptosis or hypoglobus) may occur as the eye sinks inferiorly. This displacement is sometimes easiest to demonstrate in photographs, using a straight edge to line up the medial canthus or lateral canthus and comparing the globe position on each side relative to the straight edge.

Extraocular motility often is restricted in patients who have orbital floor blowout fractures with corresponding diplopia. With orbital floor fractures, restriction of upgaze, downgaze, or both is common (Fig. 10). With medial wall fractures, restriction is less common and usually occurs in horizontal gaze. Some discomfort with extraocular movements is common after a fracture, but severe pain with eye movement or nausea and vomiting should alert the clinician to possible muscle entrapment in a trapdoor fracture, which may require urgent intervention.

Suggested readings

Basic and clinical science course: orbits, eyelids, and lacrimal system. Section 7. San Francisco: The Foundation of the American Academy of Ophthalmology; 2000.

McCord CD Jr, Tannenbaum M, Nunery WR, editors. Oculoplastic surgery. 3rd edition. New York: Raven Press; 1995.

Nesi FA, Lisman RD, Levine MR, editors. Smith's ophthalmic plastic and reconstructive surgery. 2nd edition. St. Louis (MO): Mosby-Year Book; 1998.

Stewart WB, editor. Surgery of the eyelid, orbit, and lacrimal system. III. In: Ophthalmology monographs 8. San Francisco: American Academy of Ophthalmology; 1995.

ELSEVIER
SAUNDERS

Otolaryngol Clin N Am
39 (2006) 923–942

OTOLARYNGOLOGIC
CLINICS
OF NORTH AMERICA

Evaluation and Management of Graves' Orbitopathy

H.B. Harold Lee, MD[a],*, I. Rand Rodgers, MD[b], John J. Woog, MD, FACS[a]

[a]Department of Ophthalmology, Mayo Clinic, 200 First St. SW, Rochester, MN 55905, USA
[b]229 E. 79th St., New York, NY 10021, USA

Graves' orbitopathy, also known as Graves' ophthalmopathy or thyroid eye disease, is a potentially progressive but generally self-limited autoimmune process associated with hyperthyroidism. It is the most common cause of proptosis and the most common orbital inflammatory disorder in adults, representing 85% of bilateral exophthalmos cases and 50% of unilateral cases [1].

Graves' disease has a strong female preponderance, with a female:male ratio of approximately 4:1. It has an incidence of 0.4% in the United States. A study of patients from the Mayo Clinic found an age-adjusted annual incidence of 16 per 100,000 for women and 3 per 100,000 for men [2]. This study found a bimodal distribution of age at presentation. Peak presentation was between the ages of 40 and 44 and 60 and 64 for women, and between 45 and 49 and 65 and 69 for men. Despite the greater prevalence of Graves' disease in women, affected men tend to progress more rapidly and severely.

Both heredity and environmental influences play a role in the pathogenesis of Graves' disease [3,4].

Genetics

Genetic factors may contribute a role in the pathogenesis of Graves' disease. Twenty percent to 60% of affected individuals have a positive family history of thyroid disease. A population-based study of Danish monozygotic twins showed a 35% concordance rate [5]. Patients with Graves'

Portions of this article are reprinted from: Bartlett JD, Rodgers IR. Evaluation and Management of Graves' Orbitopathy. In: John J. Woog, Ed. Manual of Endoscopic Lacrimal and Orbital Surgery. Philadelphia: Butterworth/Heinemann, 2004; with permission.
* Corresponding author.
E-mail address: Lee.Hui@mayo.edu (H.B. Harold).

disease also express certain human leukocyte antigens (HLA) more often than control subjects without the disease. HLA-B8, DR3, and DQA1*0501 haplotypes may increase susceptibility to the disease. HLA DR β1*07 may offer protection.

The immunopathogenesis of Graves' orbitopathy is not fully understood. One theoretic construct, however, holds that certain antigen-presenting cells (eg, macrophages and dendritic cells) that express Class II major histocompatibility complexes (MHC molecules HLA-DR, DP, DQ), bind antigen and present it to CD4 helper T cells. Activation of this T-cell cohort is dependent on the binding of antigen to the MHC molecules on the antigen-presenting cells. Thus, the HLA molecules influence the selection of antigens that can be presented to T cells. Subsequent activation of T cells results in the cascade of events leading to the autoimmune recognition of self-antigen, which may occur both within the thyroid as well as extra-thyroidal tissues such as the orbit.

The process of negative and positive selection, occurring in the thymus, ultimately determines which lymphocytes will mature and subsequently enter the circulation. Negative selection is a mechanism by which the human body can prevent an immunologic reaction toward itself. If an HLA molecule on an antigen-presenting cell (APC) binds self-antigen and then presents it to a T cell, whose receptor recognizes the HLA molecule–antigen complex, this T cell is negatively selected. However, if this process fails at any level, an autoimmune reaction may ensue. Specific HLA types (HLA-B8, DR3, and DQA1*0501) may fail to present self-antigen to the T cells in the thymus, thus permitting the cells to be released in the periphery where they can later recognize autoantigen. Similarly, HLA-DR β1*07 may predispose a patient population to protection from the autoimmune disease by promoting negative selection [6].

Pathophysiology

As reviewed above, there is evidence of genetic factors in the pathogenesis of Graves's disease and subsequent development of Graves' orbitopathy. Environmental factors may also contribute to the autoimmune disease. Thyroid surgery, smoking, radiation exposure, thyroid inflammation, and trauma have all been implicated in the genesis of Graves' disease, although the exact role of each is unclear [7,8]. Although controversial, microbial infections such as Yersinia may also contribute to disease manifestation in some patients. These pathogens may act as superantigens, resulting in overactivation of the immune response. Molecular mimicry, where crossreaction to similar epitopes from microbial and self-antigens, has also been postulated as a mechanism of autoimmunity [6].

Graves' hyperthyroidism is an autoimmune disease that may involve the binding of stimulatory autoantibodies to the thyroid-stimulating hormone (TSH) receptor (TSHr) of thyroid follicular cells. Several different TSHr-binding autoantibodies have been described. These proteins, upon binding, stimulate thyroid hormone synthesis, freeing the thyroid from pituitary negative-feedback regulation [9]. This results in the characteristically depressed TSH and elevated thyroid hormone levels. The immunologic basis for orbital findings in Graves' disease is somewhat less well understood than the thyroid processes. Graves' orbitopathy is a multifactorial disease composed of mechanical, immunologic, and cellular processes [10]. Much of the immunologic contribution stems from histologic studies of both human and animal models of Graves' orbitopathy. T- and B-cell lymphocytes, mast cells, and fibroblasts orchestrate an array of cytokines and chemokines within the confined space of the bony orbit, and local mechanical stress may further propagate the process. The TSHr is the likely autoantigenic target of the immune response seen in the eye manifestations of Graves' disease. Antigen-presenting cells within the orbit may recognize TSHr, resulting in a cell-mediated process. Alternatively, anti-TSHr autoantibodies may crossreact with orbital autoantigens at the B-cell level [10]. However, transplacental transfer of anti-TSHr antibodies fail to cause clinical neonatal Graves' orbitopathy [6]. Thus, it is likely that a cell-mediated process contributes a greater role to the orbital pathology.

Histologic studies of orbital tissue in Grave's orbitopathy demonstrate an excess of glycosaminoglycans (GAG). Hyaluronan is the predominant GAG, characterized as a large, hydrophilic, polyanionic compound. Clinical expansion of both the orbital connective tissues and extraocular muscles result from accumulation of GAGs in the retro-orbital space and within the connective tissues investing the muscle fibers [10]. Initially, muscle proteins (eg, G2s, D1, eye muscle membrane antigen) were implicated as autoimmune targets in Graves' orbitopathy. However, the extraocular muscle antibodies detected in the serum of Graves' patients may be secondary to the immune driven orbital damage. The primary role of orbital fibroblasts is the synthesis of GAG's and maintenance of the connective tissue milieu. Recent studies have shown diversity in the phenotypic expression of tissue-specific fibroblasts. Subpopulations of these cells can be identified by surface protein, carbohydrate, and ganglioside markers [6]. Specifically, orbital fibroblasts express a receptor CD 40 not found in fibroblasts from other tissue sites. Binding of this receptor with the CD 40 ligand, also known as CD 154, results in multiple events including an increase in hyaluronan synthesis, upregulation of chemokines, and maintenance of a general inflammatory response (Fig. 1) [11]. In addition, orbital fibroblasts exhibit an attenuated proteolytic environment with the lack of hyaluronidase expression [6,10]. Immunoglobulins from patients with Graves' disease may also contribute to enhanced collagen synthesis and T-cell chemotractant activity [12,13]. These phenotypically distinct characteristics contribute to the accumulation of GAGs in the orbit of Graves' patients.

In addition to oversynthesis and underdegradation of GAGs, adipose tissue expansion contributes to orbital volume overload. Preadipocyte fibroblast expression of TSHr seems to be linked to their differentiation into mature fat cells. In a recent study, endogenous ligands to a receptor on these

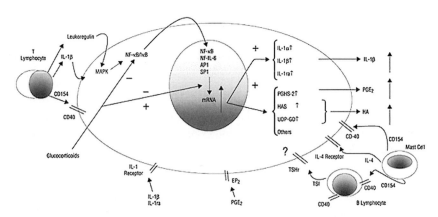

Fig. 1. Schematic diagram of the current model for the proposed immune cascade in Graves'
orbitopathy (*From* Kazim M, Goldberg RA, Smith TJ. Insights into the pathogenesis of thyroid-associated orbitopathy. Arch Ophthalmol 2002;120(3);380–6; with permission).

preadipocytes (peroxisone proliferator-activated receptor [PPAR]-γ) lead to
their maturation [14]. Increased expression of PPAR-γ and adiponectin,
produced in mature adipocytes, was noted in Graves' orbitopathy patients
[15]. It is likely that an imbalance of these pathways secondary to an intense
immune response ultimately favors fat production. Future therapies targeting this receptor may play a role in inhibiting excess fat production in
Graves' orbitopathy.

Clinically, inflammation associated with Graves' orbitopathy may be classified into two types [16]. Type I is characterized by orbital fat and connective
tissue involvement. Type II results in severe extraocular muscle involvement.
The two types tend to have different clinical outcomes. Patients with type I
disease have an excellent prognosis and rarely develop visual loss. Patients
with type II disease, however, have a more aggressive disease course and
are at risk for diplopia, lid retraction, and compressive optic neuropathy. Individual patients may have evidence of both type I and type II involvement.

Clinical evaluation

Clinical signs may be categorized according to Werner's classification system for thyroid ophthalmopathy, also known by the mnemonic NOSPECS,
from the first letter of each class [17,18]. The classes are organized by
increasing severity. Although this classification is a useful schema for quan-
tifying disease severity, orbitopathy does not necessarily progress in an orderly fashion. Also, there may be significant asymmetry between the two
eyes so that each may be in a different category.

Class 0 (No signs) represents subclinical disease without apparent signs or
symptoms. Early ophthalmopathy may manifest in subtle, nonspecific signs
and symptoms, such as tearing, photophobia, foreign body sensation, mild

conjunctival injection and chemosis, superficial punctate keratopathy, and increased intraocular pressure. As these are commonly found in a variety of clinical disorders, their true etiology may go unnoticed until further manifestations of Graves' ophthalmopathy develop. Recently, superior limbic keratoconjunctivitis has been recognized as a significant risk factor for the development of thyroid dysfunction and Graves' orbitopathy [19].

Class I (Only signs) consists of eyelid retraction and stare only. Elevated sympathomimetic activity or fibrosis of the lid tissues may cause lid retraction (Fig. 2). Lid lag on downgaze is also commonly seen.

Class II (Soft tissue swelling) is characterized by soft tissue involvement. Common signs include deep conjunctival injection, especially over the rectus muscle insertions. Conjunctival chemosis may be mild, only interpalpebral, or diffuse, or occasionally, hemorrhagic. Edema of the caruncle may be present. Inflammation may result in periorbital edema and erythema.

Class III (Proptosis) includes exophthalmos. Extraocular muscle inflammation and an increase in soft tissue and orbital fat volume result in axial proptosis (Fig. 3). Increased resistance to posterior displacement of the globe (retropulsion) may develop. Exophthalmos is generally measured and followed clinically with an exophthalmometer. Although normal exophthalmometric measurements vary with age, gender, and ethnicity, measurements of greater than 21 mm or a difference of greater than 2 mm between eyes is suggestive of an orbital process. Migliori and Gladstone noted the upper limits of normal were 21.7 mm for White men, 24.7 mm for Black men, 20.1 mm for White women, and 23 mm for Black women [20].

Class IV (Extraocular muscle) is characterized by extraocular muscle involvement. Muscle involvement starts with an accumulation of inflammatory cells and fluid. When the affected patient is in a supine position, fluid tends to collect. Therefore, diplopia may be worse in the morning during this initial period. Later, as muscle is replaced with fibrous tissue,

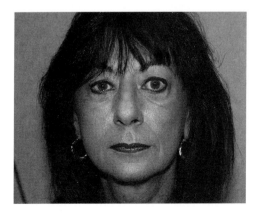

Fig. 2. This woman demonstrates a widened left palpebral fissure OS in the setting of eyelid retraction.

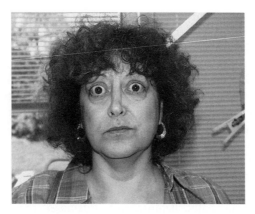

Fig. 3. The right globe is markedly proptotic. Upper and lower eyelid retraction is attributable to Müller's muscle stimulation in all four eyelids.

permanent strabismus occurs. Any extraocular muscle may be involved, although the inferior and medial rectus muscles are the most commonly affected [21]. Forced duction testing characteristically yields positive results.

Class V (Corneal exposure) includes corneal involvement. Exposure keratitis in thyroid eye disease is multifactorial. Eyelid dysfunction, proptosis, tear film abnormalities, and an inadequate Bell phenomenon secondary to muscle restriction all contribute to exposure.

Class VI (Sight loss) involves visual loss secondary to optic nerve injury Extraocular muscle enlargement and orbital fat inflammation may result in progressive proptosis. As the eye becomes more prominent, the optic nerve is stretched. However, because of its sinuous course, the nerve has several millimeters of laxity and is not initially injured. With increasingly severe degrees of proptosis, however, stretching of the optic nerve may result in optic neuropathy in some patients. Perhaps more commonly, when muscle enlargement occurs posteriorly at the orbital apex, optic nerve compression may take place. Patients with compressive optic neuropathy may not exhibit optic nerve head swelling. For this reason, it is important to evaluate visual acuity and color vision while assessing the pupils for afferent pupillary defect and obtaining visual field studies in suspected cases of optic neuropathy, in addition to performing fundoscopic examination. Serial Humphrey or Goldmann visual fields may be helpful in the evaluation of patients with evolving optic nerve compression. It should be noted, as well, that an afferent pupillary defect may be absent or difficult to detect in individuals with bilateral compressive optic neuropathy.

Orbital imaging

In general, computed tomography (CT) is the best imaging technique for evaluating Graves' orbitopathy. CT scans show extraocular muscle involvement in up to 85% of patients with thyroid eye disease. Findings on CT scanning may include muscle belly enlargement that spares the tendinous insertions, an apparent increase in orbital fat volume, lacrimal gland enlargement, and compression of the optic nerve at the orbital apex [22]. CT scanning is a sensitive test of orbital involvement, and may demonstrate muscle enlargement even in otherwise asymptomatic patients. Intravenous (IV) contrast studies are not usually necessary if the diagnosis of Graves' orbitopathy is clear. However, these studies do help to exclude other disorders, like orbital pseudotumor, that may present in a similar fashion. In considering the use of IV contrast material, it is important to remember that administration of iodine-containing contrast agents may, in the short term, preclude the use of radioactive iodine for the treatment of hyperthyroidism.

Magnetic resonance imaging (MRI) may also be a helpful imaging tool. MRI studies allow visualization of the optic nerve and extraocular muscles. In individuals with isolated inferior enlargement of the rectus muscle without other, definitive evidence of Graves' orbitopathy, sagittal MRI views may allow the clinician to distinguish between tendon involvement and tendon sparing (the latter generally encountered in the setting of Graves' disease). Limitations of MRI include the relative lack of information regarding the bony orbit and paranasal sinuses, as well as the generally higher cost of this study compared with CT scanning. Ultrasonography can also be used to evaluate the extraocular muscles. This imaging modality, however, provides relatively poor visualization of the posterior orbit and bony walls, and the degree of information provided by the study is dependent on the experience of the ultrasonographer.

Radiologic imaging studies are not required in every patient with Graves' orbitopathy. In many cases, the diagnosis of Graves' orbitopathy may be made on the basis of clinical findings alone. CT scans may be obtained when the signs and symptoms are atypical (as in the case of a patient with severe pain on eye movement) and the diagnosis is in doubt. Imaging studies may be also useful in patients with clinical evidence of Graves' orbitopathy but apparently normal thyroid function. Imaging studies may be particularly helpful when radiation therapy or decompressive surgery is planned, as they allow the degree of extraocular muscle and orbital fat involvement to be defined and sinus anatomy to be delineated clearly before intervention. Finally, the diagnosis of optic nerve compression is a clinical one and not a radiologic one.

Medical management

General considerations

From the endocrine perspective, the goal of treatment for patients with Graves' disease is the achievement of a euthyroid state. Some experts believe that patients treated with radioactive iodine may exhibit an exacerbation of orbital inflammation compared with patients treated with other modalities [23–25]. They maintain that thyroid glandular destruction by radioiodine stimulates increased antigen–antibody responses, further exacerbating the autoimmune process. Thus, some endocrinologists administer corticosteroids to decrease the possible exacerbation of Graves' ophthalmopathy in patients receiving radioiodine [26]. In any case, it is believed that patients with hyperthyroidism tend to have more severe progression of orbital involvement, reinforcing the importance of appropriate systemic management. Unfortunately, in the 6 months following iodine 131 treatment, signs and symptoms of thyroid eye disease remain the same, improve, or worsen in relatively equal percentages of patients, suggesting that the course of thyroid eye disease is independent of serum thyroid hormone levels [27]. Advocates of thyroidectomy argue that removal of the gland reduces antigenic stimulation and thus the severity of eye disease, but this has never been clinically proven [28].

Smoking, as indicated earlier, has been implicated as an important contributing factor in Graves' disease [6]. Smokers have been shown to have more severe orbital progression, and smoke further irritates inflamed orbital tissues [29]. Patients should be counseled regarding the risks of smoking and the benefits of smoking cessation.

Ophthalmic management: Local measures

Many of the early symptoms of ophthalmopathy, including tearing, injection, and photophobia, can be treated effectively by lubrication or by the placement of punctal plugs to increase the amount of moisture over ocular surfaces. Individuals requiring frequent lubricant instillation may benefit from the use of nonpreserved lubricating drops and ointments so as to avoid preservative-related inflammation. Taping the eyelids shut at night can serve a similar purpose. Sunglasses help reduce photophobia. Because orbital and eyelid edema are often worse in the morning owing to the fluid-pooling effects of a supine position, elevating the head of the patient's bed may help to minimize these symptoms.

Lid retraction, in the early phases, is primarily attributable to increased sympathetic tone. This can be treated transiently with topical adrenergic blocking agents. The most commonly used agent is guanethidine sulfate [30]. Although this medication may be employed temporarily, its use may be associated with ocular irritation, and its therapeutic effects may wane over time. Topical adrenergic blocking agents do not play a significant long-term role in the permanent treatment of lid retraction.

Functionally significant diplopia may be best corrected surgically. However, while awaiting the stabilization of symptoms that is required before surgical intervention, prisms can be used. The utility of prisms is, unfortunately, often hampered by the fact that the magnitude of the strabismus varies with the direction of gaze (noncomitant strabismus). Patching of the nondominant eye may be the only possible temporizing measure for intractable diplopia.

Corticosteroids

Steroids represent one of the principal treatments for Graves' orbitopathy. Patients with acute inflammatory disease respond best, owing to the lymphocytic and fibroblastic inhibitory effects of steroids. Therapy is instituted with prednisone, often prescribed at a dosage of 60 to 100 mg per day. Some clinicians prefer to administer this in divided doses [31]. This initial dose is continued for several days, then tapered over several weeks. Steroids are generally effective only while being administered, and inflammatory symptoms commonly rebound when treatment is tapered. However, because of the numerous, potentially dangerous side effects of prolonged steroid therapy, continuous treatment throughout the 1- to 3-year course of Graves' orbitopathy is best avoided. Repeated, short treatment courses may be used in some patients, whereas in other patients, some form of combination therapy is preferred. In the authors' experience, steroid therapy is generally prescribed only in conjunction with radiation therapy or orbital decompression surgery to control additional inflammation associated with these treatments and to achieve some level of therapeutic response while the other modalities are beginning to work.

Steroids can be very effective on a temporary basis, but both patients and physicians need to be aware of potential side effects [32]. Common side effects include weight gain and fat redistribution, which result in the characteristic cushingoid appearance that is characteristic of long-term steroid use. Steroids also can complicate glycemic control in diabetics. Sleep disturbances and emotional changes are relatively common. Steroids affect bones throughout the body and can cause spinal compression fractures and aseptic necrosis of the femoral head. Potentially fatal gastrointestinal ulceration and hemorrhage have been reported. From an ocular standpoint, corticosteroids can hasten cataract formation and exacerbate glaucoma with increased intraocular pressure. Moreover, along with suppression of orbital lymphocytes, steroids cause systemic immunosuppression, which increases the vulnerability of the patient to infections. A particular concern is reactivation of latent tuberculosis, so it may be advisable to perform appropriate skin testing before initiating steroid treatment. For these reasons, in the authors' experience, the use of systemic corticosteroids is typically limited to patients with optic nerve compression or severe acute proptosis with significant corneal exposure. Systemic steroids are not typically favored for the treatment of milder soft tissue signs of Graves' disease because of the side effects and the recurrence of inflammatory symptoms upon discontinuation of steroid therapy.

Some debate exists as to whether optic neuropathy secondary to severe, active Graves' disease should be treated initially with intravenous steroid therapy or surgery. In a recent study by Wakelkamp and colleagues [33], 15 patients with severe, active Graves' orbitopathy and optic neuropathy were randomized to either pulsed IV therapy with methylprednisolone or primary surgical decompression. The authors found that immediate surgical decompression did not preclude treatment with IV steroids. In fact, five of six (82%) of the patients in the surgery arm needed further immunosupression, while four of nine (45%) of the patients in the steroid treatment arm needed additional surgical decompression. The authors favored primary treatment with pulsed IV steroids over immediate decompression of patients with optic neuropathy due to active Graves' disease [33].

Retrobulbar steroid injections have been suggested to minimize systemic steroid effects. However, the response rate is significantly lower, and the risk of injection into a tight, inflamed orbit is significantly increased. Retrobulbar corticosteroids are rarely used. Topical steroids may be helpful in addressing ocular surface inflammation, but in the editor's experience, do not result in significant improvement of deeper orbital inflammation. Careful monitoring to prevent glaucoma and cataract formation is required.

Because of the drawbacks of steroids, other immunosuppressives have also been used in the treatment of thyroid-related ophthalmopathy. The efficacy of agents, such as methotrexate, cyclophosphamide, cyclosporin, and azathioprine, is less clear compared with corticosteroids [34,35].

Radiation therapy

Radiation therapy is the second of the three main treatment modalities for Graves' orbitopathy. Although there is no standardized protocol, therapy generally consists of delivering a low dose of 2000 to 2500 cGy (rad) in multiple fractions to the orbits, usually over a period of 2 weeks [36,37], CT scans are used to create dosimetric maps. These maps, along with lead shields, are used to limit the treatment area, which extends from the anterior edge of the lateral orbital rim to the border of the sella turcica. Radiation therapy, like steroids, is most effective in combating acute inflammation. Radiation is effective because inflammatory cells and lymphocytes, in particular, are radiosensitive. Results are typically seen within 1 to 8 weeks of treatment. Because of the cumulative dose effects, repeat treatments are relatively contraindicated. Restrictive strabismus and eyelid retraction are unlikely to be improved by radiation therapy. Some radiation therapists believe that radiation lessens the amount of proptosis, and this may, indeed, be true [36]. Evidence regarding the efficacy of radiation therapy in the management of Graves' orbitopathy is limited, owing to methodologic weaknesses of available studies.

Only recently have the first prospective, randomized, controlled studies been published [38,39]. Both studies enrolled patients with soft tissue disease. In the Mayo Clinic study, no beneficial result from radiotherapy was proven [37]; in the second study, the only beneficial effect was in improving upward gaze [39].

Complications from this low-dose radiation are uncommon and usually only occur in patients with predisposing factors [36]. Dry eye is the most common complication. There is at least a theoretic concern of accelerated cataractogenesis. Higher dose radiation exposure may cause orbital fibrosis, secondary neoplasms, and optic neuropathy. Systemic chemotherapy may potentiate radiation effects and increase the effective delivered dose. Diabetics have an increased risk for microangiopathic complications, including macular hemorrhage and exudates, capillary nonperfusion, and neovascularization, which can occur several years after radiation treatment. Other rare complications include radiation retinopathy with loss of vision, central retinal artery occlusions, encephalopathy, and premature atherosclerosis [40–44].

Surgical treatment modalities

The indications for surgical intervention in thyroid-related orbitopathy include optic neuropathy, diplopia, corneal exposure, and cosmesis. Broadly speaking, surgical procedures may be directed toward orbital decompression, strabismus repair, and the correction of eyelid malpositions. Cosmetic improvement can require any or all of these procedures. Traditionally, orbital decompression, if required, is performed initially, followed by strabismus surgery and eyelid repair. This is because the nature and degree of strabismus may change after orbital surgery, and lid position may be altered following strabismus repair [45].

The timing of surgery is of significance. Decompression may be necessary on an urgent basis for compressive optic neuropathy or severe proptosis with corneal ulceration refractory to other treatment measures. However, neuropathy can often be stabilized with steroid medical therapy. The results of surgery may be somewhat more predictable when the orbitopathy has stabilized, generally between 1 and 4 years following the onset of the disease [46].

Orbital decompression

Decompression of orbital contents can be accomplished either by removing one or more of the bony walls of the orbit, allowing prolapse of the orbital contents, or by removing orbital fat, thereby decreasing the amount of tissue in the orbit. Any of the walls of the orbit may be removed, allowing expansion into the ethmoid sinus medially, the antrum of the maxillary sinus inferiorly, the temporal fossa laterally, and the cranial cavity superiorly. Bony wall removal is perhaps most commonly performed, and can result in significant globe repositioning. Reduction in exophthalmos of up to 5 to 6 mm or more may be achieved [47,48]. The indications for surgical decompression vary from specialist to specialist and from one geographic region to the next. Decompression may be performed for relief of compressive or stretch-related optic neuropathy, proptosis with significant corneal exposure, spontaneous globe subluxation, and cosmesis [49].

The most commonly performed decompression surgeries include antral–ethmoidal decompression, lateral orbital decompression (Krönlein's operation), "three-wall decompression" (combined lateral and antral–ethmoidal decompression), and "four-wall decompression" (extension of the "three-wall decompression" to include the orbital roof (transfrontal or Naffziger's procedure) [49]. Surgical incisions useful in accessing the medial, lateral, and inferior floors of the orbit are illustrated in Fig. 4A and B. The choice of procedure may be influenced by the precise indication (or indications) for surgery, the surgeon's expectations, and patient preferences. For optic neuropathy, in which there is crowding at the orbital apex, removal of the anterior and posterior ethmoids is required. Ethmoidectomy is usually combined with removal of the floor or other walls. For aesthetic decompression, the posterior ethmoids need not be resected. The amount of globe repositioning achieved may be correlated with the degree of extraocular muscle involvement. The presence of large muscles with significant fibrosis may result in the achievement of a lesser degree of decompression than may be achieved in cases of primary fat compartment enlargement or enlarged muscles associated with a lesser degree of fibrosis.

Antral–ethmoidal decompression may be achieved using a number of surgical approaches. One approach is through the eyelid, either with a lateral canthotomy and cantholysis followed by an inferior fornix incision (Fig. 4), or via a subciliary incision [47]. The procedure can also be performed transantrally through the superior buccogingival sulcus (Caldwell-Luc approach; Fig. 5), via a transcaruncular approach, or via a transnasal endoscopic approach. Once exposure is obtained and the periosteum is elevated, rongeurs are used to create an osteotomy that includes the medial wall and orbital floor (Fig. 6). The amount of bone removed can be titrated based on the amount of decompression desired. Bony removal may be stopped at the infraorbital neurovascular bundle, or more bone can be removed by carefully stripping the bundle. It should be noted, however, that more aggressive floor resection may be associated with an increased risk of postoperative diplopia and hypoglobus, especially if the inferomedial orbital strut (maxillary buttress) is resected.

Lateral orbitotomy can be accomplished using either a canthotomy incision, a lid crease incision, or a coronal approach. After incision, muscle and periosteum are elevated to allow excision of the underlying lateral orbital wall. As with the orbital floor and medial wall, the periorbita must be incised so that the orbital structures can herniate into the osteotomy. This procedure may be performed in conjunction with orbital floor and medial wall decompression (Figs. 7, 8, and 9).

Orbital unroofing is an infrequently performed procedure that is generally accomplished using a frontotemporal craniotomy approach. Because

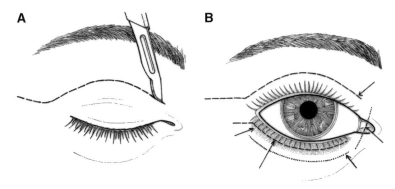

Fig. 4. (*A*) An eyelid crease incision may be used to reach the lateral orbital wall. (*B*) Multiple surgical approaches may be used to access the lateral, medial, and inferior floors of the orbit.

of the generally lesser degree of decompression achieved with this procedure and the potential for more serious complications, it is probably best used to complement the other types of operations rather than as a primary procedure.

None of these procedures is without risks and complications. The most common complication is the development or worsening of strabismus. Other complications include infraorbital nerve dysfunction, loss of vision (including permanent blindness), infection, hemorrhage, cerebrospinal fluid leakage, and nasolacrimal duct injuries. The number and severity of complications may be related to the aggressiveness of the decompressive surgery, as well as to the degree of preoperative strabismus and optic neuropathy. Complications may be limited to some degree by appropriate preoperative management. It is recommended that patients avoid preoperative

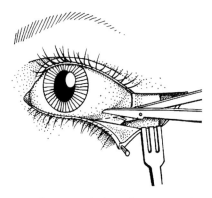

Fig. 5. The orbital floor can be accessed through a transconjunctival approach. Lateral canthotomy and cantholysis are performed, followed by an incision in the inferior fornix. (*From* Levine MR. Manual of oculoplastic surgery. 2nd edition. Boston (MA): Butterworth-Heinemann; 1996; with permission.)

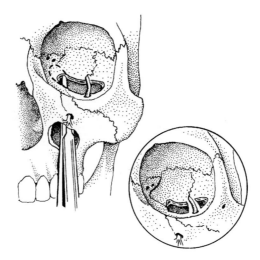

Fig. 6. A Caldwell-Luc approach may be used to access the orbital floor. (*From* Levine MR, Manual of oculoplastic surgery. 2nd edition. Boston (MA): Butterworth-Heinemann; 1996; with permission.)

use of aspirin or nonsteroidal anti-inflammatory medications, as these increase the likelihood of hemorrhage. Thyroid serum levels should be normalized to minimize general anesthetic complications, and antibiotics and steroids are often administered in the perioperative period.

Removal of orbital fat without bony resection was first performed in Europe, and is now performed in the United States as a primary procedure in selected patients, particularly those with CT evidence of orbital fat expansion. Resection of orbital fat in the inferolateral and superomedial orbit has been shown to lessen the degree of proptosis [50]. Proponents of this approach maintain that fat decompression precludes damage to the infraorbital nerve, worsening of strabismus, and the incidence of hypoglobus.

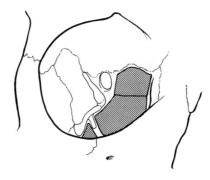

Fig. 7. Decompression of the orbital floor and medial walls is illustrated. (*From* McNab AA. Manual of orbital and lacrimal surgery. Philadelphia (PA): WB Saunders; 1998; with permission.)

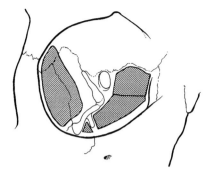

Fig. 8. The orbital bones removed in a three-wall decompression are depicted. (*From* McNab AA. Manual of orbital and lacrimal surgery. Philadelphia (PA): WB Saunders; 1998; with permission.)

Strabismus repair

The most commonly affected extraocular muscles are the inferior rectus and the medial rectus [21]. It follows then, that with restriction of these muscles, hypotropia and esotropia are the most common deviations noted in Graves' orbitopathy. Often, these deviations are worsened after decompression surgery. As the recti muscles prolapse out of the decompressed orbit, the already fibrosed and tightened muscles are further stretched, worsening restriction. For this reason, strabismus surgery is best performed after decompression, when the ocular deviation has stabilized. Similarly, because vertical muscle surgery can result in further lid retraction secondary to connective tissue attachments between these muscles and the lid musculature, lid surgery is best performed after strabismus surgery.

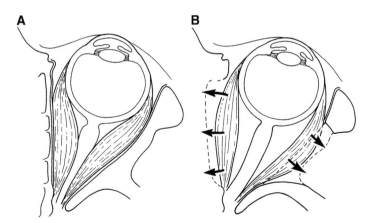

Fig. 9. (*A*) Axial section demonstrating compression of the optic nerve by edematous recti muscles. (*B*) Herniation of the orbital contents, including the recti muscles, after removal of the medial and lateral orbital walls. (*From* McNab AA. Manual of orbital and lacrimal surgery. Philadelphia (PA): WB Saunders; 1998; with permission.)

Because of the incomitant nature of strabismus in thyroid-related orbit-opathy, it is difficult and not always possible to obtain postoperative fusion in all fields of gaze. Therefore, the goal is to provide fusion in the two most important fields of gaze: primary and downgaze. It is advantageous to slightly undercorrect hypotropia and to slightly overcorrect esotropia to aid fusion in these two positions.

Before surgery, many surgeons prefer that ocular deviation measurements are stable for at least 6 months. Extraocular muscle recessions are often preferred, with marginal myotomies as an alternative. Some surgeons do perform resection surgery in the management of Graves' orbitopathy-related strabismus, as well. There is more variation in the results of strabismus surgery in this setting than with standard pediatric strabismus surgery. Reoperations are required not infrequently, and many surgeons prefer to use adjustable suture techniques to tailor surgery to individual patients.

Eyelid surgery

As previously discussed, eyelid surgery, if required, is generally best performed after orbital decompression and strabismus surgery are completed. Common eyelid procedures include lateral tarsorrhaphy, lengthening of Müller's and levator muscles, lower lid elevation, and blepharoplasty with orbital fat removal [34].

Tarsorrhaphy has the advantages that it is simple to perform and easily reversible. However, it is often not cosmetically acceptable, which may limit its utility. Furthermore, it may interfere with peripheral vision; if both the upper and lower eyelids are retracted, the tarsorrhaphy may separate.

Müller's muscle and levator surgeries involve lengthening or weakening these muscles. The surgical goal is to correct the retracted eyelid and restore a normal almond-shaped contour. The operation may be performed using local anesthetic on an outpatient basis, or it may be performed in conjunction with orbital decompression surgery. Optimally, before surgery, the eyelid position should be stable for at least 6 months, as determined on repeated measurements. However, levator-Müller's muscle surgery may be required in some cases on an urgent basis for the management of ocular surface exposure. In the upper eyelid, Müller's muscle is removed and the levator aponeurosis is weakened, either by performing marginal myotomies, by recessing the aponeurosis or Müller's muscle, or by excising Müller's muscle. Spacers, such as eye bank sclera, may be placed between the distal end of the levator aponeurosis and the superior edge of the tarsal plate to further lengthen the lid. Intraoperative adjustments are made as the patient opens and closes the eyelids. Overcorrection on the operating room table is generally desired if sclera is used, as the lid may tend to retract postoperatively.

Lower lid elevation may be accomplished through a variety of surgical techniques. The choice of procedure depends on the amount of lower eyelid retraction, the amount of fibrosis within the lower eyelid retractors, and the relationship between the globe and the underlying bony structures. For minimal amounts of retraction with a pliable lower eyelid and a nonprominent globe, a tarsal strip procedure or canthal tendon plication may suffice. For greater amounts of exposure with fibrotic lower eyelid retractors, a recession of inferior Müller's muscle and the capsulopalpebral fascia may be indicated, with or without the use of a spacer. Hard palate is often used as a lower lid spacer, as it is easily harvested, easily handled, has a mucosal surface, and demonstrates relatively little resorption. Auricular cartilage may be another option.

The success of lower eyelid surgery depends, in part, on the prominence of the globe. For individuals with relatively normal malar prominence who have undergone effective orbital decompression, lower eyelid elevation surgery is generally successful. For patients with significant proptosis, large globes, or relative malar hypoplasia who have not undergone decompression surgery, the success rate may not be quite as high.

Blepharoplasty may be performed in patients with thyroid eye disease, but certain caveats may be appropriate. Thyroid eye disease affects a disproportionate number of young women, and the disease may profoundly alter their appearance and self-image. Blepharoplasty may help improve their appearance, and may often be combined with vertical eyelid repositioning. Blepharoplasty should not be undertaken, however, during the acute phases of the disease, particularly when the patient has significant preseptal edema. The authors prefer to wait until orbitopathy is stable for at least 6 months, with no change in lid position or eyelid edema.

Blepharoplasty in patients with Graves' orbitopathy is different than a cosmetic blepharoplasty in an otherwise healthy individual. In the former case, relatively more aggressive (but still careful) resection of upper or lower eyelid fat, as well as careful sculpting of the brow fat pad, may be required to achieve the desired aesthetic result. However, it is the authors' preference, in general, to perform minimal, if any, skin resection, particularly if eyelid retraction is present or to be repaired concurrently. Individuals with Graves' orbitopathy may be at an increased risk for development of lagophthalmos and corneal irritation if significant skin resection is performed.

Future therapies

With further investigation to the pathogenesis of Graves' disease and its orbital manifestations, advances in technology and molecular science may lead to a wide array of future therapies for Graves' orbitopathy. Systemic or local treatments targeting specific cytokines, hormones, or antibodies may ultimately lead to treating not only the disease manifestations, but also the disease process.

References

[1] Dallow RL, Netland PA. Management of thyroid-associated orbitopathy (Graves' disease). In: Albert DM, Jakobiec FA, editors. Principles and practice of ophthalmology. Philadelphia (PA): WB Saunders; 2000. p. 3082.
[2] Bartley GB, Fatourechi V, Kadrmas EF, et al. The incidence of Graves' ophthalmopathy in Olmsted County, Minnesota. Am J Ophthalmol 1995;120(4):511–7.
[3] Gouch SC. The genetics of Graves' disease. Endocrinol Metab Clin North Am 2000;29(2): 255–66.
[4] Friedman JM, Fialkow PJ. Genetics of Graves' disease. Clin Endocrinol Metab 1978;7(1): 47–65.
[5] Brix TH, Kyvik KO, Christensen K, et al. Evidence for a major role of heredity in Graves' disease: a population-based study of two Danish twin cohrts. J Clin Endocrinol Metab 2001; 86(2):930–4.
[6] Prabhakar BS, Bahn RS, Smith TJ. Current perspective on the pathogenesis of Graves' disease and ophthalmopathy. Endocr Rev 2003;24(6):802–35.
[7] Weetman AP, Hunt PJ. The immunogenetics of thyroid-associated orbitopathy. Exp Clin Endocrinol Diabetes 1999;107(Suppl):S149–51.
[8] Nunery WR, Martin RT, Heinz GW, et al. The association of cigarette smoking with clinical subtypes of ophthalmic Graves' disease. Ophthalmic Plast Reconstr Surg 1993;9(2): 77–82.
[9] Clague R, Mukhtar ED, Pyle GA, et al. Thyroid-stimulating immunoglobulins and the control function. J Clin Endocrinol Metab 1976;43:550.
[10] Bahn RS. Pathophysiology of Grave's ophthalmopathy: the cycle of disease. J Clin Endocrinol Metab 2003;88(5):1939–46.
[11] Kazim M, Goldberg RA, Smith TJ. Insights into the pathogenesis of thyroid-associated orbitopathy. Arch Ophthalmol 2002;120(3):380–6.
[12] Rotella CM, Zonefrati R, Toccafondi R, et al. Ability to monoclonal antibodies to the thyrotropin receptor to increase collagen synthesis in human fibroblasts: an assay which appears to measure exophthalmogenic immunoglobulins in Graves' sera. J Clin Endocrinol Metab 1986;62(2):357–67.
[13] Pritchard J, Horst N, Cruikshank W, et al. Igs from patients with Graves' disease induce the expression of T cell chemoattractants in their fibroblasts. J Immunol 2002;168(2):942–50.
[14] Valyasevi RW, Harteneck DA, Dutton CM, et al. Stimulation of adipogenesis, peroxisome proliferatr-activated receptor-γ (PPARγ), and thyrotropin receptor by PPARγ agonist in human orbital preadipocyte fibroblasts. J Clin Endocrinol Metab 2002;87(5):2352–8.
[15] Kumar S, Leontovich A, Coenen MJ, et al. Gene expression profiling of orb ital adipose tissue from patients with Graves' ophthalmopathy: a potential role for secreted frizzles-related protein-1 in orbital adipogenesis. J Clin Endocrinol Metab 2005;90(8):4730–5.
[16] Nunery WR. Ophthalmic Graves' disease: a dual theory of pathogenesis. Ophthalmol Clin North Am 1991;4:73–88.
[17] Werner SC. Classification of the eye changes of Graves' disease. J Clin Endocrinol Metab 1969;29(7):982–4.
[18] Werner SC. Modification of the classification of the eye changes of Graves' disease: recommendations of the Ad Hoc Committee of the American Thyroid Association. J Clin Endocrinol Metab 1977;44(1):203–4.
[19] Kadrmas EF, Bartley GB. Superior limbic keratoconjunctivitis. A prognostic sign for severe Graves' ophthalmopathy. Ophthalmology 1995;102(10):1472–5.
[20] Migliori ME, Gladstone GJ. Determination of the normal range of exophthalmometric values for black and white adults. Am J Ophthalmol 1984;98:438.
[21] Feldon SE, Weiner JM. Clinical significance of extraocular muscle volumes in Graves' ophthalmopathy: a quantitative computed tomography study. Arch Ophthalmol 1982;100: 1266–9.

[22] Char DH, Norman D. The use of computed tomography and ultrasound in the evaluation of orbital masses. Surv Ophthalmol 1982;27(1):49–63.
[23] Wall JR, How J. Graves' ophthalmopathy. Boston (MA): Blackwell Scientific; 1990.
[24] Bahn RS, Gorman CA. Choice of therapy and criteria for assessing treatment outcome in throid-associated ophthalmopathy. Endocrinol Metab Clin North Am 1987;16:391–407.
[25] Prummel MF. Graves' ophthalmopathy: diagnosis and management [editorial]. Eur J Nucl Med 2000;27(4):373–6.
[26] Bartalena L, Marcocci C, Bogazzi F, et al. Use of corticosteroids to prevent progression of Graves' ophthalmopathy after radioactive iodine therapy for hyperthyroidism. N Engl J Med 1989;321:1349–52.
[27] DeGroot LJ, Gorman CA, Pinchera A, et al. Therapeutic controversies: radiation and Graves' ophthalmopathy. J Clin Endocrinol Metab 1995;80:339–49.
[28] Boyle IT, Grieg WR, Thompson JA, et al. Effect of thyroid ablation on dysthyroid exophthalmos. Proc R Soc Med 1969;62:19–23.
[29] Bartalena L, Marcocci C, Tanda ML, et al. Cigarette smoking and treatment outcomes in Graves' ophthalmopathy. Ann Intern Med 1998;129:632–5.
[30] Cartlidge NE, Crombie A, Anderson J, et al. Critical study of 5% guanethidine in ocular manifestations of Graves' disease. BMJ 1969;4(684):645–7.
[31] Leone CR. The management of ophthalmic Graves' disease. Ophthalmology 1984;91(7): 770–9.
[32] Physicians' Desk Reference. 55th ed. Montvale (NJ): Medical Economics Co. Inc.; 2001. p. 2110–1.
[33] Wakelkamp IM, Baldeschi L, Saeed P, et al. Surgical or medical decompression as a first-line treatment of optic neuropathy in Graves' ophthalmopathy? A randomized controlled trial. Clin Endocrinol (Oxf) 2005;63(3):323–8.
[34] Prummel MF, Weirsinga WM. Immunomodulatory treatment of Graves' ophthalmology. Thyroid 1998;8(6):545–8.
[35] Wiersinga WM. Immunosuppressive treatment of Graves' ophthalmopathy. Thyroid 1992; 2(3):229–33.
[36] Brennan MW, Leone CR Jr, Janaki L. Radiation therapy for Graves' disease. Am J Ophthalmol 1983;96(2):195–9.
[37] Hurbli T, Char DH, Harris J, et al. Radiation therapy for thyroid eye diseases. Am J Ophthalmol 1985;99(6):633–7.
[38] Gorman CA, Garrity JA, Fatourechi V. A prospective, randomised, double-blind, placebo controlled study of radiotherapy for Graves' ophthalmopathy. Ophthalmology 2001;108(9): 1523–34.
[39] Mouritis MP, van Kempen-Harteveld ML, Garcia MBG, et al. Radiotherapy for Graves' orbitopathy: randomised, placebo controlled study. Lancet 2000;355:1505–9.
[40] Parsons JT, Bova FJ, Fitzgerald CR, et al. Radiation optic neuropathy after megavoltage external-beam irradiation: analysis of time-dose factors. Int J Radiat Oncol Biol Phys 1994;30:755–63.
[41] Al-Mefty O, Kersh JE, Routh A, et al. The long-term side effects of radiation therapy for benign brain tumors in adults. J Neurosurg 1990;73:502–12.
[42] Capo H, Kupersmith MJ. Efficacy and complications of radiotherapy of anterior visual pathway tumors. Neuro-ophthalmology 1991;9:179–203.
[43] Goldsmith BJ, Rosenthal SA, Wara WM, et al. Optic neuropathy after irradiation of meningioma. Radiology 1992;185:71–6.
[44] Cheng SWK, Ting ACW, Wu PH, et al. Accelerated progression of carotid stenosis in patients with previous external neck irradiation. J Vasc Surg 2004;39:409–15.
[45] Shorr N, Seiff S. The four stages of surgical rehabilitation of the patient with dysthyroid ophthalmopathy. Ophthalmology 1986;93:476–83.
[46] Tarrus-Montaner S, Lucarelli MJ, Lemke BN, et al. The surgical treatment of Graves' orbitopathy: a decade of progress. Ophthalmol Clin North Am 2000;13(4):693–704.

[47] Antoszyk JH, Tucker N, Codere F. Orbital decompression for Graves' disease: exposure through a modified blepharoplasty incision. Ophthalmic Surg 1992;23(8):516–21.

[48] Fatourechi V, Garrity JA, Bartley GB, et al. Graves' ophthalmopathy. Results of transantral orbital decompression performed primarily for cosmetic indications. Ophthalmology 1994; 101(5):938–42.

[49] McCord CD. Current trends in orbital decompression. Ophthalmology 1985;92(1):21–33.

[50] Olivari N. Transpalpebral decompression of endocrine ophthalmopathy (Graves' disease) by removal of intraocular fat: experience with 147 operations over 5 years. Plast Reconstr Surg 1991;87(4):627–41.

ELSEVIER
SAUNDERS

Otolaryngol Clin N Am
39 (2006) 943–958

OTOLARYNGOLOGIC
CLINICS
OF NORTH AMERICA

Endoscopic Orbital and Optic Nerve Decompression

Steven D. Pletcher, MD[a],
Raj Sindwani, MD, FACS, FRCS[b],
Ralph Metson, MD[c,d],*

[a]*Department of Otolaryngology–Head and Neck Surgery, University of California,
San Francisco, San Francisco, CA, USA*
[b]*Department of Otolaryngology–Head and Neck Surgery, Saint Louis University School
of Medicine, Saint Louis, MO, USA*
[c]*Department of Otology and Laryngology, Harvard Medical School, Boston, MA, USA*
[d]*Department of Otolaryngology, Massachusetts Eye and Ear Infirmary, Boston, MA, USA*

For more than 100 years, surgical decompression of the orbit has been used to treat the severe proptosis and optic neuropathy associated with Graves' disease. Although decompression techniques involving removal each of the four walls of the orbit have been described [1–4], the Walsh-Ogura decompression [5] described in the 1950s was favored by most otolaryngologists. This operation uses the familiar Caldwell-Luc approach to remove the inferior and medial orbital walls, allowing the enlarged orbital fat and muscles to decompress into the ethmoid and maxillary sinus cavities.

Soon after the introduction of transnasal endoscopic sinus surgery in the mid 1980s, surgeons began to experiment with endoscopic orbital surgery. Endoscopic orbital decompression was first described by Kennedy [6] and Michel [7] in the early 1990s. Enhanced visualization of key anatomic landmarks allowed for safe and thorough decompression of the entire medial orbital wall, as well as the medial portion of the orbital floor. This improved visualization is most notable in the region of the orbital apex, a critical area of decompression in patients with optic neuropathy. These advantages have allowed the endoscopic approach to replace the Walsh-Ogura procedure as the technique of choice for orbital decompression.

The benefits of endoscopic instrumentation for orbital decompression can be similarly applied when operating in the vicinity of the optic nerve. Decompression of the optic nerve involves complete removal of the bone

---

* Corresponding author: Zero Emerson Place, Suite 2D, Boston, MA 02114.
E-mail address: ralph_metson@meei.harvard.edu (R. Metson).

0030-6665/06/$ - see front matter © 2006 Elsevier Inc. All rights reserved.
doi:10.1016/j.otc.2006.06.003

that forms the medial wall of the optic canal. Although the indications for and surgical techniques of orbital decompression are fairly well established, controversy exists regarding both the indications and extent of surgery necessary for optic nerve decompression.

Graves' orbitopathy (dysthyroid orbitopathy)

Graves' disease is an autoimmune disorder that affects primarily the thyroid and the orbit. Thyroid manifestations are characterized by the production of autoantibodies to the TSH receptor with subsequent hyperstimulation and resultant hyperthyroidism. The thyroid manifestations of Graves' disease an be treated with thyroid-suppressive medications, radiation (I^{131}), or surgery.

The orbital manifestations of Graves' disease, known as dysthyroid orbitopathy, also represent an autoimmune process although the exact antibody target remains unclear. Inflammation associated with infiltration of T-cells and deposition of glycosaminoglycan results in enlargement of orbital fat and extraocular muscles. This increase in volume of contents within the confines of the rigid bony orbit results in increased pressure and resultant proptosis, or compression of the optic nerve. The degree of proptosis does not correlate with the overall severity of disease, as patients with poor compliance of the orbital septum may not experience significant proptosis but can have severe compression at the orbital apex and develop optic neuropathy. The orbital and thyroid manifestations of Graves' disease follow distinct and independent clinical courses.

Clinical manifestations of dysthyroid orbitopathy range from mild findings such as tearing, photophobia, and conjunctival injection to significant proptosis, diplopia, exposure keratopathy, and visual loss from optic neuropathy. The clinical course of Graves' orbitopathy can be divided into the acute phase, characterized by active inflammation, which lasts 6 to 18 months and the chronic phase, characterized by fibrosis with stabilization of proptosis. It is preferable to perform orbital decompression during the chronic phase.

Medical treatment of dysthyroid orbitopathy

Local measures such as lubrication, eyelid taping, and patching for patients with dryness and diplopia represent initial conservative treatment approaches. More aggressive treatments include the use of systemic corticosteroids and orbital radiation. Both of these treatments appear to be most effective during the acute phase of the disease. Systemic corticosteroid treatment usually results in marked improvement, but the symptoms generally recur following discontinuation of steroid treatment. Because of the deleterious side effects of long-term corticosteroid use, steroid treatment are often used as a temporizing measure or in conjunction with surgical decompression. The use of orbital radiation is controversial, and its efficacy has been challenged by two recent randomized prospective trials [8,9].

Endoscopic orbital decompression

The endoscopic technique allows for unmatched visualization of critical anatomic regions including the skull base and orbital apex and avoids external or sublabial incisions. The entire medial orbital wall as well as the medial portion of the orbital floor is removed with endoscopic decompression (Fig. 1).

Technique

The patient is positioned in the supine position, and topical vasoconstriction is achieved with topical oxymetazoline (0.05%) pledgets. The eyes are maintained within surgical field, protected with scleral shields. Image-guidance systems may be used at the surgeons discretion. Local injection of lidocaine 1% with 1:100,000 epinephrine is administered along the lateral nasal wall in the region of the maxillary line (a bony eminence that extends from the anterior attachment of the middle turbinate to the root of the inferior turbinate).

Surgery begins with an incision just posterior to the maxillary line. The uncinate process is medialized and removed, exposing the natural ostium of the maxillary sinus. With orbital decompression it is important to widely open the maxillary sinus to achieve adequate access to the orbital floor and prevent blockage of the ostium from orbital fat, which protrudes following decompression. Enlargement is performed primarily in a posterior direction as extension of the antrostomy too far anteriorly risks of damage to the

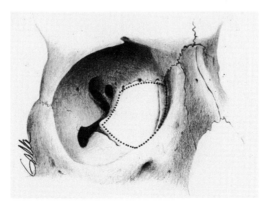

Fig. 1. Bone removed during endoscopic orbital decompression includes the medial orbital wall and the medial aspect of the orbital floor.

nasolacrimal duct. Using a 30 degree endoscope, the wide antrostomy should allow easy visualization of the infraorbital nerve as it courses along the floor of the orbit.

An endoscopic sphenoethmoidectomy is performed in standard fashion. We advocate removal of the middle turbinate during orbital decompression to optimize exposure of the medial orbital wall and facilitate postoperative cleaning. An image guidance system may be used at this point to confirm removal of all ethmoid cells along the medial orbital wall, and to ensure complete dissection to the sphenoid face and posterior skull base.

The skeletonized medial orbital wall is then carefully penetrated in a controlled fashion with a spoon curette or other blunt instrument. It should be noted that once the lamina is transgressed, orbital fat should not be visible, as long as the underlying periorbital fascia is left intact. The thin bone of the lamina papyracea is elevated while preserving the underlying periorbita. Bone fragments are removed using Blakesly forceps (Fig. 2). Bone removal proceeds superiorly toward the ethmoid roof, inferiorly to the orbital floor, and anteriorly to the maxillary line. Bone in the region of the frontal recess is left intact; if bone is removed from this region, herniated fat may obstruct drainage of the frontal sinus.

As dissection proceeds posteriorly, thick bone is encountered in the region of the orbital apex within 2 mm of the sphenoid face. This bone corresponds to the annulus of Zinn, from which the extraocular muscles originate and through which the optic nerve passes. This landmark represents the posterior limit of a standard decompression. For patients with optic neuropathy, experienced surgeons may consider continuing the decompression posteriorly into the sphenoid sinus; however, the benefits of incorporating

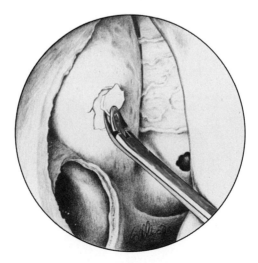

Fig. 2. Once the medial orbital wall has been exposed, Blakesly forceps are used to remove fragments of the lamina papyracea.

and optic nerve decompression into standard orbital decompression are unclear, and may lead to inadvertent injury to the nerve.

Removal of the orbital floor can be technically challenging, depending on
its thickness. Only that portion of the floor that is medial to the infraorbital
nerve is removed. A spoon curette is used to engage the orbital floor at its
medial extent and down-fracture the bone (Fig. 3). The bone of the orbital
floor is thicker than that of the medial orbital wall, and significant force may
be required for this maneuver. If the spoon curette is not sturdy enough for
this portion of the procedure the heavier mastoid curette may be used. The
bone may fracture in one large piece, typically with a natural cleavage plane
at the canal of the infraorbital nerve, or, more frequently, it fractures into
several small pieces. A 30-degree endoscope and angled forceps may facilitate bone removal while preserving the infraorbital canal as the lateral limit
of dissection.

Once the lamina papyracea and medial orbital floor have been removed,
the periorbita is fully exposed. A sickle knife is then used to open this fascial
layer. Care must be taken to avoid "burying" the tip of the sickle knife and
potentially injuring the underlying orbital contents such as the medial rectus
muscle. The periorbital incision should be initiated at the posterior limit of
decompression (just anterior to the sphenoid face) and brought anteriorly so
that prolapsing fat does not obscure visualization. Parallel incisions are performed along the ethmoid roof and orbital floor. To minimize the risk of
postoperative diplopia, a 10 mm-wide sling of fascia overlying the medial
rectus muscle may be preserved while the remainder of the periorbita is removed using angled Blakesley forceps (Fig. 4) [10]. In patients with optic
neuropathy, the fascial sling technique is not used to allow maximal

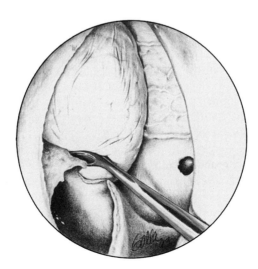

Fig. 3. A spoon curette is used to down-fracture the medial portion of the orbital floor.

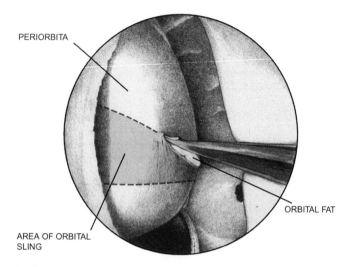

PERIORBITA

ORBITAL FAT

AREA OF ORBITAL
SLING

Fig. 4. Following bony decompression, a sickle knife is used to incise the periorbita. In patients without optic neuropathy, a sling of fascia may be preserved overlying the medial rectus muscle to minimize postoperative diplopia.

decompression. A ball-tipped probe and sickle knife may be used to identify and incise remaining fibrous bands that often course superficially between lobules of orbital fat. Upon completion of the procedure, a generous pro-lapse of fat into the opened ethmoid and maxillary cavities should be ob-served (Fig. 5). The globe may be blotted to encourage maximal fat herniation and confirm a decrease in retropulsive resistance.

Depending on the clinical scenario and desired degree of decompression, a subsequent lateral decompression may be performed through an external approach. When performed immediately following medial decompression, the orbital contents are easily retracted in a medial direction, allowing for excellent exposure of the lateral bony wall. Bilateral decompressions may be performed concurrently or in a staged procedure.

Nasal packing is avoided to ensure maximal decompression and avoid compression of exposed orbital contents. The patient is discharged the morning after surgery with a prescription for oral antistaphylococcal antibi-otics and instructions to begin twice daily nasal saline irrigations. At the first postoperative visit 1 week following surgery, crusts and debris are cleaned from the surgical site under endoscopic guidance.

For patients with severe comorbidities, a strong preference for local an-esthesia, or in whom surgery is being performed on an only seeing eye, de-compression may be performed under local anesthesia with sedation [11]. This approach allows the surgeon to monitor the patient's vision throughout the procedure. Sedation may be achieved with an intravenous bolus of pro-pofol (0.4–0.8 mg/kg) before injection of local anesthesia, followed by an in-fusion of 75 to 95 µg/kg during the procedure. Local anesthesia is

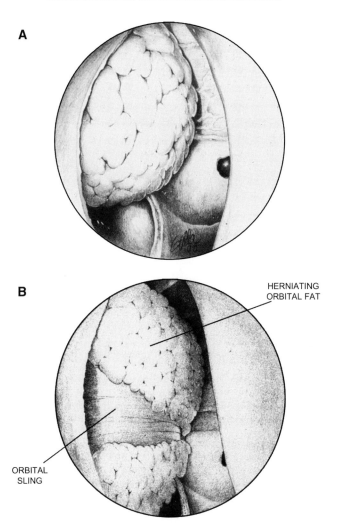

Fig. 5. Following decompression, orbital fat protrudes into the ethmoid and maxillary spaces (*A*). With the ortbital sling technique, a strip of periorbita remains to support the medial rectus muscle and minimize postoperative diplopia (*B*).

administered initially with 4% cocaine pledgets followed by injection of lidocaine 1% with 1:100,000 epinephrine. Patients may report discomfort during removal of the lamina papyracea. This sensation may be relieved by infiltration of a small amount of additional anesthetic solution along the medial orbital wall.

Results

The goals of orbital decompression vary depending upon the indication for the procedure. In patients with compressive optic neuropathy, restoration of visual deficits is the key outcome, while in patients with corneal exposure or severe proptosis, ocular recession may be the primary end point. The reported incidence of improvement following endoscopic orbital decompression for Graves' orbitopathy ranges from 22% to 89% [6,12,13]. This wide variation in results reflects the diverse patient populations and definitions of improvement. Postoperative deterioration of visual acuity occurs in less than 5% of patients [7,12,13]. Ocular recession as a result of endoscopic decompression alone averages 3.5 mm (range 2–12 mm). The addition of concurrent lateral decompression to the endoscopic procedure provides an additional 2 mm of globe recession [13].

Complications

Diplopia is not an uncommon occurrence following orbital decompression with 15% to 63% of postoperative patients reporting new-onset diplopia or worsening of preexisting symptoms [7,11,13–16]. This complication is believed to be a result of a change in the vector of pull of the extraocular muscles. Decompressive surgery rarely alleviates preexisting diplopia. Patients who have diplopia following decompressive surgery often require strabismus surgery for correction. All patients should be informed of the possibility of postoperative double vision, as well as the potential need for further surgical intervention if this persists.

Several methods to decrease postoperative diplopia have been reported. Multiple authors have described the preservation of a strut of inferomedial bone between the decompressed floor and medial wall [12,17]. When this strut is maintained, however, it is technically difficult to remove the orbital floor through a purely endoscopic technique. The maintenance of a facial sling in the region of the medial rectus has also been demonstrated to decrease the incidence of postoperative diplopia [10]. This technique provides similar support as the medial strut technique, but allows for endoscopic access to decompress the medial orbital floor. The concept of a balanced decompression (concurrent medial and lateral decompression) has also been suggested as a means to decrease postoperative diplopia [14,18,19]. When operating for compressive optic neuropathy, techniques designed to limit diplopia may also limit the extent of decompression, and postoperative diplopia is often accepted as a concession to improved visual acuity.

Postoperative bleeding following decompression is best managed through endoscopic identification and direct cauterization of the bleeding site. Nasal packing is generally not used to avoid pressure on the exposed orbital apex and optic nerve. Postoperative infection is minimized through the use of postoperative antibiotics with staphylococcal coverage. A large maxillary antrostomy and limited bone removal in the frontal recess region minimize the risk of developing postoperative sinusitis. Epiphora may develop if the maxillary antrostomy is extended too far anteriorly with transection of the nasolacrimal duct. This complication is treated with an endoscopic dacryocystorhinostomy. Leakage of cerebrospinal fluid and blindness are very rare complications that have been reported following nonendoscopic decompression techniques.

Optic nerve decompression

Historically the most common, and perhaps most controversial, indication for optic nerve decompression has been traumatic optic neuropathy (TON). The efficacy of decompression in this setting remains unclear. Endoscopic and nonendoscopic techniques of optic nerve decompression have also been used for a variety of nontraumatic causes of compressive optic neuropathy such as benign tumors and inflammatory or fibroosseus lesions [20]. It is in these patients with nontraumatic, compressive optic neuropathy that endoscopic optic nerve decompression appears to be most successful.

Controversy regarding the treatment of TON exists because the two mainstays of therapy, corticosteroids and surgical decompression, have not shown definitive clinical benefit when compared with observation alone [14,21]. To address this issue the International Optic Nerve Trauma Study (IONTS) was undertaken. The initial goal of a randomized, controlled trial was abandoned when patient recruitment was insufficient to support this study design. Thus, a comparative nonrandomized interventional study with concurrent treatment groups was performed with 127 patients [14]. No clear benefit was found for either corticosteroid therapy or surgical optic canal decompression. The authors discussed numerous published uncontrolled studies, and their overall recommendation based on the IONTS and their literature review was that treatment should be determined on an individual patient basis.

Several retrospective studies subsequent to the IONTS have suggested improvement in visual acuity with optic nerve decompression following failure of visual improvement with steroids [22–24]. The uncontrolled nature of these studies, however, must be taken into account when considering surgical decompression for traumatic optic neuropathy.

Surgical anatomy

The optic nerve may be divided into three segments: the intraorbital, the intracanalicular, and the intracranial segment. Optic nerve decompression aims to relieve compressive forces within the intracanalicular portion of the nerve. The canal of the optic nerve is formed by the two struts of the lesser wing of the sphenoid and carries both the optic nerve and the ophthalmic artery. At the orbital apex is the fibrous annulus of Zinn.

Pathophysiology

Compression on the optic nerve may result from neoplastic, inflammatory, or traumatic processes. Initial theories of vascular compromise from external compression with resultant injury to the optic nerve have been largely discarded. Manual compression resulting in conduction block and focal demyelination from compression are the favored pathophysiologic explanations for compressive optic neuropathy. Rapid recovery following decompression results from relief of the manual compression block while a delayed recovery may occur over a period of weeks to months as a result of remyelination [25].

Traumatic optic neuropathy may be divided into two categories: indirect and direct. Direct TON results from a penetrating injury with projectiles or other sharp objects. In these cases the intraorbital portion of the optic nerve is generally injured and decompression is not recommended. Indirect TON results from blunt trauma to the head. This injury can occur with or without associated fractures of the orbital canal. The pathophysiology of visual loss in these cases is frequently unclear, and may include intraneural edema, hematoma, shearing injury to the microvasculature or axons, altered cerebrospinal fluid circulation, and interruption of direct axonal transport. If there is evidence of complete disruption of the optic nerve, decompression is not indicated, as the optic nerve will not recover from such injury. In cases where edema, hematoma, or moderate bony compression is suggested, however, decompression may be considered.

Evaluation and treatment

Compressive optic neuropathy may have an insidious onset resulting in delayed diagnosis. Patients' initial symptoms are often vague including mild blurry or "fuzzy" vision without significant loss of visual acuity and with normal fundoscopic examination. More rigorous examination often reveals variable, limited visual field defects, a decrease in color vision, and an afferent papillary defect on the affected side. Unfortunately, these symptoms may go unnoticed until the more advanced stages of compression result in decreased visual acuity. Thus, careful ophthalmologic examination is essential in discovering early signs of compression and, if abnormal, should be evaluated with an MRI scan. Once a compressive optic neuropathy is diagnosed, surgical decompression is considered based upon the pathology and extent of the compressive lesion. Systemic corticosteroids frequently provide temporary improvement and may be considered while awaiting definitive treatment.

Patients with suspected TON generally have sustained significant blunt force trauma and should be evaluated by a trauma team for evidence of multisystem injury. As soon as TON is suspected, examination by an ophthalmologist is mandatory. Visual acuity should be determined as soon as possible and closely monitored. Patients should be tested for an afferent pupillary defect, which may be the only sign of TON in unconscious patients. If possible, formal visual field testing and color vision testing should be performed as abnormalities of color and peripheral vision typically precede decreased visual acuity in the progression of optic neuropathy. Evaluation of ocular pressure and fundoscopic exam may also yield important information. A fine cut CT scan through the orbit and optic canal should be obtained to look for fractures and bone displacement in the orbital apex.

Observation and treatment with corticosteroids are both reasonable medical approaches to traumatic optic neuropathy. Steroid dosing is controversial, and in the IONTS steroid dosing did not correlate with clinical outcome. Frequently a loading dose of methylprednisone (30 mg/kg bolus) followed by a continuous infusion of 5.4 mg/kg/h is given for 48 hours. This regimen is based upon studies of spinal cord injury.

Endoscopic optic nerve decompression

Traditional surgical approaches for optic nerve decompression include transorbital, extranasal transethmoid, transantral, intranasal microscopic, and craniotomy approaches. Endonasal endoscopic decompression of the optic nerve offers many advantages over these approaches, including excellent visualization, preservation of olfaction, rapid recovery time, a lack of external scars, and less operative stress in patients who may be suffering from multisystem trauma.

Technique

Patients are prepared for surgery in a similar manner to those undergoing orbital decompression. A standard sphenoethmoidectomy is performed. The sphenoid face is widely opened and the bulge of the optic canal is identified along the lateral wall of the sphenoid sinus, superior to the carotid artery. In some patients, the optic canal may be initially identified in a posterior ethmoid or Onodi cell, which can be seen on preoperative CT scan [26]. Identification and opening of the Onodi cell is important to provide adequate surgical exposure and allow full access to the optic canal.

Following exposure of the medial orbital wall, a spoon curette is used to fracture the lamina papyracea approximately 1 cm anterior to the optic canal. The lamina is then carefully removed in a posterior direction to expose the annulus of Zinn and the optic canal. Care must be taken to avoid penetration of the periorbita, as subsequent herniation of orbital fat will obscure the surgical field. As the optic canal is approached, the thin lamina will be replaced with the thick bone of the lesser wing of the sphenoid. This bone must be thinned before removal. A long-handled drill with a diamond burr is used to methodically thin the medial wall of the optic canal (Fig. 6). While drilling, care must be taken to prevent contact of the drill bit with the prominence of the carotid artery, which is located just inferior and posterior to the optic nerve. Care should also be taken to avoid excess generation of heat while drilling this bone as thermal damage to the optic nerve may result. After the bone is appropriately thinned, a microcurette

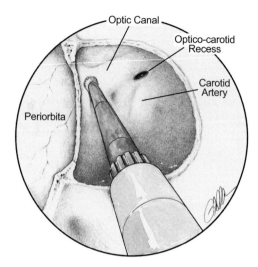

Fig. 6. Endoscopic view of the right posterior nasal cavity following wide sphenoidotomy. The lamina papyracea has been removed to reveal periobita near the orbital apex. A diamond burr is used to thin the bone of the optic canal.

is used to fracture the thinned bone in a medial direction, away from the optic nerve (Fig. 7). Bone fragments are then removed from the decompressed nerve using blakesly forceps (Fig. 8), with resultant medial decompression of the optic nerve (Fig. 9).

Controversy exists regarding the length of optic canal that should be decompressed as well as the necessity for decompression of the optic sheath. With compressive optic neuropathy secondary to neoplasms, the extent of decompression is dictated by the size and location of the neoplasm. For

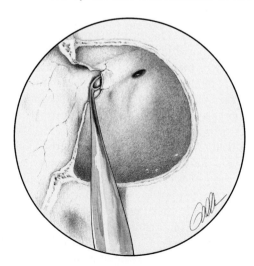

Fig. 7. A microcurette is used to elevate thinned bone of the optic canal.

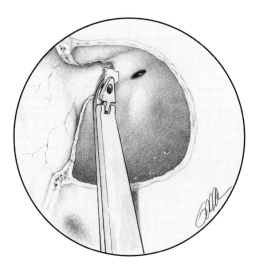

Fig. 8. Blakesly forceps are used to remove bone fragments and expose the underlying optic nerve.

cases of TON and dysthyroid orbitopathy, removal of bone for a distance of 1 cm posterior to the face of the sphenoid sinus is generally thought to be sufficient [27].

Incision of the sheath has been advocated by some authors to further de-compress the nerve itself; however, this maneuver may be unnecessary and risks damage to the underlying nerve fibers and ophthalmic artery as well as cerebral spinal fluid (CSF) leak, with resultant risk of meningitis. With clear

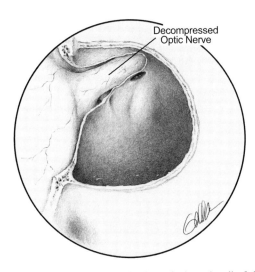

Fig. 9. The decompressed optic nerve is visible along the lateral wall of the sphenoid sinus.

risks and an absence of data to suggest benefit for sheath decompression, we do not advocate this maneuver for most patients undergoing optic nerve decompression.

Results

Most patients who undergo optic nerve decompression for compressive nontraumatic optic neuropathy will have significant improvement in visual acuity. An immediate improvement in visual acuity is frequently observed, probably from relief of a mechanical conduction block. Further improvement may occur over a period of weeks to months as remyelination of the nerve leads to more efficient conduction [25].

The efficacy of optic nerve decompression in traumatic optic neuropathy is unclear. Much of the difficulty in determining the success of surgical intervention arises from the relatively high rate of spontaneous recovery from TON. Thus, well-controlled studies with significant power are required to delineate the efficacy of surgical intervention. Unfortunately, such studies have not been possible due to the rarity of this condition.

In cases of nontraumatic, compressive optic neuropathy, however, the natural course of disease is not one of spontaneous resolution. Thus, it is reasonable to conclude that visual improvement following surgical decompression is a direct result of the procedure. In our recent experience of endoscopic optic nerve decompressions for nontraumatic optic neuropathy, improved visual acuity was noted following 8 of 10 decompressions. One patient required multiple decompressions due to progression of her fibrous dysplasia with recurrent impingement upon the optic nerve [20].

Complications

The risk of CSF leak, meningitis, and visual loss with optic nerve decompression appears to be higher than with standard endoscopic sinus surgery or orbital decompression. Although several studies with 20 to 45 patients report no complications, the IONTS and another recent study reported several cases of CSF leak, some with associated meningitis and visual decompensation [14,23]. In the IONTS, it is unclear whether the complications occurred in patients who underwent endoscopic decompression representing less than 40% of patients in their series, or an external approach.

Summary

With excellent visualization of the orbital apex and optic canal, the endoscopic transnasal approach is well suited for both orbital and optic nerve decompression. This operation is an advanced endoscopic technique, and should be performed only by surgeons experienced in endoscopic nasal surgery. Although the indications and expected results for orbital decompression are well established, those for optic nerve decompression continue to evolve.

References

[1] Kronlein R. Zur Pathologie und operativen Behandlung der Desmoid Cysten der Orbita. Beitr Klin Chir 1889;4:149–63.
[2] Sewall E. Operative control of progressive exophthalmos. Arch Otolaryngol Head Neck Surg 1936;24:621–4.
[3] Hirsch O. Surgical decompression of exophthalmos. Arch Otolaryngol Head Neck Surg 1950;51:325–31.
[4] Naffziger HC. Progressive exophthalmos. Ann R Coll Surg Engl 1954;15:1–24.
[5] Walsh TE, Ogura JH. Transantral orbital decompression for malignant exophthalmos. Laryngoscope 1957;67:544–68.
[6] Kennedy DW, Goodstein ML, Miller NR, et al. Endoscopic transnasal orbital decompression. Arch Otolaryngol Head Neck Surg 1990;116:275–82.
[7] Michel O, Bresgen K, Russmann W, et al. Endoscopically-controlled endonasal orbital decompression in malignant exophthalmos. Laryngorhinootologie 1991;70:656–62.
[8] Gorman CA, Garrity JA, Fatourechi V, et al. A prospective, randomized, double-blind, placebo-controlled study of orbital radiotherapy for Graves' ophthalmopathy. Ophthalmology 2001;108:1523–34.
[9] Mourits MP, van Kempen-Harteveld ML, Garcia MB, et al. Radiotherapy for Graves' orbitopathy: randomised placebo-controlled study. Lancet 2000;355:1505–9.
[10] Metson R, Samaha M. Reduction of diplopia following endoscopic orbital decompression: the orbital sling technique. Laryngoscope 2002;112:1753–7.
[11] Metson R, Shore JW, Gliklich RE, et al. Endoscopic orbital decompression under local anesthesia. Otolaryngol Head Neck Surg 1995;113:661–7.
[12] Schaefer SD, Soliemanzadeh P, Della Rocca DA, et al. Endoscopic and transconjunctival orbital decompression for thyroid-related orbital apex compression. Laryngoscope 2003; 113:508–13.
[13] Metson R, Dallow RL, Shore JW. Endoscopic orbital decompression. Laryngoscope 1994; 104:950–7.
[14] Shepard KG, Levin PS, Terris DJ. Balanced orbital decompression for Graves' ophthalmopathy. Laryngoscope 1998;108:1648–53.
[15] Wright ED, Davidson J, Codere F, et al. Endoscopic orbital decompression with preservation of an inferomedial bony strut: minimization of postoperative diplopia. J Otolaryngol 1999;28:252–6.
[16] Eloy P, Trussart C, Jouzdani E, et al. Transnasal endoscopic orbital decompression and Graves' ophtalmopathy. Acta Otorhinolaryngol Belg 2000;54:165–74.
[17] Goldberg RA, Shorr N, Cohen MS. The medical orbital strut in the prevention of postdecompression dystopia in dysthyroid ophthalmopathy. Ophthal Plast Reconstr Surg 1992;8:32–4.
[18] Unal M, Leri F, Konuk O, et al. Balanced orbital decompression combined with fat removal in Graves' ophthalmopathy: do we really need to remove the third wall? Ophthal Plast Reconstr Surg 2003;19:112–8.
[19] Graham SM, Brown CL, Carter KD, et al. Medial and lateral orbital wall surgery for balanced decompression in thyroid eye disease. Laryngoscope 2003;113:1206–9.
[20] Pletcher SD, Metson R. Endoscopic optic nerve decompression for non-traumatic optic neuropathy. American Rhinologic Society combined otolaryngologic spring meeting, Chicago, Il, 2006.
[21] Cook MW, Levin LA, Joseph MP, et al. Traumatic optic neuropathy. A meta-analysis. Arch Otolaryngol Head Neck Surg 1996;122:389–92.
[22] Kountakis SE, Maillard AA, El-Harazi SM, et al. Endoscopic optic nerve decompression for traumatic blindness. Otolaryngol Head Neck Surg 2000;123:34–7.

[23] Rajiniganth MG, Gupta AK, Gupta A, et al. Traumatic optic neuropathy: visual outcome following combined therapy protocol. Arch Otolaryngol Head Neck Surg 2003;129:1203–6.

[24] Li KK, Teknos TN, Lai A, et al. Traumatic optic neuropathy: result in 45 consecutive surgically treated patients. Otolaryngol Head Neck Surg 1999;120:5–11.

[25] McDonald WI. The symptomatology of tumours of the anterior visual pathways. Can J Neurol Sci 1982;9:381–90.

[26] Allmond L, Murr AH. Clinical problem solving: radiology. Radiology quiz case 1: opacified Onodi cell. Arch Otolaryngol Head Neck Surg 2002;128:596, 598–599.

[27] Luxenberger W, Stammberger H, Jebeles JA, et al. Endoscopic optic nerve decompression: the Graz experience. Laryngoscope 1998;108:873–82.

ELSEVIER
SAUNDERS

Otolaryngol Clin N Am
39 (2006) 959–977

OTOLARYNGOLOGIC
CLINICS
OF NORTH AMERICA

Evaluation and Management of Congenital Nasolacrimal Duct Obstruction

Mitesh K. Kapadia, MD, PhD[a,b,c], Suzanne K. Freitag, MD[a,d,*], John J. Woog, MD, FACS[e,f]

[a]*Department of Ophthalmology, Boston Medical Center,*
720 Harrison Avenue Boston, MA 02118, USA
[b]*Department of Ophthalmology, Tufts University School of Medicine,*
136 Harrison Avenue, Boston, MA 02111, USA
[c]*New England Eye Center, Tufts-New England Medical Center,*
750 Washington Street, NEMC #450, Boston, MA 02111, USA
[d]*Department of Ophthalmology, Boston University School of Medicine,*
715 Albany Street, Boston, MA 02118, USA
[e]*Department of Ophthalmology, Mayo Clinic College of Medicine,*
200 First Street SW, Rochester, MN 55905, USA
[f]*Department of Ophthalmology, Mayo Clinic, 200 First Street SW,*
Rochester, MN 55905, USA

Congenital nasolacrimal obstruction is a common disorder in infants that results in persistent tearing and may lead to infections, such as dacryocystitis, orbital cellulitis, and bacterial conjunctivitis. The true incidence of this disorder in healthy newborns remains controversial. The most frequently quoted number of 6% comes from a study of 200 consecutive live births in the 1940s in which nasolacrimal patency was assessed by the presence or absence of discharge on compression of the lacrimal sac [1]. Estimates from other studies, which often use different criteria for diagnosis, vary considerably from 1.2% to 30% [1–6]. The incidence of the disorder is higher in children who have

Portions of this article are reprinted from: Freitag SK, Woog JJ. Evaluation and Management of Congenital Dacryostenosis. In: John J. Woog, Ed. Manual of Endoscopic Lacrimal and Orbital Surgery. Philadelphia: Butterworth/Heinemann, 2004; with permission.
* Corresponding author.
E-mail address: suzanne.freitag@bmc.org (S.K. Freitag).

oto.theclinics.com

craniofacial disorders and Down's syndrome [7]. This article reviews the causes and treatment of congenital nasolacrimal obstruction.

Anatomy

The lacrimal drainage system begins with the superior and inferior puncta, which lead to the superior and inferior canaliculi (Fig. 1). In adults, the canaliculi are oriented vertically for 2 mm, turn horizontally, and extend 8 to 10 mm before entering the lacrimal sac. In approximately 90% of individuals, the superior and inferior canaliculi fuse to form a common canaliculus for 2 to 3 mm before entering the sac.

The lacrimal sac lies within the lacrimal sac fossa formed by the maxillary and lacrimal bones. The superior portion of the sac lies above the medial canthal tendon, which splits into anterior and posterior crura to surround the sac. This tendon is the main support structure that anchors the eyelids to the medial face and must be preserved during lacrimal surgery. In adults, the lacrimal sac averages about 10 mm long and 4 mm wide and connects to a 12-mm nasolacrimal duct, which opens into the nose below the inferior turbinate. A membrane formed at the junction of the lacrimal and nasal mucosa, the valve of Hasner, helps to prevent reflux of nasal material into the lacrimal duct. The lack of a patent opening through this membrane into the nose is the most frequent anatomic cause of congenital nasolacrimal obstruction.

The development of the lacrimal outflow system begins with a thickened ridge of cells of surface ectoderm at the naso-optic fissure. In the 12-week embryo, these cells dive into the surrounding mesoderm to form a solid cord of cells, elongating in a direction from the future medial canthus

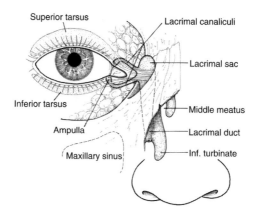

Fig. 1. Anatomy of the lacrimal outflow system. (*From* Rose JG, Lucarelli MJ, Lemke BN. Lacrimal, orbital and sinus anatomy. In: John J. Woog, Ed. Manual of Endoscopic Lacrimal and Orbital Surgery. Philadelphia: Butterworth/Heinemann, 2004; with permission.)

toward the primitive nasal cavity. The canalization of the solid rod to form a hollow tube proceeds progressively in a direction from the medial canthus to the nose and should be complete during the sixth month of gestation. The canaliculi open into the eyelid margin during the seventh month, just before the eyelids separate.

The canalization of the ectodermal rods should be complete during the sixth month, but a persistent membrane often remains at the junction of the tubes, and is believed to represent the embryologic basis of congenital nasolacrimal duct obstruction (CNLDO). Postnatal sucking and respiration probably play an important role in the rupture of many persistent membranes. A study found that more than 70% of stillborn infants have CNLDO at birth [8], many times higher than that seen in normal newborns.

Other anomalies of the nasolacrimal system may arise from problems at any stage of the development process. Agenesis of portions of the system may result from failure of parts of the surface ectoderm to invaginate. Incomplete separation of the ectoderm from the surface may result in additional puncta or external lacrimal fistula. Partial canalization may result in a loss of patency or stenosis at any point in the system, including the puncta, lacrimal sac, and lacrimal duct.

Evaluation of the tearing infant

Symptoms of congenital nasolacrimal obstruction are observed often within the first few weeks of life and may be unilateral or bilateral. Epiphora is the most common, but least specific presenting sign. More specific signs include the presence of high tear meniscus and mucoid discharge that causes crusting of the eyelid margins. Regurgitation of mucopurulent material on compression of the lacrimal sac may be observed. Because the presence of these symptoms is variable, a thorough assessment of the eye and lacrimal system is important to rule out other causes of tearing and avoid subjecting infants unnecessarily to the risks of general anesthesia.

The first step in the evaluation of an infant who has epiphora is to determine whether excess tearing is a result of tear overproduction or outflow obstruction. Excess tear production may be caused by almost any factor that causes ocular irritation, including trichiasis, foreign body, corneal abrasion, or abnormal eyelid position. Any child who has epiphora and photophobia must be evaluated for congenital glaucoma.

The patency of the lacrimal outflow system is assessed using the modified fluorescein dye disappearance test. Fluorescein mixed with topical anesthetic is placed into the lower conjunctival fornix of each eye and excess solution and tears are blotted with a tissue. After 5 minutes the child is examined while seated in the parent's lap. Light passed through a cobalt blue filter helps to identify residual fluorescein, which should not be present [9]. In a prospective study of 80 infants, MacEwen and Young [10] found this test to be 90% sensitive and 100% specific for the presence of nasolacrimal obstruction.

Causes of congenital nasolacrimal obstruction

Congenital nasolacrimal duct obstruction

The most common cause of congenital nasolacrimal obstruction is an imperforate membrane at the valve of Hasner, at the opening of the lacrimal duct into the inferior meatus of the nose. Because this disorder is so common, most patients with signs and symptoms of lacrimal outflow obstruction are treated empirically without the use of imaging studies or confirmatory tests, unless the patient's history or physical examination suggests an alternate cause.

In this article, CNLDO refers specifically to obstruction that results from an imperforate membrane at the valve of Hasner, whereas the more general term "congenital nasolacrimal obstruction" refers to an obstruction anywhere in the lacrimal outflow system. Because CNLDO is by far the most common cause of congenital nasolacrimal obstruction and most patients are treated empirically, the terms often are used interchangeably in the literature and in the studies that are described in this article.

The presence of acute dacryocystitis is strongly suggestive of nasolacrimal obstruction. Typically, erythema, pain, and tenderness to palpation are observed around the medial canthus of the affected eye. Purulent discharge often is noted on compression of the lacrimal sac. Cellulitis, fever, and malaise also may be present.

The underlying cause of dacryocystitis remains controversial. One argument states that obstruction is the primary cause, which leads to the accumulation of tears and cellular debris with secondary infection. An alternative argument is that infection is the primary event with secondary obstruction from fibrosis and inflammation.

Bacterial cultures may have a role in the modification of initial antibiotic therapy, but do not seem to be a reliable indicator of whether or not obstruction or infection is present. MacEwen and colleagues [11] cultured 334 infants who did and did not have CNLDO; the incidence of bacterial growth was 21% and 23%, respectively. No correlation was found between the presence of purulent discharge on examination and the growth of bacteria in cultures; the discharge often was composed of sterile debris, mucus, and epithelial cells. Furthermore, no correlation was found between the status of bacterial cultures and the rate of spontaneous resolution of symptoms.

The most common organisms that are identified from children who have CNLDO are *Staphylococcus aureus*, *Streptococcus pneumoniae*, *Haemophilus influenzae*, *Moraxella* spp, *Pseudomonas* spp, *Streptococcus* spp, *Pasteurella* spp, and *Acinetobacter Iwoffi* [11]. Initial treatment includes topical as well as systemic antibiotics, and, if present, drainage of lacrimal abscesses. Fever, orbital cellulitis, or severe preseptal cellulitis warrants hospital admission for intravenous antibiotics. The definitive treatment for dacryocystitis is dacryocystorhinostomy (DCR), preferably following or in conjunction with antibiotic treatment of the acute infection.

Lacrimal fistula

Lacrimal fistula, which may be congenital or acquired, occur in approximately 1 in 2000 live births [12]. Internal fistula connect the lacrimal sac to the nasal mucosa and are diagnosed rarely. External fistula connect the lacrimal system to the skin and are located most commonly inferomedial to the medial canthus. Occasionally, lacrimal fistula may be bilateral, have more than one opening, or end in a blind pouch.

Histologically, lacrimal fistula resemble the normal canalicular structure— a hollow tube lined by nonkeratinized, stratified squamous epithelium. Fistula may cause epiphora if the normal superior or inferior canaliculus is replaced or may be asymptomatic if the fistula forms a supernumerary canalicular structure. A fistula may become infected or cause local dermatitis from chronic drainage. The condition usually is sporadic, but a single family that demonstrates autosomal dominance inheritance was described [13]. Lacrimal fistulae have been reported in conjunction with several other abnormalities, including nasolacrimal duct obstruction, mucocele, absent canaliculus, contralateral absent punctum, and total agenesis of the lacrimal system.

Surgical management of symptomatic patients may include cautery, simple closure of the fistula opening, excision of the entire fistula tract, DCR, silicone tube intubation, or common canalicular dissection.

Congenital dacryocystocele

Congenital dacryocystocele presents around the time of birth as a blue- or pink-colored mass inferior to the medial canthus that represents a sterile, dilated lacrimal sac. The etiology of this condition is believed to be related to simultaneous proximal and distal obstruction of the lacrimal system. The distal obstruction is at the junction of the nasolacrimal duct and nose, as seen in typical CNLDO, whereas the proximal obstruction occurs at the junction of the common canaliculus and lacrimal sac. The proximal obstruction may function as a one-way valve, which allows for the accumulation of mucus, tears, and cellular debris.

Complications of dacryocystocele include dacryocystitis, preseptal cellulitis, cutaneous fistula formation, formation of nasal cysts, and induced astigmatism from mass effect with possible resultant amblyopia.

Dacryocystocele is unilateral in 86% to 100% of cases [14–17]. Dacryocystitis is common, occurs in 14% to 75% of cases [14–17], and warrants surgical intervention. Conservative treatment with warm compresses, massage, and topical antibiotics may be attempted if there is no evidence of infection. The rate of successful resolution with conservative treatment ranges from 17% to 80% in different studies [15–17].

Most investigators recommend probing as an initial surgical intervention. In a series by Mansour and colleagues [15], probing was attempted in 83% of 54 dacryocystoceles, including 36 cases that were complicated by dacryocystitis. Successful resolution was seen in 78% of patients. Unsuccessful attempts at probing may require repeated probings, silicone tube intubation, or DCR.

Congenital dacryocystocele also is referred to as dacryocele, mucocele, and lacrimal sac cyst. In a particular form of this condition, known as amniotocele, the sac is believed to fill with amniotic fluid in utero [18].

Lacrimal duct cysts

Nasolacrimal duct obstruction associated with cyst formation was described first by Raflo and colleagues [19] in 1982. Dilated lacrimal duct cysts may obstruct the airways of infants, who are preferential nose breathers, which leads to respiratory distress that requires urgent surgical intervention [20–26]. Although rare, this entity should be considered in the differential diagnosis of neonatal airway obstruction.

Mass lesions simulating nasolacrimal duct obstruction

Several mass lesions may cause compression of the lacrimal outflow system and mimic nasolacrimal duct obstruction, including meningoencephalocele, capillary hemangioma, dermoid cyst, sudoriferous cyst, nasal glioma, lymphangioma, lacrimal sac tumors, rhabdomyosarcoma, anterior ethmoiditis, and pneumatocele. Most of these disorders present with a mass in the medial canthal region that does not have the typical appearance of a dacryocystocele. Radiologic imaging is helpful to make the correct diagnosis and to plan surgical or nonsurgical treatment.

Radiologic imaging

Most cases of congenital nasolacrimal obstruction are managed without the need for diagnostic imaging; however, patients who fail treatment or have atypical presentations may warrant imaging studies to guide further management.

Dacryocystography (DCG), the earliest radiologic method of evaluating the lacrimal system, is performed by injecting contrast material directly into the lacrimal system using a blunt cannula [27]. Radiographs are taken with the patient supine and in Waters position as contrast is injected. DCG provides sufficient detail to localize areas of stenosis, diverticulae, or fistulae within the lacrimal system and to visualize bony landmarks; however, it provides poor detail of surrounding soft tissues. Hurwitz and Welham [28] studied the results of DCG on 80 children who had CNLDO at the time of initial probing. They found that the success of probing could be correlated with the site of obstruction seen radiologically. Patients with lower duct obstruction had a high cure rate, whereas patients with obstructions in the common canaliculus or lacrimal sac had a much lower cure rate.

Radionuclide DCG, also known as dacryoscintigraphy, is a noninvasive method to evaluate the functioning of the lacrimal system. It was described originally in adults [29] and adapted to children [30,31]. Technetium-99 pertechetate solution is placed on the surface of the globe and pictures are taken with a gamma tracer as the material works its way through the lacrimal system. Unlike DCG, there is no visualization of surrounding bony structures. Several technical factors make the test difficult to perform in children. Patients are required to maintain an upright position for 20 minutes and crying can cause the radioisotope to overflow onto the cheeks, rather than pass to through the lacrimal system. Manually blinking the eyelids of sedated children is needed to activate the lacrimal pump and to allow drainage of the lacrimal sac.

DCG has been used in conjunction with CT scanning by Ashenhurst and colleagues [32] and Zinreich and colleagues [33] in adult patients. Because of the fast acquisition times, the test may be possible to perform in children with minimal to no sedation. One disadvantage of CT-DCG over standard DCG is that assessment of the entire lacrimal outflow system requires evaluation of many sections; areas of stenosis between slices may be difficult to appreciate. Freitag and colleagues [34] developed a technique whereby axial slices are reconstructed into a three-dimensional image, which allows the surgeon to visualize the entire lacrimal system simultaneously at high resolution. The three-dimensional image can be rotated at a computer workstation to aid in visualizing areas of pathology [34,35]. CT-DCG also may be used to examine the causes of failed DCR surgery [36].

MRI also has been used to image the lacrimal system in adult patients. The technique offers better soft tissue visualization compared with CT imaging, but less detail of bony structures [37,38]. Manfre and colleagues [39] performed MR-DCG and CT-DCG on patients who had epiphora and found equal efficacy in identifying stenotic areas of the lacrimal outflow system. Because of long image acquisition times, the test requires sedation in children, but it has the advantage of being free of radiation.

Ultrasound may be useful in imaging the upper lacrimal system and in postoperative assessment of the osteotomy after DCR surgery [40–43]; however, the dense echogenicity of bone makes it difficult to visualize the lower lacrimal outflow system. The technique also may be useful in evaluating the lacrimal pump [44]. Because ultrasound can be performed at the bedside with fast acquisition times and no radiation, the technique may be particularly well suited for use in children.

Radiologic evaluation of the lacrimal outflow system is discussed further elsewhere in this issue in the article by Kousoubris.

Treatment

Conservative treatment

The natural history of congenital nasolacrimal duct obstruction is that a large percentage of children improves spontaneously without treatment or with conservative therapy that consists of topical antibiotics and lacrimal sac massage. Crigler [45] first described lacrimal sac massage in 1923. In his original description, the technique involved placing one finger over the common canaliculus to block upward flow and then stroking downward along the lacrimal sac to increase hydrostatic pressure and attempt to break a membrane at the opening of the nasolacrimal duct into the nose. Parents occasionally report a popping sensation as the obstruction is relieved followed by complete resolution of symptoms.

Kushner [46] randomized 175 eyes of 132 children to the Crigler technique of lacrimal massage, upward massage, or no massage for at least 1 month. Thirty-one percent of eyes had resolution of symptoms with the Crigler technique, whereas success in other groups reached only 7% to 9%. Most studies, which follow patients for a longer period of time, report success rates of between 85% and 95% for lacrimal massage with or without topical antibiotics [16,47–49].

Probing and irrigation

Most investigators recommend probing and irrigation as the next intervention after conservative management. Because of the high success rate of conservative therapy, there is considerable controversy about how long patients should be treated conservatively and when additional intervention should be initiated.

Probing may be performed under general anesthesia, or in selected patients, in the office using a restraint device. Irrigation may be performed at the start of the procedure to confirm the presence of nasolacrimal obstruction if the diagnosis is uncertain. The procedure begins with examination of the puncta. The lower punctum is widened using a punctual dilator. A Bowman probe is passed vertically through the dilated lower punctum and is advanced horizontally into the lacrimal sac until the "hard stop" of the lacrimal sac fossa is felt. The probe is angled inferior and slightly posterior and advanced through the nasolacrimal duct into the nose. A popping sensation may be felt as the probe passes through a membrane at the end of the nasolacrimal duct and into the inferior meatus of the nose. Irrigation can be repeated to confirm a patent nasolacrimal system. Some investigators advocate repeating the procedure with progressively larger probes to maximize the size of the newly created opening into the nose and to relieve any stenotic portions of the nasolacrimal system.

The most common complication of the procedure is the creation of false passages. To avoid this complication, care must be taken to advance the probe slowly and to abort the procedure if a "soft stop" is encountered, which indicates severe stenosis or a proximal obstruction in the nasolacrimal system.

There are clear advantages and disadvantages to early and late probing, with early intervention usually defined as before the age of 1 year. Clearly, early intervention may lead to earlier relief of symptoms. Although many children do not seem to be bothered by tearing and discharge, these symptoms often are a significant source of worry for parents; early treatment may help to alleviate this anxiety. Complications of nasolacrimal obstruction, such as the development of acute dacryocystitis, conjunctivitis, and cellulitis, also might be avoided with early intervention. Chronic, low-grade infection can lead to fibrosis and scarring of the nasolacrimal system that makes further treatment more difficult.

One of the most compelling reasons for early intervention is that probing that is done at a young age—typically less than 6 to 8 months—often can be done in the office using a papoose restraint and obviates the need for general anesthesia. Although office restraint may involve psychologic trauma to parents and children, it is not clear that this is more traumatic than a trip to the operating room that involves breathing through a mask, placement of an intravenous line, and postoperative nausea and irritability. Ninety-five percent of parents who were surveyed after office probing stated that the procedure was easier than expected, and 81% were happy with the decision to initiate early intervention [50,51]. The main disadvantage to early probing is that it requires surgical intervention in patients who might have complete resolution of symptoms with additional conservative management.

Many investigators who are not advocates of office probing at 6 or 7 months recommend probing under general anesthesia soon after a child's first birthday, citing studies that demonstrate that the success of probing declines with increasing age. Table 1 summarizes studies of 50 or more patients that have examined this issue. Most of the studies show a trend toward decreasing efficacy of the probing procedure with increasing age, but the extent of this decline varies significantly between studies. Several investigators suggest that the decrease in efficacy for probing in older children is due to the presence or development of more complex forms of obstruction, such as canalicular stenosis or abnormalities that involve the lacrimal sac [52,53].

When probing fails and symptoms recur, there are several options for additional treatment. One option is to repeat the probing procedure; however, as children get older additional probings may be less successful. A large study of 1748 patients who were up to 4 years of age found resolution of symptoms in 100% of patients with additional probing procedures, but this result is not typical of other studies. Katowitz and Welsh [55] found a success rate of 54% for second probings in 18- to 24-month old children, but the success rate decreased to 33% in children who were older than 2 years. Additional procedures at the time of second probing, such as infracture of the inferior turbinate, balloon catheter dilation, nasal endoscopic examination, or silicone tube intubation, may increase the success rate.

Table 1
Success rates for initial nasolacrimal probing by patient age

Investigation	Age and probing success
Stager et al (n = 2369) [51]	<9 mo = 94%
	>9 mo = 84%
Katowitz and Welsh (n = 572) [55]	<1 y = 96%
	1–2 y = 69%
	>2 y = 33%
Mannor et al (n = 142) [54]	<1 y = 92%
	1–2 y = 89%
	2–3 y = 80%
	3–4 y = 71%
	4–5 y = 42%
Zwaan (n = 110) [56]	<1 y = 97%
	1–2 y = 88%
	2–3 y = 93%
Robb (n = 303) [57]	1–2 y = 92%
	2–3 y = 96%
	3+ y = 93%
Kashkouli et al (n = 207) [58]	<1 y = 92%
	1–2 y = 85%
	2–3 y = 65%
	>3 y = 64%
Singh and Singh (n = 1748) [59]	<1 y = 100%
	1–2 y = 99%
	2–3 y = 95%
	3–4 y = 90%
Honovar et al (n = 60) [52]	2–3 y = 97%
	3–4 y = 75%
	>4 y = 43%
Maheshwari (n = 83) [60]	1–2 y = 88%
	>2 y = 80%

Silicone tube intubation

A common practice after a failed probing is to repeat the probing procedure and intubate the lacrimal system with silicone tubing. The tubing helps
to prevent the formation of granulation tissue–related obstruction along the
newly patent tract after the probing procedure, and it has the additional advantages of dilating stenotic segments of the lacrimal outflow system. The
technique was described first by Quickert and Dryden [61] in 1970.

The procedure is performed most commonly under general anesthesia. The
nose is packed with vasoconstricting agents, such as cocaine or neosynephr-
ine. A single piece of silicone tubing, which is attached to metal probes at both
ends, is cannulated through the upper and lower puncta and advanced into
the nose; each end is retrieved using a metal hook. After the metal probes
are cut off, the tubing is tied and allowed to retract into the nasal cavity or
sutured to the lateral wall of the nose. A small loop of tubing is visible between the upper and lower puncta and typically does not cause discomfort.

Common complications of this procedure include breakage of the tubing that allows contact with the cornea, which may lead to corneal abrasion and possible corneal ulceration. A broken tube also may be extruded through the nose or possibly aspirated. Other complications include the creation of false passages, erosion or slitting of the punctum, and the formation of pyogenic granulomas.

The timing of tube removal has been the subject of considerable debate. Most investigators advocate leaving the tube for 3 to 6 months, but good success has been found with removal of tubes as early as 6 weeks [62]. The tubing may be removed by blowing it out of the nose or pulling the tubing out through the puncta.

Overall, the success rate of silicone tube intubation ranges from 77% to 100% in different studies [62–67]. Because of the preservation of normal anatomy, this procedure typically is recommended before more invasive surgery.

Alternate surgical techniques also have been described. Mauffray and colleagues [68] describe a technique of double bicanalicular intubation, whereby two loops of tubing are passed through the lacrimal system to create a functionally larger stent. Complete resolution of symptoms was observed in 8 of 10 patients, all of whom had failed previous probing.

An alternative to bicanalicular intubation, is monocanalicular intubation through the superior punctum only with a Monoka tube. The advantage of this technique is that this type of tube is easier to remove in an office setting; however, the success rate of 79% in one study is less than the success of bicanalicular intubation in most studies, and almost half of all tubes fell out prematurely [69].

Infracture of the inferior turbinate

The goal of inferior turbinate infracture is to move the inferior turbinate away from the ostium of the nasolacrimal duct to avoid physical obstruction that might lead to closure of a newly patent opening. The original procedure, described by Jones and Wobig [18], is performed by placing an instrument (eg, Freer elevator) in the nose and pushing the inferior turbinate medially until a sensation of movement is felt. An alternate technique is to grasp the inferior turbinate with a hemostat and rotate the turbinate inward by 90°. Havins and Wilkins [70] reported an 88% success rate among 24 patients for a second probing combined with inferior turbinate infracture after a failed first probing.

Balloon catheter dilation

Another alternative after a failed probing is to dilate the distal nasolacrimal duct with a balloon catheter, a procedure that was described first by Becker and colleagues [71] in 1996. The investigators reported an overall success rate of 95% in 61 eyes, including a 94% success rate in 34 lacrimal systems that had failed previous procedures, including probing or silicone tube intubation. Tao and colleagues [72] reported an overall success rate of 77% in 73 eyes, including 75% of 39 patients who had failed previous procedures. The procedure seemed to be more successful in older patients. Yuksel and colleagues [73] reported a success rate of 83% in 24 eyes, most of which had not had previous procedures. The success seems especially promising given that the mean patient age was 44 months, a group in which primary probing has poor results in most studies.

Nasal endoscopy

Probing failures may be due to the passage of a probe under the nasal mucosa without perforation into the nasal vestibule or impaction of the opening into the nose by the inferior turbinate. Nasal endoscopy allows visual confirmation that the probe has entered the nose, as well as observation of the anatomic relationship of the opening to surrounding structures, such as the inferior turbinate.

Several studies examined the role of nasal endoscopy in nasolacrimal probing. Choi and colleagues [74] reported visualization of a false passage in the submucosal space in 5 of 11 probings. Redirection of the probe resulted in a successful outcome in 4 of the 5 children, who would have been expected to fail the procedure without endoscopic guidance. MacEwen and colleagues [75] performed nasal endoscopy in 52 lacrimal systems of 40 children during probing and found the formation of false passages in 15%. Wallace and colleagues [76] performed nasal endoscopy during probing of 87 lacrimal systems. They reported a success rate of 100% in 58 lacrimal systems in which the obstruction was at the distal nasolacrimal duct. None of seven patients with obstruction or stenosis in the upper lacrimal outflow system achieved a successful result, which demonstrates the limitation of simple probing for proximal nasolacrimal disease. Gardiner and colleagues [77] studied 47 children who had failed initial probing to compare probing with nasal endoscopy with probing with silicone tube intubation. An equal success rate of 85% to 90% was observed in both groups.

Dacryocystorhinostomy

DCR is a procedure that creates a bypass fistula between the lacrimal sac and the nose to provide an alternative pathway for lacrimal outflow. An osteotomy is created adjacent to the middle meatus of the nose followed by an anastomosis of the lacrimal sac and nasal mucosa. The procedure may be performed through an external skin incision near the medial canthus, or through the nose with endoscopic visualization. Nasolacrimal intubation with silicone tubes is performed frequently with both procedures.

External dacryocystorhinostomy

The external DCR procedure was described originally in adults by Toti [78] in 1904; most procedures are performed in adults. The procedure is performed through a skin incision that starts approximately 10 mm medial to the medial canthus and extends inferiorly after packing the nose with a vasoconstrictor, such as cocaine. The periosteum is opened and blunt dissection is carried posteriorly to expose the lacrimal sac. An osteotomy is created through the lacrimal and maxillary bones to expose the underlying nasal mucosa, and a fistula is formed between the lacrimal sac and nasal mucosa by incising both structures to create anterior and posterior flaps. The flaps may be sutured to the corresponding flap from the other tissue (ie, posterior nasal mucosa to posterior lacrimal sac) or left open. Frequently, silicone tube intubation is performed by passing tubing through the proximal lacrimal system and into the nose through the fistula where the ends of the tubing are cut and tied.

Overall, the success rate for DCR in children is about 85% to 95%, similar to the success rate in adults (Table 2). Welham and Hughes [79] reported an overall success rate of 84% in 160 pediatric DCRs that were performed for several indications, including CNLDO, dacryocystitis, and trauma. The success rate increased to 93% when only patients who had CNLDO were considered. Nowinski and colleagues [80] reported an 83% success rate in 34 pediatric patients overall, and an 88% success rate in 17 patients who had CNLDO. Hakin and colleagues [81] reported an 88% success rate in 258 cases overall, and a 96% success rate in 177 cases when patients who had canalicular stenosis were excluded. Barnes and colleagues [82] reported complete resolution of symptoms in 96% of 134 cases for CNLDO or mucocele.

The main disadvantage to the external approach is the presence of a cutaneous incision with the possibility of cutaneous scarring. Surveys of adult patients demonstrated a low rate of dissatisfaction with postoperative scars. Caesar and colleagues [87] surveyed 161 patients who underwent external DCR; 67% of patients rated the scar as invisible and 97% of patients found the scar "acceptable." In a separate study of 296 external DCRs, 79% of scars were rated as invisible with only 11% rated greater than 1 on a scale of 1 to 5 [88]. The investigators of both studies found a trend toward

Table 2
Success rates for pediatric dacryocystorhinostomy

Investigators	Technique	Number of procedures	Percent success
Welham and Hughes [79]	External	160	84%
Nowinski et al [80]	External	34	83%
Hakin et al [81]	External	258	88%
Barnes et al [82]	External	134	96%
Overall	External	586	88%
Cunningham and Woog [83]	Endoscopic	4	100%
Wong et al [84]	Endoscopic	6	83%
Vanderveen et al [86]	Endoscopic	22	88%
Kominek and Cervenka [85]	Endoscopic	34	82%
Overall	Endoscopic	66	85%

increasing patient dissatisfaction in younger patients. The authors are un-
aware of studies that have examined parents' perceptions of external
DCR scars in pediatric patients.

Endoscopic dacryocystorhinostomy

Early descriptions of lacrimal surgery through the nose came from Caldwell [89] in 1893, West [90] in 1910, and Mosher [91] in 1921. Recent im-
provements in endoscopic equipment have led to a resurgence of interest
in this technique. Surgical technique is described elsewhere in this issue.
In short, a fiber optic light pipe is passed through the canalicular system
and into the lacrimal sac. The light from the pipe passes through bone
and mucosa and is visualized in the nose using an endoscope. The mucosa
is removed with a blade or Holmium:Yag laser and an osteotomy is
performed.

Cunningham and Woog [83] reported resolution of symptoms in four pediatric patients using the endoscopic technique. Wong and colleagues [84]
reported success in five of six procedures. Vanderveen and colleagues [86]
reported an 88% success rate in 22 ducts of 17 children. Kominek and Cervenka reported success in 28 of 34 cases [85]. Five of the six failed procedures achieved success after a single, endoscopic revision. Overall, the
success of endoscopic and external DCR surgery in children seems to be
similar in published reports; however, differences in inclusion criteria between studies make a direct comparison of results difficult.

Upper lacrimal system surgery

Congenital anomalies of the canalicular system may be managed by re-
constructing anomalous structures or bypassing them. If a focal segment
of the canaliculus is stenotic or obstructed, the involved area may be excised
with anastomosis of the free ends of the canaliculus over a stent. An alternative technique, described by Dutton and Holck [92], is direct ablation of
involved tissue using a holmium laser intubated into the lacrimal system.

Primary conjunctivodacryocystorhinostomy (CDCR), the creation of
a direct bypass tract between the medial canthus and the nose, is performed
in cases of canalicular agenesis, multiple failed DCRs, or when areas of canalicular stenosis are too large for primary repair. The beginning of the procedure is identical to a DCR. A skin incision is used to expose the lacrimal
sac and create an osteotomy into the nose. Next, the caruncle is incised and
a needle is passed from the medial canthus into the osteotomy. A glass tube
is fitted into the bypass tract and left in place. Tears pass from the medial
canthus, through the tube, and into the nose. The original technique was described by Jones [93] in 1962 in a series of 500 adult patients; it involved
a tube with a smooth glass surface. Recently, a frosted glass tube has
been developed to increase friction with the surrounding tissues and possibly
reduce the risk for tube extrusion [94].

Reports of the use of this technique in children are limited. Welham and Hughes [79] reported success in all 5 patients who had punctual and canalicular agenesis. Hakin and colleagues [81] reported success in 10 of 11 patients who had an unspecified mix of traumatic and congenital malformations.

The most frequent complication of CDCR is extrusion of the tube medially or laterally into the nose; less common complications include granuloma formation and infection. Although the tube position can be manipulated in an office setting in adults, extrusion or movement of the tube in young children usually requires manipulation under general anesthesia. Therefore, the surgery often is delayed until the age of about 10 years, unless the child is extremely symptomatic.

Summary

Congenital nasolacrimal obstruction is a common disorder in the pediatric age group and it affects approximately 6% of all newborns. The most common site of obstruction is an imperforate membrane at the valve of Hasner, at the opening of the nasolacrimal duct into the nose. Approximately 90% of cases resolve within the first year of life with lacrimal sac massage, but persistent obstruction beyond the age of 1 year usually warrants intervention.

Typically, probing is the first intervention performed. The success rate of probing is around 90% when performed at the age of 1 year, but there is a trend toward decreasing efficacy in older patients. A second probing usually is performed after a failed first attempt, often with an additional procedure, such as silicone tube intubation, infracture of the inferior turbinate, nasal endoscopy, or balloon catheter dilation. Continued obstruction usually warrants DCR, which may be performed endoscopically through the nose or through an external incision.

Obstructions at other points within the lacrimal outflow system are less common. Radiologic imaging procedures, such as radiographs, CT, MRI, or ultrasound, may be used to localize the site of atypical obstructions and guide further management. Obstructions of the upper lacrimal outflow system are treated by primary anastomosis of functional tissues or the creation of a direct fistula between the medial canthus and the nose.

References

[1] Guerry D, Kendig EL. Congenital impatency on the naso-lacrimal duct. Arch Ophthalmol 1948;39:193–204.
[2] Stephenson S. A preliminary communication on the affections of the tear passages in newly born infants. Medical Press and Circular 1899;119:103–4.
[3] Cassady J. Dacryocystitis in infancy. Am J Ophthalmol 1948;31:773–80.
[4] MacEwen CJ, Young JD. Epiphora during the first year of life. Eye 1991;5(Pt 5):596–600.
[5] Ffookes O. Dacryocystitis in infancy. Br J Ophthalmol 1962;46:422–34.
[6] Sevel D. Development and congenital abnormalities of the nasolacrimal apparatus. J Pediatr Ophthalmol Strabismus 1981;18(5):13–9.

[7] Berk AT, Saatci AO, Ercal MD, et al. Ocular findings in 55 patients with Down's syndrome. Ophthalmic Genet 1996;17(1):15–9.

[8] Cassady J. Developmental anatomy of nasolacrimal duct. Arch Ophthalmol 1952;47: 141–58.

[9] Zappia RJ, Milder B. Lacrimal drainage function. 2. The fluorescein dye disappearance test. Am J Ophthalmol 1972;74(1):160–2.

[10] MacEwen CJ, Young JD. The fluorescein disappearance test (FDT): an evaluation of its use in infants. J Pediatr Ophthalmol Strabismus 1991;28(6):302–5.

[11] MacEwen CJ, Phillips MG, Young JD. Value of bacterial culturing in the course of congenital nasolacrimal duct (NLD) obstruction. J Pediatr Ophthalmol Strabismus 1994;31(4): 246–50.

[12] Francois J, Bacskulin J. External congenital fistulae of the lacrimal sac. Ophthalmologica 1969;159(4):249–61.

[13] Jones L, Wobig JL. Surgery of the eyelids and lacrimal system. Birmingham (AL): Aesculapius Publishing Co.; 1976.

[14] Boynton JR, Drucker DN. Distention of the lacrimal sac in neonates. Ophthalmic Surg 1989; 20(2):103–7.

[15] Mansour AM, Cheng KP, Mumma JV, et al. Congenital dacryocele. A collaborative review. Ophthalmology 1991;98(11):1744–51.

[16] Petersen RA, Robb RM. The natural course of congenital obstruction of the nasolacrimal duct. J Pediatr Ophthalmol Strabismus 1978;15(4):246–50.

[17] Sullivan TJ, Clarke MP, Morin JD, et al. Management of congenital dacryocystocoele. Aust N Z J Ophthalmol 1992;20(2):105–8.

[18] Jones LT, Wobig JL. The Wendell L. Hughes Lecture. Newer concepts of tear duct and eyelid anatomy and treatment. Trans Sect Ophthalmol Am Acad Ophthalmol Otolaryngol 1977;83(4 Pt 1):603–16.

[19] Raflo GT, Horton JA, Sprinkle PM. An unusual intranasal anomaly of the lacrimal drainage system. Ophthalmic Surg 1982;13(9):741–4.

[20] Berkowitz RG, Grundfast KM, Fitz C. Nasal obstruction of the newborn revisited: clinical and subclinical manifestations of congenital nasolacrimal duct obstruction presenting as a nasal mass. Otolaryngol Head Neck Surg 1990;103(3):468–71.

[21] Denis D, Saracco JB, Triglia JM. Nasolacrimal duct cysts in congenital dacryocystocele. Graefes Arch Clin Exp Ophthalmol 1994;232(4):252–4.

[22] Divine RD, Anderson RL, Bumsted RM. Bilateral congenital lacrimal sac mucoceles with nasal extension and drainage. Arch Ophthalmol 1983;101(2):246–8.

[23] Grin TR, Mertz JS, Stass-Isern M. Congenital nasolacrimal duct cysts in dacryocystocele. Ophthalmology 1991;98(8):1238–42.

[24] Mazzara CA, Respler DS, Jahn AF. Neonatal respiratory distress: sequela of bilateral nasolacrimal duct obstruction. Int J Pediatr Otorhinolaryngol 1993;25(1–3):209–16.

[25] Righi PD, Hubbell RN, Lawlor PP Jr. Respiratory distress associated with bilateral nasolacrimal duct cysts. Int J Pediatr Otorhinolaryngol 1993;26(2):199–203.

[26] Yee SW, Seibert RW, Bower CM, et al. Congenital nasolacrimal duct mucocele: a cause of respiratory distress. Int J Pediatr Otorhinolaryngol 1994;29(2):151–8.

[27] Ewing A. Roentgen ray demonstration of the lacrimal abscess cavity. Am J Ophthalmol 1909;24:1.

[28] Hurwitz JJ, Welham RA. The role of dacryocystography in the management of congenital nasolacrimal duct obstruction. Can J Ophthalmol 1975;10(3):346–50.

[29] Rossomondo RM, Carlton WH, Trueblood JH, et al. A new method of evaluating lacrimal drainage. Arch Ophthalmol 1972;88(5):523–5.

[30] Foster JA, Katowitz JA, Heyman S. Results of dacryoscintigraphy in massage of the congenitally blocked nasolacrimal duct. Ophthal Plast Reconstr Surg 1996;12(1):32–7.

[31] Heyman S, Katowitz JA, Smoger B. Dacryoscintigraphy in children. Ophthalmic Surg 1985; 16(11):703–9.

[32] Ashenhurst M, Jaffer N, Hurwitz JJ, et al. Combined computed tomography and dacryocystography for complex lacrimal problems. Can J Ophthalmol 1991;26(1):27–31.

[33] Zinreich S, Miller NR, Freeman LN, et al. Computed tomographic dacryocystography using topical contrast media for lacrimal system visualization. Preliminary investigations. Orbit 1990;9:79–87.

[34] Freitag SK, Woog JJ, Kousoubris PD, et al. Helical computed tomographic dacryocystography with three-dimensional reconstruction: a new view of the lacrimal drainage system. Ophthal Plast Reconstr Surg 2002;18(2):121–32.

[35] Luchtenberg M, Kuhli C, du Mesnil de Rochemont R, et al. Three-dimensional rotational dacryocystography for imaging of the lacrimal draining system and adjacent anatomical structures. Ophthalmologica 2005;219(3):136–41.

[36] Gokcek A, Argin MA, Altintas AK. Comparison of failed and successful dacryocystorhinostomy by using computed tomographic dacryocystography findings. Eur J Ophthalmol 2005; 15(5):523–9.

[37] Rubin PA, Bilyk JR, Shore JW, et al. Magnetic resonance imaging of the lacrimal drainage system. Ophthalmology 1994;101(2):235–43.

[38] Goldberg RA, Heinz GW, Chiu L. Gadolinium magnetic resonance imaging dacryocystography. Am J Ophthalmol 1993;115(6):738–41.

[39] Manfre L, de Maria M, Todaro E, et al. MR dacryocystography: comparison with dacryocystography and CT dacryocystography. AJNR Am J Neuroradiol 2000;21(6):1145–50.

[40] Stupp T, Pavlidis M, Busse H, et al. Presurgical and postsurgical ultrasound assessment of lacrimal drainage dysfunction. Am J Ophthalmol 2004;138(5):764–71.

[41] Jedrzynski MS, Bullock JD. Lacrimal ultrasonography. Ophthal Plast Reconstr Surg 1994; 10(2):114–20.

[42] Dutton JJ. Standardized echography in the diagnosis of lacrimal drainage dysfunction. Arch Ophthalmol 1989;107(7):1010–2.

[43] Montanara A, Mannino G, Contestabile MT. Macrodacryocystography and echography in diagnosis of disorders of the lacrimal pathways. Surv Ophthalmol 1983;28(1):33–41.

[44] Pavlidis M, Stupp T, Grenzebach U, et al. Ultrasonic visualization of the effect of blinking on the lacrimal pump mechanism. Graefes Arch Clin Exp Ophthalmol 2005;243(3): 228–34.

[45] Crigler L. The treatment of congenital dacryocystitis. JAMA 1923;81:21–4.

[46] Kushner BJ. Congenital nasolacrimal system obstruction. Arch Ophthalmol 1982;100(4): 597–600.

[47] Nelson LB, Calhoun JH, Menduke H. Medical management of congenital nasolacrimal duct obstruction. Pediatrics 1985;76(2):172–5.

[48] Nucci P, Capoferri C, Alfarano R, et al. Conservative management of congenital nasolacrimal duct obstruction. J Pediatr Ophthalmol Strabismus 1989;26(1):39–43.

[49] Paul TO. Medical management of congenital nasolacrimal duct obstruction. J Pediatr Ophthalmol Strabismus 1985;22(2):68–70.

[50] Goldblum TA, Summers CG, Egbert JE, et al. Office probing for congenital nasolacrimal duct obstruction: a study of parental satisfaction. J Pediatr Ophthalmol Strabismus 1996; 33(4):244–7.

[51] Stager D, Baker JD, Frey T, et al. Office probing of congenital nasolacrimal duct obstruction. Ophthalmic Surg 1992;23(7):482–4.

[52] Honavar SG, Prakash VE, Rao GN. Outcome of probing for congenital nasolacrimal duct obstruction in older children. Am J Ophthalmol 2000;130(1):42–8.

[53] Kashkouli MB, Beigi B, Parvaresh MM, et al. Late and very late initial probing for congenital nasolacrimal duct obstruction: what is the cause of failure? Br J Ophthalmol 2003;87(9): 1151–3.

[54] Mannor GE, Rose GE, Frimpong-Ansah K, et al. Factors affecting the success of nasolacrimal duct probing for congenital nasolacrimal duct obstruction. Am J Ophthalmol 1999; 127(5):616–7.

[55] Katowitz JA, Welsh MG. Timing of initial probing and irrigation in congenital nasolacrimal duct obstruction. Ophthalmology 1987;94(6):698–705.

[56] Zwaan J. Treatment of congenital nasolacrimal duct obstruction before and after the age of 1 year. Ophthalmic Surg Lasers 1997;28(11):932–6.

[57] Robb RM. Success rates of nasolacrimal duct probing at time intervals after 1 year of age. Ophthalmology 1998;105(7):1307–9 [discussion 1309–10].

[58] Kashkouli MB, Kassaee A, Tabatabaee Z. Initial nasolacrimal duct probing in children under age 5: cure rate and factors affecting success. J AAPOS 2002;6(6):360–3.

[59] Singh Bhinder G, Singh Bhinder H. Repeated probing results in the treatment of congenital nasolacrimal duct obstruction. Eur J Ophthalmol 2004;14(3):185–92.

[60] Maheshwari R. Results of probing for congenital nasolacrimal duct obstruction in children older than 13 months of age. Indian J Ophthalmol 2005;53(1):49–51.

[61] Quickert MH, Dryden RM. Probes for intubation in lacrimal drainage. Trans Am Acad Ophthalmol Otolaryngol 1970;74(2):431–3.

[62] Migliori ME, Putterman AM. Silicone intubation for the treatment of congenital lacrimal duct obstruction: successful results removing the tubes after six weeks. Ophthalmology 1988;95(6):792–5.

[63] al-Hussain H, Nasr AM. Silastic intubation in congenital nasolacrimal duct obstruction: a study of 129 eyes. Ophthal Plast Reconstr Surg 1993;9(1):32–7.

[64] Dortzbach RK, France TD, Kushner BJ, et al. Silicone intubation for obstruction of the nasolacrimal duct in children. Am J Ophthalmol 1982;94(5):585–90.

[65] Durso F, Hand SI Jr, Ellis FD, et al. Silicone intubation in children with nasolacrimal obstruction. J Pediatr Ophthalmol Strabismus 1980;17(6):389–93.

[66] Leone CR Jr, Van Gemert JV. The success rate of silicone intubation in congenital lacrimal obstruction. Ophthalmic Surg 1990;21(2):90–2.

[67] Welsh MG, Katowitz JA. Timing of silastic tubing removal after intubation for congenital nasolacrimal duct obstruction. Ophthal Plast Reconstr Surg 1989;5(1):43–8.

[68] Mauffray RO, Hassan AS, Elner VM. Double silicone intubation as treatment for persistent congenital nasolacrimal duct obstruction. Ophthal Plast Reconstr Surg 2004;20(1):44–9.

[69] Kaufman LM, Guay-Bhatia LA. Monocanalicular intubation with Monoka tubes for the treatment of congenital nasolacrimal duct obstruction. Ophthalmology 1998;105(2): 336–41.

[70] Havins WE, Wilkins RB. A useful alternative to silicone intubation in congenital nasolacrimal duct obstructions. Ophthalmic Surg 1983;14(8):666–70.

[71] Becker BB, Berry FD, Koller H. Balloon catheter dilatation for treatment of congenital nasolacrimal duct obstruction. Am J Ophthalmol 1996;121(3):304–9.

[72] Tao S, Meyer DR, Simon JW, et al. Success of balloon catheter dilatation as a primary or secondary procedure for congenital nasolacrimal duct obstruction. Ophthalmology 2002; 11:2108–11.

[73] Yuksel D, Ceylan K, Erden O, et al. Balloon dilatation for treatment of congenital nasolacrimal duct obstruction. Eur J Ophthalmol 2005;15(2):179–85.

[74] Choi WC, Kim KS, Park TK, et al. Intranasal endoscopic diagnosis and treatment in congenital nasolacrimal duct obstruction. Ophthalmic Surg Lasers 2002;33(4):288–92.

[75] MacEwen CJ, Young JD, Barras CW, et al. Value of nasal endoscopy and probing in the diagnosis and management of children with congenital epiphora. Br J Ophthalmol 2001;85(3): 314–8.

[76] Wallace EJ, Cox A, White P, et al. Endoscopic-assisted probing for congenital nasolacrimal duct obstruction. Eye 2005;Sep 2: [Epub ahead of print].

[77] Gardiner JA, Forte V, Pashby RC, et al. The role of nasal endoscopy in repeat pediatric nasolacrimal duct probings. J AAPOS 2001;5(3):148–52.

[78] Toti A. Nuovo metodo conservatore dicura radicale delle sopperazioni croniche del sacco lacrimale (dacriocistotinostomia). Clin Moderna 1904;10:385–7.

[79] Welham RA, Hughes SM. Lacrimal surgery in children. Am J Ophthalmol 1985;99(1):27–34.

[80] Nowinski TS, Flanagan JC, Mauriello J. Pediatric dacryocystorhinostomy. Arch Ophthalmol 1985;103(8):1226–8.

[81] Hakin KN, Sullivan TJ, Sharma A, et al. Paediatric dacryocystorhinostomy. Aust N Z J Ophthalmol 1994;22(4):231–5.

[82] Barnes EA, Abou-Rayyah Y, Rose GE. Pediatric dacryocystorhinostomy for nasolacrimal duct obstruction. Ophthalmology 2001;108(9):1562–4.

[83] Cunningham MJ, Woog JJ. Endonasal endoscopic dacryocystorhinostomy in children. Arch Otolaryngol Head Neck Surg 1998;124(3):328–33.

[84] Wong JF, Woog JJ, Cunningham MJ, et al. A multidisciplinary approach to atypical lacrimal obstruction in childhood. Ophthal Plast Reconstr Surg 1999;15(4):293–8.

[85] Kominek P, Cervenka S. Pediatric endonasal dacryocystorhinostomy: a report of 34 cases. Laryngoscope 2005;115(10):1800–3.

[86] Vanderveen DK, Jones DT, Tan H, Petersen RA. Endoscopic dacryocystorhinostomy in children. J AAPOS 2001;5(3):143–7.

[87] Caesar RH, Fernando G, Scott K, et al. Scarring in external dacryocystorhinostomy: fact or fiction? Orbit 2005;24(2):83–6.

[88] Sharma V, Martin PA, Benger R, et al. Evaluation of the cosmetic significance of external dacryocystorhinostomy scars. Am J Ophthalmol 2005;140(3):359–62.

[89] Caldwell G. Two new operations for obstruction of the nasal duct, with preservation of the canaliculi and an incidental description of a new lachrymal probe. Am J Ophthalmol 1893; 10:189–92.

[90] West J. A window resection of the nasal duct in cases of stenosis. Trans Am Acad Ophthalmol Soc 1910;12:654–7.

[91] Mosher H. Mosher-Toti operation on the lacrimal sac. Laryngoscope 1921;31:284–6.

[92] Dutton JJ, Holck DE. Holmium laser canaliculoplasty. Ophthal Plast Reconstr Surg 1996; 12(3):211–7.

[93] Jones LT. The cure of epiphora due to canalicular disorders, trauma and surgical failures on the lacrimal passages. Trans Am Acad Ophthalmol Otolaryngol 1962;66:506.

[94] Dailey RA, Tower RN. Frosted jones pyrex tubes. Ophthal Plast Reconstr Surg 2005;21(3): 185–7.

**ELSEVIER
SAUNDERS**

Otolaryngol Clin N Am
39 (2006) 979–999

OTOLARYNGOLOGIC
CLINICS
OF NORTH AMERICA

Acquired Nasolacrimal Duct Obstruction

David M. Mills, MD*, Dale R. Meyer, MD, FACS

*Ophthalmic Plastic Surgery, Lions Eye Institute, Albany Medical Center,
1220 New Scotland Avenue, Suite 302 Slingerlands, NY 12159, USA*

The lacrimal system is essentially a system of fluid pools and channels connecting them. The eye is one pool, the lacrimal sac is another pool, and the nose is the final pool. Lacrimal secretion flows first into the eye pool. From there a channel system called the canalicular system carries the tears to the lacrimal sac pool. A second channel called the nasolacrimal duct carries the tears from the lacrimal sac to the nose, where they are reabsorbed or evaporated.

The causes of tearing can be classified into one of three main categories: hypersecretion, lacrimal pump failure, and lacrimal drainage obstruction. Each main category has its own subcategories. Lacrimal secretion and drainage imbalance can lead to accumulation of too much lacrimal fluid in the lacrimal pools resulting in bothersome symptoms. Although this discussion will focus mainly on nasolacrimal duct obstruction, a brief background discussion of tearing in general will provide a useful framework to better understand the role of nasolacrimal duct obstruction within the lacrimal system.

Hypersecretion may be primary or reflex. The etiology of primary hypersecretion is unknown at this time. It can be associated with eating, the so-called, "crocodile-tears syndrome." Also known as gustatory hyperlacrimation, gustatory epiphora, or the gustolacrimal reflex, it may be congenital (presumed innervation of the lacrimal gland by efferent fibers of the facial nerve), or follow facial palsy, infection, or trauma. Some surgeons are successfully using botulinum toxin injections into the lacrimal gland to treat this condition [1–3]. Reflex hypersecretion is more common than primary hypersecretion, and is usually found in response to ocular surface irritation either primarily or as a result of some other process or recent surgery. Common causes include trichiasis, superficial foreign bodies, eyelid malpositions,

No funding support received by any author. No authors have any disclosures to report.

* Corresponding author.

E-mail address: davidmills4186@msn.com (D.M. Mills).

doi:10.1016/j.otc.2006.07.002
oto.theclinics.com

eyelid margin disease, tear deficiency or instability, and trigeminal nerve irritation [4]. Primary and reflex hypersecretion can be delineated with Schirmer's lacrimal secretion testing to differentiate baseline lacrimal secretion levels from reflex secretion levels.

Lacrimal pump failure from a number of causes including punctal or eyelid ectropion, orbicularis oculi weakness, and facial nerve palsy may fail to push the tears to the drain system. This is an especially important consideration with the increasing number of botulinum toxin injections and the toxin's effect on the medial eyelids. The weakening effect of botulinum toxin can lead to decreased orbicularis oculi contraction and, therefore, decreased lacrimal pump function. However, this effect may be therapeutic in some cases. In fact, in a study by Sahlin and colleagues [5], botulinum toxin was injected into the medial portion of the lower eyelids of normal patients and patients with dry eyes. Three weeks after injection, the mean blink output was reduced to 64% and 70% of the baseline values in the normal and dry eye patients, respectively. This reduction was more dramatic (38% of baseline) in another set of dry eye patients who also had botulinum toxin injected into the medial aspect of the upper eyelids. Of the patients with dry eyes, six of nine reported improved eye comfort with lower eyelid injections, and seven of ten reported improved eye comfort with injections into both the upper and lower eyelids illustrating that botulinum toxin injection may be used to treat patients with dry eye conditions.

Lacrimal drainage obstruction includes upper system obstructions, such as punctal or canalicular obstruction stenosis that lead to a lack of flow from the eye pool to the sac pool. It also includes lower lacrimal drainage obstructions, such as nasolacrimal duct obstruction, in which the fluid cannot move from the sac pool to the nose pool. Last, obstructions within the lacrimal sac itself such as tumors or dacryoliths are possible. However, these in essence lead to upper or lower level obstructions by interfering with flow into or out of the lacrimal sac.

The canals that carry tears between the lacrimal pools can be affected by functional or anatomic obstructions. A simplified system for thinking about the obstructed patient is as follows: functional obstructions are ones that can be overcome with forceful irrigation, and anatomic obstructions are ones that cannot be overcome with forceful irrigation. It is important to note the, "forceful" simply implies more force than the usual lacrimal pump creates; the clinician need not use exuberant or extreme force when irrigating. Understanding the basic schema outlined above allows the clinician to appropriately place the pathology identified within the system, which leads clinical decision making regarding therapy.

Nasolacrimal duct obstruction

The focus of this article is acquired nasolacrimal duct obstruction, which is a common problem and can lead to bothersome epiphora or dacryocystitis. The two types of acquired nasolacrimal duct obstruction are primary and secondary. Primary acquired nasolacrimal duct obstruction (PANDO) is the most common cause of lacrimal obstruction in adults [6] and has the highest incidence in the fifth to sixth decades. Females are more frequently affected than males by a ratio of 3 to 1.

Investigators have attempted to explain the female preponderance by analysis of the nasolacrimal duct itself. In a study by Groessl, Sires, and Lemke [7], the mean minimum diameter of the bony nasolacrimal canal was 3.70 mm in a control group of 50 men, 3.35 in a control group of 50 women, and 3.0 in a group of 19 patients with primary acquired nasolacrimal duct obstruction. The differences between the patient group and control groups were significant, and the authors concluded that a small diameter of the bony canal appeared to be one of the etiologic factors in PANDO. Others have made similar observations that the osseous nasolacrimal canal is longer and narrower in women than in men [8,9], and in Whites than in other races. Others have proposed that hormonal fluctuations and a heightened immune status may contribute to the disease process. Such changes are known to elicit a generalized deepithelialization in the body and may caused sloughing within the lacrimal sac and duct, which may occlude more easily in patients with already narrow ducts. Studies have also demonstrated an association between sinus disease and nasolacrimal duct obstruction [10]. Mucosal thickening may also lead to obstruction more easily in patients starting with narrower nasolacrimal ducts. However, Whitnall reported marked variation in the canal within a series of normal skulls. As such, the exact role of the size of the osseous canal or nasolacrimal duct opening in the etiology of acquired obstruction or as an explanation for the female preponderance is controversial.

Clinical presentation and examination

Chief complaint

Tearing is by far the most common presenting complaint of patients with nasolacrimal duct obstruction. It is important, however, to distinguish welling of tears in the eye from frank epiphora and to inquire about any mucoid discharge or dacryocystitis either separately from or in combination with the tearing. The majority of the history and physical is dedicated to determining whether the cause of the patient's tearing is nonobstructive (hypersecretion or pump failure) or obstructive.

History of present illness

The onset, severity, consistency, and frequency of the tearing, along with the nature of any discharge, relationship to environmental factors, and any alleviating or aggravating factors are important to ascertain. Recurrent symptoms are more suggestive of obstruction than a single or initial episode.

Morning mucus, dry eye symptoms, and ocular burning or itching are more consistent with reflex tearing, and may be associated with chronic topical or systemic medication usage, which may lead to direct irritation or indirect drying of the ocular surface. The patient should be asked about pain and the nature, location, severity, and so on, of the pain should be elucidated. Although bloody tears may be idiopathic [11], in general, any patient with bloody tears should receive a workup for lacrimal obstruction, specifically neoplasm.

Past medical history

The past medical history should be reviewed for previous eye or eyelid surgery or trauma, previous orbital or facial trauma or surgery, facial nerve palsy, paranasal sinus disease or surgery, malignancy, or irradiation. Bell's palsy in particular can be associated with either aberrant regeneration leading to "crocodile tears" or orbicularis oculi weakness (with or without frank ectropion) and subsequent pump failure. Either of these can lead to nonobstructive tearing. One should inquire about conditions or treatments that may sometimes cause lacrimal outflow obstruction, such as chemotherapy, or antiviral eye drops (both may cause canalicular obstruction), radiation (may cause obstruction anywhere along the system), lymphoma, Wegener's granulomatosis, sarcoidosis, ocular cicatricial pemphigoid, Kawasaki disease, scleroderma, sinus histiocytosis, and parasitic infections (can lead to nasolacrimal duct obstruction).

Clinical examination

The diagnosis of nasolacrimal duct obstruction can often be made by careful clinical examination. First, the examiner performs an external examination looking for other causes of epiphora such as hypersecretion or lacrimal pump failure, specifically ectropion of the eyelid(s) or punctum(ae), entropion, trichiasis, eyelid retraction, or lagophthalmos. Lacrimal pump function may be assessed by evaluating the dynamic eyelid functions, position of the eyelids, and their movements with both natural and forced blinking. The normal movement of the lower punctum with natural blinking is a medial translation and inward rotation, thereby dunking the punctum into the tear lake. This can be evaluated by manually elevating the ipsilateral upper eyelid and asking the patient to blink. If the lower punctum shows decreased medial and inward movement, one should consider the diagnosis of lacrimal pump failure. The maximal strength of forced closure can also be assessed. Decreased closure strength, as with a facial palsy, may also indicate pump failure.

By slit lamp examination, the height of the tear lake is measured (1 mm being the "normal" tear lake height), and the patency and position of the punctum relative to the tear lake is assessed to rule out punctal ectropion or stenosis, the latter of which is actually a form of obstruction. A tear lake higher than 2 mm is suggestive of outflow obstruction. Besides the tear lake height, the tear breakup time and tear film distribution are also useful in examining a tearing patient. Tear breakup time is the time from completion of a blink until the tear film begins to show breakup following instillation of fluorescein dye. Normal breakup time is 15 to 30 seconds. A time of 10 seconds or less is considered abnormal and indicates rapid drying of the ocular surface, which may lead to reflex hypersecretion and cause epiphora.

The eyelid, conjunctiva, cornea, and anterior chamber should be inspected for evidence of inflammation (eg, blepharitis or iritis), disease (eg, angle-closure glaucoma), or infection (eg, viral keratitis). Blepharitis, iritis, and angle closure may be associated with reflex hypersecretion. The treatment of viral keratitis may include topical antiviral drops, which may occasionally be associated with canalicular obstruction.

The medial canthal region should be examined closely only after slit-lamp examination, as palpation of the lacrimal sac may cause fluid reflux and alter the tear lake and tear film assessments made during slit-lamp examination. A distended lacrimal sac usually feels like a fluctuant tender mass over the medial canthal area, and is consistent with dacryocystitis or distal lacrimal drainage system obstruction. Palpation of the lacrimal sac can reveal the presence of a mass or elicit reflux from the lacrimal punctae when the valve of Rosenmüller at the junction of the common canaliculus and lacrimal sac is incompetent. Reflux of purulent fluid is diagnostic for nasolacrimal duct obstruction. However, one should note that the absence of reflux with manual sac compression does not rule out obstruction. Palpation of a firm mass near the medial canthus may be suggestive of a neoplastic process. Specifically, any mass above the medial canthal tendon should raise a strong suspicion of a lacrimal sac neoplasm, as dacryocystitis rarely occurs in this location. Hypervascularity of the overlying medial canthal skin and lower eyelid edema are also features suggestive of neoplasm. Lacrimal sac neoplasms can cause either partial or complete lacrimal obstruction.

Nasal examination

It is important that intranasal examination be performed on all patients with presumed acquired nasolacrimal duct obstruction to rule out neoplastic, inflammatory, or structural disorders of the nasal passages that could lead to nasolacrimal duct obstruction [12]. This can be done with a standard nasal speculum and a headlight or with an endoscope. Allergic rhinitis may also occasionally cause obstruction by mucosal thickening. Furthermore, a preoperative assessment of the nasal passages aids in surgical planning. The approach for and effectiveness of external dacryocystorhinostomy, endonasal dacryocystorhinostomy, or conjunctivodacryocystorhinostomy (with Jones tube placement) can be affected by intranasal anatomy.

Office testing

If mucoid or purulent discharge is elicited with manual pressure on the lacrimal sac, it can be sent for Gram stain, culture, and sensitivity testing. In some cases Giemsa stain, KOH (for fungus), and anticytoplasmic antibodies (for Wegener's granulomatosis), and other special studies may be helpful.

Schirmer testing can measure basal and stimulated tear secretion and, when combined with the other aspects of a complete lacrimal exam, can be useful in distinguishing between primary hypersecretion, reflex hypersecretion, and nasolacrimal duct obstruction. It is performed either with or without topical anesthesia by blotting dry the inferior cul de sac and then resting a commercially available Schirmer filter paper strip in the inferior cul de sac at the lateral aspect of the palpebral aperture. The amount of wetting at a certain time point indicates stimulated tear secretion if performed without topical anesthesia and basal tear production if performed with topical anesthesia. Without anesthesia, normal stimulated tear production is 10 to 30 mm of wetting on the Schirmer paper at 5 minutes. Less than 10 mm of wetting after 5 minutes indicates hyposecretion or dry eye, which may be associated with intermittent episodes of reflex hypersecretion leading to epiphora [13]. With anesthesia, normal basal secretion is greater than 10 mm of wetting at 5 minutes. This basal tear production test following the instillation of topical anesthesia is most useful to rule out primary hypersecretion as the cause of epiphora. Primary hypersecretion will show wetting of nearly the entire strip. The results of these tests must be applied within the context of the complete examination to yield maximum information.

The most important office tests to diagnose nasolacrimal duct obstruction, however, are the fluorescein dye disappearance, Jones' I, and Jones' II tests. When combined with canalicular probing and irrigation, these tests are generally successful in determining whether lacrimal drainage obstruction exists as well as the level of the obstruction, if any [14]. They should be performed in sequential order and can be done in the office exam room under topical anesthesia. The tests are low risk with potentially high benefit, making them valuable tools in the assessment of the tearing patient.

The fluorescein dye disappearance test was initially described by Zappia and Milder [15]. They recommended placing 1 drop of 2% fluorescein ophthalmic solution in each eye and instructing the patient to blink normally, taking care not to squeeze the lids. The amount of dye remaining in the tear lake after 5 minutes was then graded. Their system was later simplified by Meyer and colleacute [16] to yield a grading system of 0, + 1, or +2 to indicate no or only trace residual dye, intermediate or minimal residual dye, and marked residual dye, respectively. In this system, a positive test result indicates an abnormal situation.

The microreflux test (MRT) can be performed before canalicular irrigation. In this technique described by Camara and colleagues [17], two drops of fluorescein dye are instilled into the inferior cul de sac and the patient is asked to blink five times to activate the lacrimal pump. This technique obviously depends on an intact lacrimal pump and patent upper lacrimal punctum. The excess dye is then blotted away with tissue paper and the lacrimal punctum is examined under cobalt blue slit lamp magnification while digital pressure is exerted over the lacrimal sac. The initial pressure is allowed to empty the inferior canaliculus without being recorded as positive reflux. However, continued reflux of fluorescein-stained tears with continued massage is considered an indication of complete nasolacrimal duct obstruction. In Camara's study of this technique, the MRT was found to be a reliable screening test for the presence of complete nasolacrimal duct obstruction by sensitivity, specificity, positive- and negative-predictive value calculations. Realize, however, that massage on the lacrimal sac may also force some dye inferiorly and alter the validity of the Jones' I test as described below.

The Hornblass saccharine test is another method to investigate nasolacrimal drainage obstruction. In this test, saccharine drops are instilled into one eye and chloramphenicol drops are instilled into the other. The ability of the patient to detect the sweet taste of the saccharine and the bitter taste of the chloramphenicol indicates a patent drainage system [18]. The availability of these type drops, however, is somewhat limited, and this test is generally not in widespread use.

The Jones' I test [19,20] is a test for functional tear drainage obstruction [21], in which fluorescein dye is instilled into the tear lake, and an attempt is made to recover the dye on a cotton-tipped applicator placed under in the ipsilateral inferior turbinate 5 minutes later.

The Jones' II test is a test for anatomic tear drainage obstruction. Immediately following the Jones' I test, clear saline is used to irrigate the lacrimal system with a 23- or 27-guage blunt lacrimal cannula. If the patient's head is leaned forward, the drainage will drip from the nose and should be recovered with a tissue to prevent staining of the patient's clothes. More commonly, the test is performed with the head leaned back, and the eye surface is inspected for fluid reflux while the patient is instructed to notify the examiner if he/she detects/tastes the saline fluid in the naso- or oropharynx. If fluid can be passed into the nose, the system is anatomically patent. This test is done with a pressure greater than what the lacrimal pump usually creates. This can overcome, and in fact indicate, a functional obstruction. If no fluid can be detected in the nose or oropharynx, and the examiner notes all irrigation solution refluxing into the eye, then an anatomic lacrimal obstruction exists. The examiner should pay careful attention to the location of fluid reflux. Although irrigating the lower canaliculus, for example, if fluid returns from the upper punctum, obstruction beyond the canaliculus, most likely of the nasolacrimal duct, is suspected. If, however, fluid refluxes from the lower canaliculus around the irrigating cannula, then canalicular obstruction is most likely. The examiner may also feel a "soft stop" in cases of canalicular obstruction, making it difficult to fully advance the lacrimal cannula. In any of the above cases of suspected stenosis, lacrimal imaging may be considered to further characterize the nature of the obstruction.

Lacrimal imaging

A variety of lacrimal imaging studies exist. Each physician should communicate with his or her local radiologists to discuss what studies are available.

Dacryoscintigraphy with technetium-99m is a radioisotope scan to assess tear flow. A gamma camera is used to image the lacrimal system for 5 minutes following placement of a drop of a radioisotope such as technetium-99m into the inferior cul de sac. Complete nasolacrimal duct obstruction and physiologic pump failure can be elucidated with this technique. It is more sensitive for incomplete blocks of the upper drainage system and less invasive than dacryocystography. However, it does not provide as much detailed anatomic imaging as contrast dacryocystography, and precise localization of an obstruction is not usually possible.

Dacryocystography (DCG) allows visualization of anatomic details of the internal lumen of the entire lacrimal drainage system using a low-viscosity radiopaque contrast agent. A cannula must be inserted into the canaliculus to deliver the contrast agent. The patient's head is then imaged using Caldwell's view. A digital subtraction dacryocystography (DS-DCG) is a DCG in which a computer subtracts the surrounding bone and other tissues on the imaging study. This allows the outline of the radiopaque dye, which appears black as opposed to its usual white color on standard DCG, to be seen more clearly. On conventional DCG and DS-DCG, the lacrimal sac and duct are smooth, with the sac measuring 4 to 8 mm and the duct measuring 1 to 4 mm in diameter [22]. Lacrimal sac dilatation is assumed if greater than 1 to 2 mm size asymmetry from the fellow side exists. Inflammatory changes are typically manifest by irregularities in contour with concentric areas of soft tissue density. DCG may reveal normal findings in patients with functional or partial obstructions. The accuracy of DCG is technique-dependent, and contrast flow must overcome the lacrimal system ductal flow capacitance to illustrate functional obstruction. Observation of the ductal contrast column in at least two planes is helpful in delineating a true stenosis. The ductal contrast column may abruptly terminate or taper over a long segment on DCG [23]. Dilatation above any stenosis is a sign that the obstruction is functionally significant. Neoplasms and dacryoliths of the sac and duct generally present as filling defects with varying radiologic features. On DCG, they are commonly seen as stable, dark, and irregularly shaped objects within bright contrast dye. Air bubbles may also be seen, but are typically rounded, sharply demarcated, and change in size and shape. The detailed imaging that DCG provides can help in determination of the surgical plan based on localization of the obstruction.

CT or MRI scanning are used when traumatic, neoplastic, or mechanical secondary acquired nasolacrimal duct obstruction is suspected [21,24,25]. Combined CT- DCG facilitates visualization of the lacrimal drainage system via three-dimensional reconstruction. Furthermore, it offers the advantage of demonstrating a DCG filling defect while providing CT information on the density of the lesion and surrounding architecture. Special imaging equipment and software are required for CT-DCG testing. The sac–duct junction is the most common site of obstruction in the adult patient, which may manifest as filling of the lumen with soft tissue density on CT-DCG. CT-DCG is considered superior to MRI-DCG for canalicular visualization, but the lacrimal sac and duct are equally well visualized with both techniques [26]. MRI is probably less useful than CT overall due to its poor imaging of bony erosion or obstruction.

When deciding which test to order, or whether imaging is even indicated, the additional cost, time, and limited availability in some areas of special lacrimal imaging equipment should be considered and weighed against the additional information obtained from the test. In most patients, straightforward office examination and testing is sufficient.

Rhinoscopy also falls within the lacrimal imaging arena and is useful both pre- and postoperatively in evaluating tearing patients. As stated earlier, the nose should be inspected before undertaking any lacrimal surgery.

Pathophysiology and etiology of acquired nasolacrimal duct obstruction

The nasolacrimal duct is the site of most cases of primary acquired nasolacrimal duct obstruction in adults [27,28]. Acquired nasolacrimal duct obstruction may be primary or secondary.

Primary obstructions are associated with a fibroinflammatory process of unknown etiology. Many lacrimal surgeons have analyzed the process of primary acquired nasolacrimal duct obstruction. Linberg and McCormick [29] analyzed biopsies obtained during routine dacryocystorhinostomy (DCR) surgeries and concluded that obstructive fibrosis secondary to chronic inflammation of the membranous nasolacrimal duct is the usual cause. They observed chronic lymphoplasmacytic inflammation in the "periductal connective tissues." The degree of inflammation and fibrosis seen on histopathology roughly correlated with the clinical history in terms of duration of symptoms. Fibrotic obstruction of the lumen of the nasolacrimal duct accompanied longer standing disease. Acute inflammation was rarely seen. Additionally, infection was not observed in any of the specimens. They postulated that tear stasis and inflammation were involved in the pathogenesis of chronic nasolacrimal duct obstruction (NLDO). Paulsen and colleagues [30] performed histologic and immunohistochemical studies comparing tissue specimens from the nasolacrimal ducts of patients undergoing endonasal dacryocystorhinostomy for postinflammatory dacryostenosis with signs of chronic inflammation to specimens from cadaver donors. They found that organized lymphoid tissue with the cytomorphologic features of mucosa-associated lymphoid tissue was found in more than one-third of the donor specimens, but in only a few of the endo-DCR specimens. They concluded that this tear duct-associated lymphoid tissue is a common feature in normal nasolacrimal ducts. Because it seems to be lost with the scarring of symptomatic dacryostenosis, it is unlikely to be the cause of this scarring.

Dacryocystitis is inflammation of the lacrimal sac. It may present as an acute or chronic process [31–33]. It generally occurs in association with partial or complete NLDO. The bimodal incidence of dacryocystitis tends to parallel the incidence of NLDO. Acute dacryocystitis is usually bacterial in origin, representing fulminant infection of the lacrimal sac [34]. In the presence of tear stasis, such as that seen with NLDO, conditions favor the overgrowth of bacteria, and acute infection can ensue if a virulent organism is inoculated into the lacrimal sac or the host's immune system is compromised or suppressed. Acute dacryocystitis presents with marked distention of the lacrimal sac with erythema and pain. If left untreated, the sac may rupture, usually anteriorly through the overlying skin. Infection may also spread to the face, eyelids (preseptal cellulitis), orbit (orbital cellulitis), or sinuses. Before the advent of antibiotics, spread of infection through the valveless veins of the orbit into the cavernous sinus was commonly lethal. Common organisms responsible for acute bacterial dacryocystitis include *Staphylococcus* (*aureus* and *epidermidis*), *Streptococcus* (*pneumococci*, alpha- and beta- hemolytic), *Haemophilus influenzae*, *Pseudomonas*, *Pasteurella*, and *Enterobacter* species. Fungal organisms such as *Aspergillus* and *Candida* have been cultured, but their causative role has not been well defined. Histologic analyses of lacrimal sac specimens obtained during DCR for dacryocystitis-associated NLDO typically show inflamed epithelium with a mixture of proliferation and necrosis.

Chronic dacryocystitis represents a more indolent form of lacrimal sac inflammation and infection. It differs from acute dacryocystitis in that the process is usually less destructive. Lacrimal sac specimens obtained during DCR in these cases reveal thickening of the lacrimal sac walls and distention of the lacrimal sac lumen with the mucosa thrown into folds. The epithelium may be hyperplastic with occasional areas of necrosis or ulceration, and the underlying stroma typically has a lymphoplasmacytic infiltrate.

Primary inflammatory disorders of the lacrimal system generally lead to obstructed outflow. Inflammation may occur with or without infection, and can complicate preexisting obstruction from other causes. In a study by DeAngelis and colleagues [35] in 2001, histopathologic analysis of nasolacrimal sac and bone specimens obtained during external DCR revealed bony inflammatory changes in 14% and lacrimal sac inflammatory changes in 94% of patients with known nasolacrimal duct obstruction. In their study, the inflammatory changes were felt to be independent of gender, symptom duration, dacryocystitis history, lacrimal sac mucocele, obstruction location, or lacrimal sac calculi. Paulsen and colleagues [36] performed a comparative autopsy study on patients with a history of primary acquired nasolacrimal duct obstruction status post endonasal dacryocystorhinostomy, in which tissue specimens were analyzed by histologic studies and electron microscopy. They concluded from correlating the duration of symptoms to the level of inflammation seen in each specimen that descending inflammation from the eye or ascending inflammation from the nose initiates swelling of the mucous membrane, connective tissue fiber remodeling, subepithelial cavernous body malfunction, and temporary lacrimal passage obstruction. Repeated dacryocystitis occurrences may lead to total fibrous closure of the lumen or to a nonfunctional lacrimal passage segment.

There are multiple possible etiologies for secondary obstruction, as categorized by Bartley in his classification system for secondary acquired lacrimal drainage obstruction [37–39]. The general categories include infectious, inflammatory, neoplastic, traumatic, and mechanical. Topical ocular antihypertensive medications and radiation therapy [40,41] have also been reported to cause nasolacrimal duct obstruction. Less common causes of secondary obstruction include primary lacrimal system neoplasia, dacryolithiasis, sarcoidosis [42], Wegener's granulomatosis [43], foreign bodies, and melanin casts [44]. A series from Denmark reported secondary causes to be dacryocystitis (79%), dacryolithiasis (7.9%), tumor (4.5%), trauma (3.0%), congenital malformation (1.4%), canaliculitis (1.2%), and granulomatous inflammation (1.2%) [45]. It should be noted that most authorities consider dacryocystitis a secondary consequence of lacrimal obstruction rather than a cause of it. Lacrimal biopsy and imaging studies may prove valuable in diagnosing these disorders.

Dacryoliths or dacryocystoliths (lacrimal stones) can also cause acquired nasolacrimal duct obstruction. They are composed of laminated amorphous seromucous material, lipid, and inflammatory cells. Infrared spectroscopy and gas chromatography performed on 15 dacryoliths by Kominek and colleagues [46] revealed the chemical composition to be proteinaceous. The reported incidence in patients with primary acquired nasolacrimal duct obstruction was 10.4% in a study by Yazici, Hammad, and Meyer [47]. Relative risk factors for the development of dacryoliths in their study included male gender and initial presentation with lacrimal sac distention. Age, duration of epiphora, history of acute dacryocystitis, and previous use of topical ocular antihypertensive medications had no association with dacryolith formation. Hawes [48] reported a separate series of patients with dacryoliths showing the incidence to be 14% in patients undergoing dacryocystorhinostomy. The typical patient in this series was exemplified by a 4.8-year history of intermittent epiphora, at least one episode of acute dacryocystitis, and the ability to irrigate with some fluid getting into the nasopharynx. DCR patients with a history of acute dacryocystitis had a nine times higher likelihood of having a dacryolith than DCR patients without a history of acute dacryocystitis in this series. Andreou and Rose [49] similarly found that patients with dacryoliths were more likely to have a history of dacryocystitis when compared with dacryolith-free patients. In addition, they reported that patients with stones sought treatment earlier than stone-free patients. They reported no age or gender difference between lacrimal stone and stone-free patients. Piaton and colleagues [50] reported a series of patients undergoing lacrimal surgery for epiphora in which the incidence of dacryolithiasis was 6.9%. They proposed a mechanism of stone formation in which anatomic abnormalities of the valve of Hasner are thought to be responsible for stone formation. Seven hundred ninety-seven patients were examined with preoperative nasal videoendoscopy. Mucopurulent discharge was visualized in 45.8% of stone patients and 5.8% of stone-free patients. Anatomic abnormalities of the Hasner valve were visualized in 83.3% of the stone patients and in 11.4% of the stone-free patients. Typical abnormalities included a narrow valve (<2 mm), a long valve (>15 mm), or both. Other associated factors were younger age (48.2 years in the stone group and 59.1 years in the control group), a history of acute non-infectious dacryocystic retention, and partial obstruction of the lacrimal pathway. They suggested that when dacryolithiasis is suspected, a nasal videoendoscopic evaluation must be done to seek Hasner valve abnormalities and mucopurulent discharge at the valve. They also proposed that the association of mucopurulent discharge with a patent lacrimal system has a high specificity. This is consistent with a review of 89 years worth of pathology reports from the Eye Pathology Institute in Denmark, in which Marthin and colleagues [45] reported that microorganisms (especially Gram-positive rods) were seen in 87% of cases with dacryoliths, but in only 9% of cases with dacryocystitis.

Another serious, but less common, cause of secondary nasolacrimal obstruction is neoplasm, which may be a primary lacrimal sac tumor or secondary extension from the eyelids (basal cell and squamous cell being most common), nasal cavity, paranasal sinuses, or orbit. Metastatic spread is extremely rare, but has been reported with breast and prostate cancer. Although bloody tears may be idiopathic [11], in general, any patient with bloody tears should receive a workup for lacrimal neoplasm. Pseudotumors (idiopathic inflammatory mass) commonly arise within the lacrimal system comprising about 25% of lacrimal sac tumors. A series of cases reported by Duke-Elder found 26 cases of pseudotumor within 117 cases of lacrimal sac tumors [51]. Primary lacrimal sac malignancies are considered rare. However, early diagnosis is important as a high percentage (typically 50–70%) prove to be malignant or show malignant potential [45,52]. The vast majority of lacrimal sac tumors are epithelial (squamous or transitional cell), followed by sarcomas, melanomas, neural tumors, lymphomas [53,54], and other rare tumors [55]. Gao and colleagues [56] noted that as of 2005, all expired or recurrent cases of primary lymphoma of the lacrimal drainage system occurred in women, and suggested that sex was a prognostic factor in this disease. Lacrimal system neoplasm is an unusual cause of tearing, but should be suspected in patients with known systemic disease such as leukemia or lymphoma [57]. A high index of suspicion is indeed important for any potentially lethal disease and may lead surgeons to routinely perform lacrimal sac biopsies in patients undergoing DCR surgery. However, the value of routine biopsy is debated. Bernardini and colleagues [58] reported that of 302 specimens obtained during "routine" DCR, the only 10 specimens revealing "positive" histopathologic findings had a history of systemic disease or grossly abnormal-appearing lacrimal sacs during surgery. They recommended only performing lacrimal sac biopsy in these two groups of patients. After a series of 202 lacrimal sac biopsies from patients undergoing DCR for primary acquired nasolacrimal duct obstruction revealed 0 tumors, Lee-Wing and Ashenhurst [59] suggested that a lacrimal sac biopsy should only be performed when there is suspicion of a neoplasm based on the clinical, historic, or intraoperative findings.

Infections may also lead to nasolacrimal duct obstruction. Bacteria, viruses, fungi, and parasites have all been implicated as causes of infectious lacrimal drainage obstruction. *Actinomyces, Propionibacterium, Fusobacterium, Bacteroides, Mycobacterium, Chlamydia* (trachoma), *Nocardia, Enterobacter, Aeromonas, Treponema pallidum,* and *Staphylococcus aureus* are possible bacterial causes [4,60,61]. Fungi, such as *Aspergillus, Candida, Pityrosporum,* and *Trichophyton,* may be related to dacryolith formation or form other obstructive casts. Parasitic obstruction is rare, but has been reported with *Ascaris lumbricoides,* which can enter the system through the Hasner valve. In a series of 114 patients undergoing routine external DCR, direct biopsy and culture from the sac–duct junction revealed 44.7% of patients to have positive culture results, with the majority (78.5%) being Gram-positive organisms; 76.5% of the Gram-positive organisms were *Staphylococcus* sp., and the presence of a positive culture result was independent of a history of dacryocystitis or the presence of a mucocele [62].

Midface trauma such as fractures of the medial maxilla [63] can lead to scarring of the nasolacrimal duct with subsequent obstruction. Other trauma leading to lacrimal drainage obstruction usually involves the canaliculus and lacrimal sac in addition to the nasolacrimal duct. Early repair of traumatic nasolacrimal injuries with silicone tubing intubation has been advocated to prevent subsequent scarring, which often leads to obstruction. Late repair generally requires dacryocystorhinostomy.

Pseudotumor can also cause obstruction, as can granulomatous disease such as sarcoidosis [12,64] and Wegener's granulomatosis [65]. Lacrimal drainage obstruction may be the initial manifestation of sarcoidosis [42], and once the diagnosis is made, systemic steroids have been reported in some cases to reverse the obstruction.

Sinus or nasal surgery, especially endoscopic sinus surgery [66,67], are other potential causes. The nasolacrimal duct lies anterior to the usual site of and is vulnerable during enlargement of the nasal ostium of the maxillary sinus. It is also possible to injure the duct with nasolacrimal probing. However, this is rare.

Irradiation can also lead to lacrimal obstruction. External beam radiation in the medial canthal/orbital region may be associated with canalicular stenosis. Shepler and colleagues [68] reported nasolacrimal duct obstruction following ^{131}I therapy for thyroid carcinoma. A thyrogen scan after ^{131}I therapy indicated a focus of uptake initially suspected to be a metastasis. Probing and irrigation revealed complete blockage of the nasolacrimal duct. However, histopathology following DCR in this case revealed foreign-body reaction and fibrosis with no malignant cells.

Treatment

The treatment of nasolacrimal duct obstruction, or epiphora caused by lacrimal outflow obstruction in general, begins with an understanding of lacrimal flow between the pools as described above. Surgical techniques for obstructive epiphora are designed to either reestablish the natural channels of flow between the pools or establish new channels.

Initial treatment of nasolacrimal duct obstruction may include measures to reestablish the natural flow such as topical or oral antibiotics and antiinflammatory medications along with office-based canalicular probing and lacrimal irrigation. A review by Mauriello [69] of 75 patients with complete primary acquired nasolacrimal duct obstruction treated with conservative management consisting of oral and topical antibiotics followed by appropriately timed office lacrimal drainage system irrigation showed that this approach may be considered in a select group of patients. However, the majority of patients with lacrimal sac mucocele or history of acute dacryocystitis opted for early lacrimal surgical intervention in this study. More severe or chronic infections may require systemic antibiotics. This becomes especially important in the treatment of preseptal cellulitis, which may develop from infectious dacryocystitis and fester into orbital cellulitis with abscess formation. The choice of antibiotic depends on the suspected or known agents based on initial culture and sensitivity results. Of note, *Actinomyces* infections, which can cause canalicular obstructions, commonly necessitate complete removal of canalicular stones despite their documented sensitivity to penicillin.

Unlike congenital NLDO, primary acquired NLDO in an adult generally responds poorly to probing. Although probing with silicone tubing intubation or balloon dacryoplasty has been reported to successfully treat a subset of acquired NLDO in adults, the treatment of choice for primary acquired NLDO remains DCR, which bypasses the usual site of obstruction in the distal nasolacrimal duct. The success rate of external DCR for primary acquired NLDO is nearly 95% [70]. However, one recent study reported a more favorable success rate with endoscopic DCR at 84% than with external DCR at 77% [71]. The 77% success rate of external DCR in this study is below the success rate commonly found in the literature, however. Some authors have delineated their success rates based on "presac" or "postsac" delays, as evidenced by preoperative lacrimal scintigraphy or other imaging. One such study reported a 91% success rate of DCR for postsac delays and a 67% success rate of DCR for presac delays at 3.6 months postop. This difference was still noted at 3 years postop with a postsac success rate of 80% and a presac success rate of 47%, suggesting that external DCR with silicone tubing intubation has a higher success rate in the setting of a postsac obstruction [72].

External versus endonasal DCR

In general, it is difficult to make definitive evidence-based determinations about the relative efficacy of endonasal and external DCR because of deficiencies in the reported literature. As of 2001, the published literature contained two reports of clinical trials that compared endonasal with external DCR with a 1-year follow-up. The success rate was 91% for the external group in both reports and 63% and 75% for the endonasal groups, defined by patency to irrigation. However, other studies with lesser "strength of evidence" ratings suggest that endonasal DCR is a viable option for primary or revisional correction of acquired nasolacrimal duct obstruction in select patients. Complications of endonasal DCR generally do not appear to be greater in frequency or magnitude than those associated with external DCR [73].

External surgery

External DCR is considered an effective procedure for NLDO regardless of the etiology. As the current gold standard for lacrimal bypass surgery, its success rate is reported in several studies to be greater than 95% and does not seem to be affected by gender, presenting symptoms, duration of symptoms preoperatively, or silicone tubing insertion [74]. Associated canalicular stenosis may affect the outcome of external DCR if severe enough, and should be ruled out before proceeding with external DCR. External DCR is considered effective even for partial nasolacrimal duct obstruction. It allows identification, biopsy, and removal of dacryoliths and lacrimal sac tumors as needed.

Endoscopic surgery

In addition to an external approach, one may also perform a DCR using an endoscopic approach. The main advantages of endoscopic surgery promoted by its proponents include lack of external scar and relatively "less invasive" nature. Disadvantages include preferred use/need of general anesthesia by many surgeons, high cost of equipment, and the steep learning curve for the procedure, as well as a lower success rate in most studies.

Augmented/alternative lacrimal surgery

People have attempted to improve the success rates of lacrimal surgery by using balloon catheters, lasers, and antimetabolites. Endoscopic balloon dacryoplasty provides complete relief or substantial improvement in a significant number of patients with incomplete (partial) NLDO, and may be considered an appropriate treatment option [75].

Laser-assisted DCR, performed either through an endocanalicular, transconjunctival, or endonasal approach, yields the advantages of less bleeding, faster recovery, and elimination of a skin incision/scar. Moore, Bentley, and Olver [76] compared endosurgical DCR and endolaser (Holmium:yttrium-aluminum-garnet [YAG] laser) DCR. All patients underwent silicone tubing intubation, and results were obtained at least 6 months after surgery and at least 3 months after removal of the silicone tubes. They reported success rates of 83% after endosurgical DCR and 71% after endolaser DCR.

Some surgeons have advocated the use of antimetabolites such as mitomycin C and 5-fluorouracil to augment dacryocystorhinostomy surgery. Liao and colleagues [77] performed a prospective randomized controlled study in which 88 DCR surgeries were divided randomly into conventional (no mitomycin C) or mitomycin C (0.2 mg/mL applied to osteotomy site for 30 minutes) groups. Postoperative assessments were made objectively and subjectively. Within the mitomycin C group, 95.5% of patients remained asymptomatic compared with 70.5% in the conventional group. This was found to be a significant difference, but the 70.5% success rate of conventional DCR in this study is below the success rate commonly found in the literature. However, importantly, no significant complications such as abnormal bleeding, mucosal necrosis, or infection were reported. One patient in the mitomycin C group did show delayed wound healing without sequelae. They concluded that mitomycin C application was successful in increasing the success rate of DCR surgery in standard PANDO with no significant complications. Other studies have also shown favorable results with mitomycin C even with shorter applications. Camara, Bengzon, and Henson [78] showed a 9.6% improvement in success rate with 5 minutes of application of 0.5 mg/mL solution of mitomycin C in endonasal endoscopic laser-assisted dacryocystorhinostomy over a control group. In contrast, other studies have shown less favorable results with antimetabolite augmentation. The success rate with 5-fluorouracil augmented endonasal laser dacryocystorhinostomy was reported to be 63.6% (versus 94.7% for external DCR in the same study) by Watts and colleagues [79]. Endoscopic radiofrequency-assisted dacryocystorhinostomy with double stent and the use of a Griffiths collar button has been reported as an another augmented approach with a success rate of 98% [80].

Light and electron microscopic techniques have been used to examine lacrimal tissue obtained during revisions for failed DCR following antimetabolite-augmented DCR. Hypo- and acellular areas were identified by light microscopy, and fragmentation and necrosis of the fibroblast nuclei along with scanty cytoplasm poor in organelles were identified by electron microscopy. Tissues from the control group (not treated with antimetabolites at the initial surgery) showed increased numbers of active fibroblasts with cytoplasm containing numerous organelles by light and electron microscopy [81].

An alternative treatment to dacryocystorhinostomy is retrograde placement of a hollow polyurethane nasolacrimal duct stent. The stent is placed under fluoroscopic guidance over a guide wire facilitated by use of a Ritleng probe through the upper lacrimal punctum. After passing the probe beyond the obstruction, a guidewire is passed through the probe and the stent can be placed into the lacrimal sac and duct bridging the sac–duct junction. The overall success rate of this procedure was reported to be 82% in 2001 [82]. A later paper [83], in 2004, however, stated that although epiphora could be relieved using polyurethane stent implantation if meticulous technique was employed, overall, nasolacrimal polyurethane stent implantation has a low success rate in the treatment of primary acquired nasolacrimal duct obstruction. Inflammation and fibrosis may be induced by stent placement leading to further difficulties in subsequent lacrimal surgery.

Conjunctivodacryocystorhinostomy

Conjunctivodacryocystorhinostomy is generally reserved for cases of high grade canalicular stenosis. Typically, this is performed with placement of a Pyrex glass Jones tube to act as conduit for tear flow from the medial lacrimal cul de sac into the nose. The tubes require periodic irrigation and sometimes need to be exchanged. Migration or extrusion of the tubes may also occur.

Summary

In summary, proper evaluation of the tearing patient is necessary to determine the cause of tearing. Nasolacrimal duct stenosis is the most common cause of lacrimal obstruction leading to epiphora, and fortunately, treatment generally has a high success rate.

References

[1] Rodrigues Pereira R, Arts WF. Crying upon eating: the crocodile-tears syndrome. Ned Tijdschr Geneeskd 2005;149(3):144–5.
[2] Hofmann RJ. Treatment of Frey's syndrome (gustatory sweating) and "crocodile tears" (gustatory epiphora) with purified botulinum toxin. Ophthal Plast Reconstr Surg 2000; 16(4):289–91.
[3] Montoya FJ, Riddell CE, Caesar R, et al. Treatment of gustatory hyperlacrimation (crocodile tears) with injection of botulinum toxin into the lacrimal gland. Eye 2002;16(6):705–9.
[4] Camara JG, Bengzon AU. Nasolacrimal duct, obstruction. http://www.emedicine.com/oph/topic465.htm 2005.
[5] Sahlin S, Chen E, Kaugesaar T, et al. Effect of botulinum toxin injection on lacrimal drainage. Am J Ophthalmol 2000;129(4):481–6.
[6] Bartley GB. Acquired lacrimal drainage obstruction: an etiologic classification system, case reports and a review of the literature. Part I. Ophthal Plast Reconstr Surg 1992;8: 237–42.

[7] Janssen AG, Mansour K, Bos JJ, et al. Diameter of the bony lacrimal canal: normal values and values related to nasolacrimal duct obstruction: assessment with CT. AJNR Am J Neuroradiol 2001;22(5):845–50.

[8] Weber AL, Rodriguez-DeVelasquez A, Lucarelli MJ, et al. Normal anatomy and lesions of the lacrimal sac and duct. In: Weber AL, editor. Neuroimaging clinics of North America: imaging of the globe, orbit, and visual pathway, Vol. 6. Philadelphia (PA): WB Saunders; 1996. p. 205–6.

[9] Groessl SA, Sires BS, Lemke BN. An anatomic basis for primary acquired nasolacrimal duct obstruction. Arch Ophthalmol 1997;115(1):71–4.

[10] Kallman JE, Foster JA, Wulc AE, et al. Computed tomography in lacrimal outflow obstruction. Ophthalmology 1997;104:676–82.

[11] Ho VH, Wilson MW, Linder JS, et al. Bloody tears of unknown cause: case series and review of the literature. Ophthal Plast Reconstr Surg 2004;20(6):442–7.

[12] Fergie N, Jones NS, Downes RN, et al. Dacryocystorhinostomy in nasolacrimal duct obstruction secondary to sarcoidosis. Orbit 1999;18(3):217–22.

[13] Ugurlu S, Bartley GB, Woog JJ. Evaluation and management of acquired dacryostenosis. In: Woog JJ, editor. Manual of endoscopic lacrimal and orbital surgery. Philadelphia (PA): Butterworth-Heinemann; 2004. p. 49.

[14] Meyer DR. Evaluation and management of lacrimal disorders. In: Stephenson CM, editor. Ophthalmic plastic, reconstructive, and orbital surgery. Boston (MA): Butterworth-Heinemann; 1997. p. 49.

[15] Zappia RJ, Milder B. Lacrimal drainage function. 2. The fluorescein dye disappearance test. Am J Ophthalmol 1972;74:160.

[16] Meyer DR, Antonello A, Linberg JV. Assessment of tear drainage after canalicular obstruction using fluorescein dye disappearance. Ophthalmology 1990;97:1370.

[17] Camara JG, Santiago MD, Rodriguez RE, et al. The Micro-Reflux Test: a new test to evaluate nasolacrimal duct obstruction. Ophthalmology 1999;106(12):2319–21.

[18] Hornblass A. A simple test for lacrimal obstruction. Arch Ophthalmol 1973;90(6):435–6.

[19] Jones LT, Wobig JL. Surgery of the eyelids and lacrimal system. Birmingham (AL): Aesculapius; 1976.

[20] Jones LT. An anatomical approach to problems of the eyelids and lacrimal apparatus. Arch Ophthalmol 1961;166:111.

[21] Dutton JJ. Diagnostic tests and imaging techniques. In: Linberg JV, editor. Lacrimal surgery. New York: Churchill Livingstone; 1988. p. 19.

[22] Malik SRK, Gupta AK, Chaterjee S, et al. Dacryocystography of normal and pathological lacrimal passages. Br J Ophthalmol 1969;53:174–9.

[23] Francis IC, Kappagoda MB, Cole IE, et al. Computed tomography of the lacrimal drainage system: retrospective study of 107 cases of dacryostenosis. Ophthalmic Plast Reconstr Surg 1999;15(3):217–26.

[24] Flanagan JC, Zolli CL. Lacrimal sac tumors: surgical management. In: Linberg JV, editor. Lacrimal surgery. New York: Churchill Livingstone; 1988. p. 203.

[25] Russell EJ, Czervionke L, Huckman M, et al. CT of the inferomedial orbit and the lacrimal drainage apparatus: normal and pathologic anatomy. Am J Radiol 1985;145:1147.

[26] Caldemeyer KS, Stockberger SM, Broderick LS. Topical contrast-enhanced CT and MR dacryocystography: imaging the lacrimal drainage apparatus of healthy volunteers. AJR 1998; 171:1501–4.

[27] Duke-Elder S. Normal and abnormal development. Part 2. Congenital deformities. In: Duke-Elder S, editor. System of ophthalmology, Vol. 3. St. Louis (MO): Mosby; 1963. p. 911.

[28] Thomas A, Sujatha S, Ramakrishnan PM, et al. Malignant melanoma of the lacrimal sac. Arch Ophthalmol 1975;3:84.

[29] Linberg JV, McCormick SA. Primary acquired Nasolacrimal duct obstruction: a clinicopathologic report and biopsy technique. Ophthalmology 1986;93:1055.

[30] Paulsen FP, Schaudig U, Maune S, et al. Loss of tear duct-associated lymphoid tissue in association with the scarring of symptomatic dacryostenosis. Ophthalmology 2003;110(1): 85–92.

[31] Font RL. Eyelids and lacrimal drainage system. In: Spencer WH, editor. Ophthalmic pathology. Philadelphia (PA): Saunders; 1986. p. 2312.

[32] Meyer DR, Linberg JV. Acute dacryocystitis: diagnosis and management. In: Linberg JV, editor. Oculoplastic and orbital emergencies. East Norwalk (CT): Appleton & Lange; 1989. p. 29.

[33] Sood NN, Ratnaraj A, Balarman G, et al. Chronic dacryocystitis: a clinicobacteriological study. All India Ophthalmol Soc 1967;15:107.

[34] Meyer DR, Wobig JL. Acute dacryocystitis due to *Pasteurella multocida*. Am J Ophthalmol 1990;110:444.

[35] DeAngelis D, Hurwitz J, Oestreicher J, et al. The pathogenesis and treatment of lacrimal obstruction: the value of lacrimal sac and bone analysis. Orbit 2001;20(3):163–72.

[36] Paulsen FP, Thale AB, Maune S, et al. New insights into the pathophysiology of primary acquired dacryostenosis. Ophthalmology 2001;108(12):2329–36.

[37] Bartley GB. Acquired lacrimal drainage obstruction: an etiologic classification system, case reports, and a review of the literature. Part 1. Ophthal Plast Reconstr Surg 1992;8(4):237–42.

[38] Bartley GB. Acquired lacrimal drainage obstruction: an etiologic classification system, case reports, and a review of the literature. Part 2. Ophthal Plast Reconstr Surg 1992;8(4):243–9.

[39] Bartley GB. Acquired lacrimal drainage obstruction: an etiologic classification system, case reports, and a review of the literature. Part 3. Ophthal Plast Reconstr Surg 1993;9(1):11–26.

[40] Yeatts RP. Acquired nasolacrimal duct obstruction. In: Bradley EA, Bartley GB, Garrity JA, editors. Oculoplastic surgery update: Ophthalmology Clinics of North America. Philadelphia (PA): WB Saunders; 2000. p. 13:719–29.

[41] Spaeth GL. Nasolacrimal duct obstruction caused by topical epinephrine. Arch Ophthalmol 1967;77:355–7.

[42] Chapman KL, Bartley GB, Garrity JA, et al. Lacrimal bypass surgery in patients with sarcoidosis. Am J Ophthalmol 1999;127(4):443–6.

[43] Hardwig PW, Bartley GB, Garrity JA. Surgical management of nasolacrimal duct obstruction in patients with Wegener's granulomatosis. Ophthalmology 1992;99(1):133–9.

[44] Dryden RM, Wulc AE. Pseudoepiphora from cerebrospinal fluid leak: case report. Br J Ophthalmol 1986;70(8):570–4.

[45] Marthin JK, Lindegaard J, Prause JU, et al. Lesions of the lacrimal drainage system: a clinicopathological study of 643 biopsy specimens of the lacrimal drainage system in Denmark 1910–1999. Acta Ophthalmol Scand 2005;83(1):94–9.

[46] Kominek P, Cervenka S, Doskarova S, et al. Dacryolithiasis—analysis of 15 cases. Cesk Slov Oftalmol 2002;58(3):205–11.

[47] Yazici B, Hammad AM, Meyer DR. Lacrimal sac dacryoliths: predictive factors and clinical characteristics. Ophthalmology 2001;108(7):1308–12.

[48] Hawes MJ. The dacryolithiasis syndrome. Ophthal Plast Reconstr Surg 1988;4(2):87–90.

[49] Andreou P, Rose GE. Clinical presentation of patients with dacryolithiasis. Ophthalmology 2002;109(8):1573–4.

[50] Piaton JM, Keller P, Sahel JA, et al. Dacryolithiasis: diagnosis using nasal endoscopy. J Fr Ophtalmol 2003;26(7):685–98.

[51] Duke-Elder S. Tumors of the lacrimal passages. In: Duke-Elder S, editor. System of ophthalmology, Vol. 5. St. Louis (MO): Mosby; 1952. p. 5346.

[52] deBree R, Scheeren RA, Kummer A, et al. Nasolacrimal duct obstruction caused by an oncocytoma. Rhinology 2002;40(3):165–7.

[53] Buc D, Travade P, Kemeny JL, et al. A case of primary non-Hodgkin lymphoma of the lacrimal sac. J Fr Ophtalmol 2002;25(9):931–5.

[54] Mori T, Tokuhira M, Mori S, et al. Primary natural killer cell lymphoma of the lacrimal sac. Ann Hematol 2001;80(10):607–10.

[55] Sutula FC. Tumors of the lacrimal gland and sac. In: Albert DM, Jakobiec FA, editors. Principles and practice of ophthalmology. Philadelphia (PA): WB Saunders; 1994. p. 1952–67.

[56] Gao HW, Lee HS, Lin YS, et al. Primary lymphoma of nasolacrimal drainage system: a case report and literature review. Am J Otolaryngol 2005;26(5):356–9.

[57] Yip CC, Bartley GB, Habermann TM, et al. Involvement of the lacrimal drainage system by leukemia or lymphoma. Ophthal Plast Reconstr Surg 2002;18(4):242–6.

[58] Bernardini FP, Moin M, Kersten RC, et al. Routine histopathologic evaluation of the lacrimal sac during dacryocystorhinostomy: how useful is it? Ophthalmology 2002;109(7):1214–7 [discussion 1217–8].

[59] Lee-Wing MW, Ashenhurst ME. Clinicopathologic analysis of 166 patients with primary acquired nasolacrimal duct obstruction. Ophthalmology 2001;108(11):2038–40.

[60] McCormick SA, Linberg JV. The pathology of nasolacrimal duct obstruction: clinicopathologic correlates of lacrimal excreting system disease. In: Linberg JV, editor. Lacrimal surgery. New York: Churchill Livingstone; 1988. p. 91.

[61] Katowitz JA, Kropp TM. Mycobacterium fortuitun as a cause for nasolacrimal obstruction and granulomatous eyelid disease. Ophthalmic Surg 1987;18:97.

[62] DeAngelis D, Hurwitz J, Mazzulli T. The role of bacteriologic infection in the etiology of nasolacrimal duct obstruction. Can J Ophthalmol 2001;36(3):134–9.

[63] Harris GJ, Fuerste FH. Lacrimal intubation in the primary repair of midfacial fractures. Ophthalmology 1987;94:242.

[64] Harris GJ, Williams GA, Clarke GP. Sarcoidosis of the lacrimal sac. Arch Ophthalmol 1981; 99:1198.

[65] Haynes BF, Fishman ML, Fauci AS, et al. The ocular manifestations of Wegener's granulomatosis: fifteen years' experience and review of the literature. Am J Med 1977;63:131.

[66] Corey JP, Bumsted R, Panje W, et al. Orbital complications in functional endoscopic sinus surgery. Otolaryngol Head Neck Surg 1993;109(5):814–20.

[67] Serdal CL, Berris CE, Chole RA. Nasolacrimal duct obstruction after endoscopic sinus surgery. Arch Ophthalmol 1990;108:391.

[68] Shepler TR, Sherman SI, Faustina MM, et al. Nasolacrimal duct obstruction associated with radioactive iodine therapy for thyroid carcinoma. Ophthal Plast Reconstr Surg 2003;19(6): 479–81.

[69] Mauriello JA Jr, Guzman C. Oral and topical antibiotic therapy of complete, primary acquired nasolacrimal duct obstruction in adults. Ophthal Plast Recontr Surg 1999;15(5): 363–5.

[70] Dressner SA, Klussman K, Meyer DR, et al. Outpatient dacryocystorhinostomy. Ophthalmic Surg 1991;22:1.

[71] Ben Simon GJ, Joseph J, Lee S, et al. External versus endoscopic dacryocystorhinostomy for acquired nasolacrimal duct obstruction in a tertiary referral center. Ophthalmology 2005; 112(8):1463–8.

[72] Delaney YM, Khooshabeh R. External dacryocystorhinostomy for the treatment of acquired partial nasolacrimal obstruction in adults. Br J Ophthalmol 2002;86(9):1068.

[73] Woog JJ, Kennedy RH, Custer PL, et al. Endonasal dacryocystorhinostomy: a report by the American Academy of Ophthalmology. Ophthalmology 2001;108(12):2369–77.

[74] Kashkouli MB, Parvaresh M, Modarreszadeh M, et al. Factors affecting the success of external dacryocystorhinostomy. Orbit 2003;22(4):247–55.

[75] Couch SM, White WL. Endoscopically assisted balloon Dacryoplasty treatment of incomplete nasolacrimal duct obstruction. Ophthalmology 2004;111(3):585–9.

[76] Moore WM, Bentley CR, Olver JM. Functional and anatomic results after two types of endoscopic endonasal dacryocystorhinostomy: surgical and holmium laser. Ophthalmology 2002;109(8):1575–82.

[77] Liao SL, Kao SC, Tseng JH, et al. Results of intraoperative mitomycin C application in dacryocystorhinostomy. Br J Ophthalmol 2000;84(8):903–6.

[78] Camara JG, Bengzon AU, Henson RD. The safety and efficacy of mitomycin C in endonasal endoscopic laser-assisted dacryocystorhinostomy. Ophthal Plast Reconstr Surg 2000;16(2): 114–8.

[79] Watts P, Ram AR, Nair R, et al. Comparison of external dacryocystorhinostomy and 5-fluo-rouracil augmented endonasal laser dacryocystorhinostomy. A retrospective review. Indian J Ophthalmol 2001;49(3):169–72.

[80] Javate R, Pamintuan F. Endoscopic radiofrequency-assisted dacryocystorhinostomy with double stent: a personal experience. Orbit 2005;24(1):15–22.

[81] Yalaz M, Firinciogullari E, Zeren H. Use of mitomycin c and 5-fluorouracil in external da-cryocystorhinostomy. Orbit 1999;18(4):239–45.

[82] Yazici B, Yazici Z, Parlak M. Treatment of nasolacrimal duct obstruction in adults with polyurethane stent. Am J Ophthalmol 2001;13(1):37–43.

[83] Ozturk S, Konuk O, Ilgit ET, et al. Outcome of patients with nasolacrimal polyurethane stent implantation: do they keep tearing? Ophthal Plast Reconstr Surg 2004;20(2):130–5.

ELSEVIER
SAUNDERS

Otolaryngol Clin N Am
39 (2006) 1001–1017

OTOLARYNGOLOGIC
CLINICS
OF NORTH AMERICA

Endoscopic Dacryocystorhinostomy and Conjunctivodacryocystorhinostomy

John J. Woog, MD, FACS[a],*,
Raj Sindwani, MD, FACS, FRCS[b]

[a]Department of Ophthalmology, Mayo Clinic College of Medicine, 200 First Street SW,
Rochester, MN 55905, USA
[b]Department of Otolaryngology-Head & Neck Surgery, Saint Louis University School
of Medicine, 3635 Vista Avenue, 6th Floor FDT, Saint Louis, MO 63110, USA

Endonasal approaches to the correction of nasolacrimal duct (NLD) obstruction were described by several investigators, including Caldwell [1], West [2], and Mosher [3] in the late 1800s and early 1900s. Because of technical limitations in terms of visualization of the surgical site and effective soft tissue and bone removal, the popularity of intranasal dacryocystorhinostomy (DCR) was limited throughout most of the twentieth century; lacrimal bypass surgery was performed more commonly by way of external routes, as reported by Toti [4] and Dupuy-Dutemps and Bouquet [5]. With the advent of the rigid fiberoptic endoscope and its use in paranasal sinus surgery, there has been renewed interest over the past decade in endoscopic surgery for the correction of primary [6–8] and recurrent [9–11] lacrimal obstruction.

Patient selection

Primary endoscopic DCR (EDCR) may be indicated in the management of tearing or infection that is associated with primary acquired NLD obstruction or NLD obstruction that is secondary to specific inflammatory or infiltrative disorders. Generally, this procedure is indicated when the level of obstruction is determined to be at or distal to the junction of the lacrimal sac and duct, although more proximal pathology also may be managed

Portions of this article are reprinted from: Woog JJ. Endoscopic Dacryocystorhinostomy and Conjunctivodacryocystorhinostomy. In: John J. Woog, Ed. Manual of Endoscopic Lacrimal and Orbital Surgery. Philadelphia: Butterworth/Heineman, 2004; with permission.
* Corresponding author.
E-mail address: woog.john@mayo.edu (J.J. Woog).

endoscopically. EDCR also is useful in the management of lacrimal duct injuries that are associated with sinus surgery, as well as in selected patients with a history of facial trauma. In addition, it may be appropriate in certain patients who have atypical forms of congenital dacryostenosis.

EDCR has been considered contraindicated in several settings. Most importantly, EDCR is contraindicated for patients who have a suspected neoplasm that involves the lacrimal outflow system or for those in whom such a lesion cannot be excluded. Clinical criteria that raise the possibility of a neoplasm may include (1) the presence of an indurated, noncompressible mass, possibly with fixation to the underlying bone or extension above the level of the medial canthal tendon; (2) bloody epiphora; (3) atypical age of onset of obstruction (eg, young adulthood); and (4) the presence of bony destruction or a filling defect on radiologic studies, although the latter also may occur in the setting of nonneoplastic causes of obstruction (eg, dacryolithiasis). Relative contraindications to EDCR include the presence of a large diverticulum lateral to the lacrimal sac, common canalicular stenosis, or retrieval of large lacrimal system stones.

For patients who require endoscopic sinus surgery in addition to EDCR, this procedure may be performed conveniently and efficiently using the same instrumentation, during the same setting. The endoscopic skills and instruments that are used for EDCR are the same as those used routinely for endoscopic sinus surgery by otolaryngologists. The endoscopic approach provides excellent visualization and management of intranasal structures, and may be associated with an improved outcome, because intranasal synechiae and improper placement of the rhinostomy site (eg, into an agger nasi cell or the superolateral aspect of the middle turbinate) are common causes of failure of external DCR (EXTDCR). There are no facial incisions. As a result, the risk for cutaneous fistulas, of concern in patients who had previous radiation therapy or certain granulomatous disorders, also may be reduced.

Surgical technique

Anesthesia and nasal preparation

EDCR may be performed using general or local anesthesia. If general anesthesia is used, decongestion of the nasal mucosa is achieved by placement of nasal pledgets that contain oxymetazoline 0.05% in the middle meatus, followed by endoscopic injection of 1% xylocaine containing 1:200,000 epinephrine into the lateral nasal wall and middle turbinate.

Surgery using local anesthesia begins with instillation of topical proparacaine or tetracaine in the conjunctival cul-de-sac of the operated eye. Intravenous administration of short-acting sedative-hypnotics may enhance patient comfort during subsequent anesthetic injection. A 1:1 mixture of 2% xylocaine with 1:200,000 epinephrine and 0.75% bupivacaine is administered to provide an infraorbital nerve block. Additional local anesthetic is infiltrated subcutaneously and subconjunctivally in the medial eyelids and medial canthal region. Pledgets that contain oxymetazoline and viscous xylocaine solution are placed in the middle meatus, and the local anesthetic is injected submucosally.

Lacrimal sac localization

The point of insertion of the root of the middle turbinate on the lateral nasal wall and the maxillary line are key intranasal landmarks for identifying the location of the lacrimal sac. For surgeons who are becoming familiar with intranasal anatomy and surgery in patients who have atypical anatomy or a history of sinonasal procedures, it may be helpful to introduce a 20-gauge fiberoptic endoilluminator (Fig. 1), as used in vitreoretinal surgery, through the superior or inferior canaliculus after punctal dilation. The endoilluminator is advanced gently until a hard stop that signifies the lacrimal bone medial to the lacrimal sac is identified. The location of the lacrimal sac then may be visualized endoscopically by transillumination (Fig. 2). Alternatively, a surgical navigation system may be used to localize the region of the lacrimal fossa and sac.

Mucosal incision and removal

After lacrimal sac localization, the mucosa on the lateral wall is incised using a sickle knife, blade, or electrocautery and is elevated using a Freer elevator (Fig. 3). It is helpful to place this incision well anterior to the location of the lacrimal sac to allow full exposure of the overlying bone. The incision is oriented vertically, extending from inferior to superior to minimize interference from bleeding. After the mucosa is elevated widely from the underlying bone, it is removed with Blakesley forceps. Alternatively, mucosal ablation

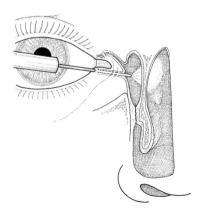

Fig. 1. The endoscopic approach to the lacrimal sac is demonstrated in this coronal section of the right lacrimal system and nasal cavity. A fiberoptic endoilluminator is introduced through the superior or inferior canaliculus into the lacrimal sac.

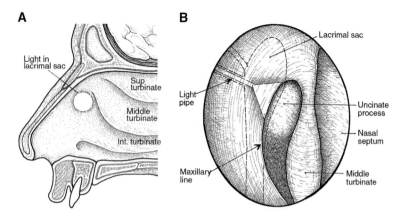

Fig. 2. (*A*) From the sagittal perspective, the lacrimal sac is noted to be anterior to the point of insertion of the root of the middle turbinate on the lateral nasal wall. (*B*) On the coronal view, the maxillary line, which originates from the middle turbinate insertion, overlies the lacrimal sac.

may be performed with KTP:YAG, holmium:YAG, or carbon dioxide lasers. Although this approach may afford enhanced hemostasis, the drawbacks of laser-based techniques include the lack of tissue availability for histopathologic examination, as well as the potential for increased scarring.

Bone removal

To expose the lacrimal sac, the bony lacrimal fossa must be uncovered. If the endoilluminator is used for surgery, the bones overlying the lacrimal sac often can be visualized by way of transillumination. When viewed endoscopically, movement of the endoilluminator within the lacrimal sac may be

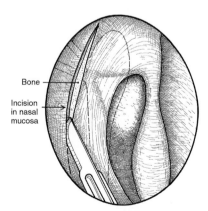

Fig. 3. The nasal mucosa is incised anterior to the maxillary line from a point superior to the turbinate insertion to the level of the midpoint of the maxillary line, a point that corresponds to the sac–duct junction. The mucosa is elevated and removed to allow full visualization of the bone overlying the lacrimal outflow system.

helpful in demonstrating the relative bony thicknesses of the thin posterior lacrimal bone versus the thick anterior maxilla. Bone removal may be achieved by using a variety of instruments, and it should commence at the maxillary line and proceed anteriorly. Although the lacrimal bone, located posterior to the maxillary line, may be taken down with minimal force, the authors recommend the use of a high-speed drill with a cutting burr (supplemented by Kerrison or pituitary rongeurs) for removal of the dense frontal process of the maxilla, which is situated anteriorly (Fig. 4). Lasers also may be used, although laser-based techniques may be inefficient because of the need for frequent mechanical char removal and may result in an increased degree of devitalized tissue.

Regardless of the technique selected, a bony rhinostomy of adequate size and location facilitates a successful outcome. It is particularly important that the bone overlying the common canaliculus is resected completely. Generally, a rhinostomy with a vertical dimension of at least 6 to 8 mm is achieved in adult patients. It is not uncommon for an anterior ethmoidectomy to be required to allow satisfactory access to the lacrimal fossa by removing prominent agger nasi cells.

Removal of the lacrimal sac mucosa

After removal of the overlying bone, the lacrimal sac is incised using a sickle knife (Fig. 5). Often, it is helpful for the assistant to "tent out" the medial wall of the lacrimal sac with lacrimal probes that are introduced through the canaliculi. The medial wall of the lacrimal sac and NLD then may be removed with Blakesley forceps and submitted for histopathologic examination. An adequate rhinostomy should permit easy passage of lacrimal probes. Removal of the medial wall of the lacrimal sac in the area of the common canaliculus also may be confirmed by direct visualization of the internal common punctum with a 0°- or 30°-endoscope.

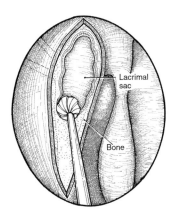

Fig. 4. The bone overlying the lacrimal sac is removed with a high-speed drill or rongeurs to allow visualization of the lacrimal sac.

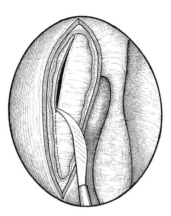

Fig. 5. The medial wall of the lacrimal sac is incised using a sickle knife.

Lacrimal system intubation

After the medial sac wall has been resected, a bicanalicular intubation set is used to intubate both canaliculi, with subsequent retrieval of the probes from the rhinostomy site endoscopically (Fig. 6). The tubing is tied in the nasal vestibule in such a way as to allow the appropriate length and tension of the silicone tubing loop in the medial commissure. Thus, the closed loop formed acts as stent for the newly created rhinostomy. The authors prefer to remove the stent 6 weeks postoperatively, but intervals for stent removal that range from 4 weeks to 6 months have been advocated by other investigators [12–14].

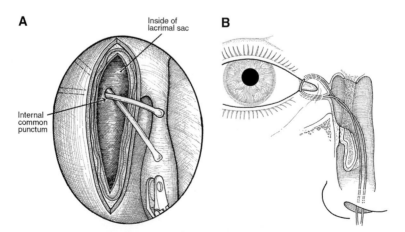

Fig. 6. (*A*) Bicanalicular silicone tubing is introduced and the probes are retrieved from the nasal cavity endoscopically. (*B*) A coronal view demonstrates placement of the silicone tubing stent within the canaliculi and intranasal rhinostomy.

Mitomycin C application and adjunctive procedures

Some surgeons elect to apply topical mitomycin C to the intranasal rhinostomy site. Mitomycin C is an antimetabolite that has been used to modulate fibrosis after glaucoma and pterygium surgery. Reports on the usefulness of mitomycin C in the prevention of postoperative fibrosis and rhinostomy closure demonstrated mixed findings. Dolman [15] recently performed an elegant prospective randomized study to address the efficacy of mitomycin C application; no difference in success rates was found between the groups that were and were not treated with mitomycin C (93% and 94% of 58 and 118 patients, respectively). If used, mitomycin C is applied intranasally in a concentration of 0.4 mg/mL using a cotton-tipped applicator, for a period of 5 minutes, after which copious saline irrigation of the rhinostomy site is performed (Fig. 7).

Concomitant ethmoidectomy may be required to provide adequate access to the anterior lacrimal sac. Other procedures, including uncinectomy, middle turbinectomy, and septoplasty, also may facilitate exposure of the lateral nasal wall. The frequency with which these procedures are performed is summarized in Table 1.

Postoperative care

Postoperatively, the patient is placed on a combination antibiotic–steroid eye drop, such as sulfacetamide-prednisolone acetate, four times a day for 2 weeks, and is instructed to perform frequent nasal saline irrigations for 4 to 6 weeks. The patient is seen 1 week postoperatively, at which time lacrimal irrigation and nasal endoscopy with debridement are performed. These procedures are repeated again as necessary. At the appropriate time after surgery, the stent is cut in the vestibule and removed endoscopically in the office.

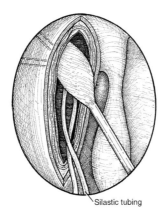

Silastic tubing

Fig. 7. Mitomycin C may be applied to the intranasal ostium.

Table 1
Endoscopic dacryocystorhinostomy adjunctive procedures

Investigators	Septoplasty (%)	Ethmoidectomy (%)	Middle turbinectomy (%)
Rice, 1990 [17]	4	52	24
Metson, 1991 [16]	NS	NS	24.5
Sadiq et al, 1996 [18]	33	33	58
Mortimore et al, 1999 [14]	5	10	20
Dolman, 2003 [15]	5	78	33

Recent technical modifications of endoscopic dacryocystorhinostomy

There have been several recent developments in terms of the under-standing of relevant surgical anatomy as well as alternative technical op-tions in the performance of EDCR. From the anatomic viewpoint, using CT and dacryocystogram studies, Wormald and colleagues [19] determined that the lacrimal sac extended, on average, 8.8 mm superior to the inser-tion of the middle turbinate along the lateral nasal wall. This led the inves-tigators to suggest that the mucosal incision that is made during intranasal DCR be carried up to this level. Similarly, Chastain and colleagues [20] demonstrated that the maxillary line, a commonly visualized landmark during endoscopic surgery, corresponds to the junction of the frontal pro-cess of the maxilla with the lacrimal bone extranasally, and the uncinate process intranasally. Approximately one half of the lacrimal sac fossa lies anterior to the location of the maxillary line; this supports the recom-mendation that the nasal mucosal incision be placed anterior to this landmark.

From the technical perspective, several investigators described their ex-perience with variations in terms of removal of bone or soft tissue, and the use of stents during surgery. Javate and Pamintuan [21] noted a success rate of 98% in 117 patients who underwent EDCR using radiofrequency instrumentation for mucosa removal, followed by mitomycin C application (0.5 mg/mL for 3 minutes), followed by placement of a double stent. Cokkeser and colleagues [22] reported success in 87% of 62 patients who underwent bone removal with a hammer and chisel technique. Ibra-him and coworkers [23] described their experience with an endoscopically guided trephination procedure, and reported success in 83% of 19 patients in their study.

The creation of nasal or lacrimal sac mucosal flaps was reported by sev-eral investigators in recent years. Wormald [24] and Tsirbas and Wormald [25] noted success rates of 95.7% and 91% in patients who underwent EDCR with nasal and lacrimal sac flaps. Massegur and colleagues [26] re-ported success in 93% of patients who underwent hammer and chisel EDCR in conjunction with lacrimal sac and posteriorly based nasal mucosal flaps.

Results

The reported outcomes of EDCR and related procedures are summarized in Table 2. As displayed, the success rates of primary EDCR in several recent series exceed those obtained in earlier reports, and in some cases match the 90% to 95% success rates that are obtained with EXTDCR. Further emphasized in Table 3, most contemporary comparisons have demonstrated similar success rates between external and nonlaser EDCR, with a tendency for patient preference for EDCR noted in several studies. The reported improvement in surgical outcomes recently may reflect a collective "learning curve"–type effect among surgeons who perform this procedure. The existence of such a learning curve is supported by a report by Onerci and colleagues [27], who noted that an EDCR success rate of 94% in the hands of experienced surgeons decreases to only 58% when the procedure is performed by inexperienced surgeons.

Recently, several groups attempted to identify other factors that may influence the success rate of EDCR in selected patients. Wormald and Tsirbas [28] noted a success rate of 97% in patients who had anatomic obstruction, but only 84% in patients who had functional outflow impairment. Yung and coworkers [29] looked at surgical success as a function of the level of obstruction and noted success rates of 93% for patients who had obstruction at the level of the lacrimal sac or NLD. The success rates decreased to 88% and 54% with obstruction at the level of the common canaliculus or canaliculi, respectively. Civantos and colleagues [30] reported the successful performance of EDCR in individuals with a history of facial radiation therapy; they suggested that this procedure may be preferable to EXTDCR in this patient population.

Table 2
Results of primary endoscopic dacryocystorhinostomy

Investigators	Outcome measures	N	Success rate (%)	Comments
Tripathi et al, 2002 [32]	Sx	46	89	Success; local anesthesia
Tsirbas and Wormald, 2003 [25]	Sx, endoscopy	44	89	Lacrimal and nasal mucosal flaps
Massegur et al, 2004 [26]		96	93	Hammer-chisel, mucosal flaps
Fayet et al, 2004 [33]	Sx	300	87	
Durvasula & Gatland, 2004 [34]		70	92	
Wormald & Tsirbas, 2004 [28]	Sx, endoscopy	70	97	Success anatomic obstruction
Javate & Pamintuan, 2005 [21]	Sx, endoscopy	117	98	Radiofrequency, double stent, mitomycin C

Table 3
External versus endoscopic dacryocystorhinostomy

Investigators	EXTDCR N/Success	EDCR N/Success	Comments
Cokkeser et al, 2000 [35]	79; 90%	51; 88%	OR time EX/EN 65/33 min
Ibrahim et al, 2001 [36]	110; 82%	53; 58%	Symptomatic relief similar
Dolman, 2003 [37]	153; 92%	201; 93%	OR time EX/EN 34.3/18.5 min
Tsirbas et al, 2004 [38]	24; 96%	31; 94%	–
Ben Simon et al, 2005 [39]	90; 70%	86; 84%	–

Complications

The most common complication of EDCR in most series is failure of the procedure with persistence of tearing or infection. This may result from fibrous occlusion of the rhinostomy site or the presence of synechiae between the lateral nasal wall and middle turbinate or nasal septum. In other cases, the ostium may be patent but too small to provide efficient tear drainage. Failure to open the inferior portion of the lacrimal sac satisfactorily may result in continued accumulation of lacrimal debris (lacrimal sump syndrome). Similarly, persistent discharge or infection may develop in a lacrimal sac diverticulum that may not have been drained completely by way of the intranasal route. Other potential problems may include bleeding and sinusitis.

Successful outcomes in DCR surgery are predicated upon proper placement of an adequate rhinostomy with particular attention to the position of adjacent intranasal structures. Sufficient bone removal inferiorly to the level of the sac–duct junction, which corresponds to an axial line drawn anteriorly through the midpoint of the maxillary line along the lateral nasal wall [20], may mitigate the accumulation of debris within the sac. A thorough preoperative evaluation and meticulous surgical technique to avoid unnecessary mucosal trauma also are important.

Endoscopic revision dacryocystorhinostomy

Patient selection

Endoscopic revision DCR is indicated in patients in whom primary EXTDCR or EDCR has failed, and who meet the criteria for primary DCR. Although a revision EDCR may be attempted in patients who failed EXTDCR that was performed for lacrimal obstruction after trauma or in the setting of common canalicular stenosis, revision EXTDCR may be more successful in these particular settings.

Surgical technique

The technique of revision EDCR is similar to that described for primary DCR, with several important modifications.

Endoscopic evaluation

At the time of surgery, the nasal cavity is decongested and the lateral nasal wall and previous rhinostomy site are examined carefully endoscopically for potential structural issues that may have contributed to failure of the initial procedure. After local anesthesia is administered, the lacrimal puncta are dilated and a lacrimal probe is introduced through the superior canaliculus and passed into the area of the rhinostomy. In most cases, a fibrous membrane is noted to occlude the previously created channel. Gentle manipulation of the probe may allow determination of the extent of the previous opening, as well as identification of residual bone that requires removal. In revision cases, adequate space between the rhinostomy site and adjacent structures, most notably the middle turbinate and septum, must be assured.

Mucosal excision and bone removal

If it is determined that enlargement of the bony opening is required, the lateral nasal mucosa is incised, elevated, and removed widely with Blakesley forceps. The bony rhinostomy is enlarged with rongeurs or a high-speed drill. In the revision procedure, it is important to create a generous bony rhinostomy that extends from above the middle turbinate attachment to the level of the midpoint of the maxillary line inferiorly.

Soft tissue excision

Fibrous tissue that occludes the ostium is identified. This fibrous tissue is "tented" into the nasal cavity with probes that are passed through both canaliculi to provide a broad soft tissue region under tension. This is incised anterior to the probes using a sickle knife, which allows probe visualization. The edge of the incised mucosa is grasped with straight or angled Blakesley forceps and removed. Because scar tissue that occludes the ostium often is tough, removal may be facilitated by using several of the available through-cutting instruments.

In revision procedures, distinct anatomic structures, including nasal mucosa, the medial wall of the lacrimal sac, the lateral portion of the lacrimal sac that contains the internal common punctum, and orbital soft tissues adjacent to the lacrimal sac, often are incorporated into a zone of cicatrix that occludes the ostium. Because it is possible to injure the common canaliculus, medial canthal tendon, or orbital fat with vigorous avulsion of this cicatrix, the authors recommend that the surgeon closely observe the medial commissure while gentle traction is placed on the tissue to be removed at the rhinostomy site. Excessive movement of the medial commissure with this maneuver may signify that deeper tissues than desired are being grasped by the forceps.

Silicone intubation and mitomycin C application

After cicatrix excision, silicone intubation is performed as noted in the discussion of primary EDCR, and mitomycin C is applied if desired. As with primary EDCR, nasal packing is not required.

Endoscopically assisted conjunctivodacryocystorhinostomy

Patient selection

Conjunctivodacryocystorhinostomy (CDCR) is a procedure by which a fistula is created from the medial commissural conjunctiva into the nasal cavity. In most cases, a Pyrex glass tube (known as a Jones' tube) is placed within this fistula to reestablish lacrimal drainage. Indications for CDCR are summarized in Box 1.

Surgical technique

Anesthesia and nasal preparation

Anesthesia and nasal preparation are achieved as described earlier. If surgery is performed under monitored local anesthesia with intravenous sedation, additional local anesthesia, consisting of a 50% mixture each of 2% lidocaine with 1:200,000 epinephrine and 0.75% bupivacaine, is infiltrated using a 30-gauge needle that is placed beneath the caruncle after application of topical proparacaine.

Caruncular excision and conjunctival dissection

A self-retaining eyelid speculum is placed to provide exposure of the medial conjunctiva. The anterior half of the caruncle is excised through a curved 15-mm incision with a No. 15 Bard-Parker blade and sharp scissors (Fig. 8). The authors prefer to leave the posterior half of the caruncle in place to protect the medial bulbar conjunctiva from inflammation that is associated with contact with the Jones' tube orifice. The anterior edge of the incision is retracted with a fine double hook, and a malleable retractor is inserted to protect the globe lateral to the incision. The soft tissues that overlie the anterior lacrimal crest and lacrimal bone are spread gently with blunt dissection to reveal the underlying bone.

Box 1. Indications for conjunctivodacryocystorhinostomy

Canalicular agenesis
Canalicular obstruction
Common canalicular obstruction
Lacrimal pump dysfunction (eg, facial nerve paresis)

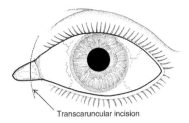

Transcaruncular incision

Fig. 8. A medial conjunctival incision is made that transects the caruncle.

Bone removal and catheter placement

A small Desmarres retractor and a malleable retractor are placed to protect the soft tissues that are located anterior, posterior, and lateral to the incision. A high-speed drill with a small cutting burr is used to remove a window of bone, approximately 8 mm in diameter and centered inferior to the location of the caruncle just posterior to the anterior lacrimal crest (Fig. 9). A 14-gauge intravenous catheter that contains an internal trocar is introduced at a 45° angle through this window, penetrating the nasal mucosa and entering the nasal cavity anterior to the middle turbinate (Fig. 10). This portion of the procedure is performed under careful endoscopic guidance. The catheter should be advanced until the end of the trocar is at least 2 mm from the lateral nasal wall but remains at least 2 mm from the nasal septum.

Jones' tube selection and placement

After satisfactory positioning of the catheter, the internal trocar is removed while the catheter is stabilized. The incision edges are allowed to return to their normal position. The catheter is grasped gently with a small hemostat just external to the conjunctival edges to allow determination of the length of the Jones' tube to be inserted. The authors prefer to use

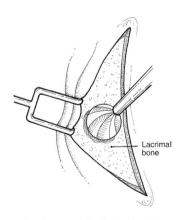

Lacrimal bone

Fig. 9. An opening is created in the lacrimal bone with a drill.

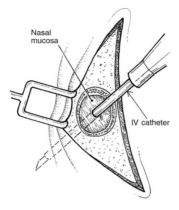

Fig. 10. A 14- to 16-gauge intravenous catheter is introduced at a 45° angle through the nasal mucosa after bone is removed using a high-speed drill.

a tube with a flange diameter of 4 mm, when possible, to maximize tear drainage, although smaller diameters are available. Other useful tube variants include angled tubes and tubes that contain a hole through which a retention suture may be passed. The soft tissue passage through which the Jones' tube is inserted may be dilated with serial placement of incrementally sized, gold-colored dilators that are included in the Jones' tube set, or with gentle spreading of the tissues using iris scissors. The goal is creation of a passage through which the tube may be inserted smoothly and without resistance. The preselected tube is placed over a lacrimal probe, which is passed through the soft tissue tract into the nasal cavity under endoscopic visualization (Fig. 11). The tube is advanced over the probe, while gentle

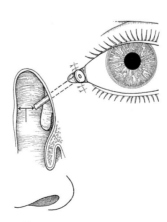

Fig. 11. A Jones' tube is inserted into the nasal cavity and secured in the medial commissure. The conjunctival incision is closed with multiple, interrupted, 6-0 plain gut sutures.

pressure is applied with a cotton-tipped applicator, until the distal end is visualized in the nose.

Jones' tube fixation, testing, and wound closure

The authors prefer to fix the Jones' tube by placing a slip-knot loop in the center of a double-armed 6-0 polyglycolic acid (Vicryl) suture that is placed around the proximal end of the tube. The tube is positioned with the proximal end just lateral to the edges of the conjunctival incision and the loop is tightened. One arm of the double-armed suture is passed from lateral to medial through the medial upper lid margin; the other arm is passed through the medial lower lid margin. The suture is tied at the medial commissure, which stabilizes the tube.

The position of the distal end of the tube is reassessed endoscopically. A fluorescein-containing saline solution, placed on the surface of the scleral shell, should drain freely through the tube into the middle meatus. The conjunctival incision is closed just medial to the end of the tube with interrupted, 6-0 plain gut suture.

Postoperatively, an oral antibiotic and a topical antibiotic–steroid eye drop are prescribed for 10 and 14 days, respectively. Nasal saline irrigation is recommended and patients are asked to refrain from vigorous nose-blowing for 6 weeks, after which they are instructed to close the operated eye and maintain gentle pressure over the Jones' tube in the medial commissure when blowing the nose or sneezing.

Results and complications

Although only limited data are available in the literature, operative time and blood loss have been reported to be slightly decreased in endoscopically assisted CDCR when compared with external CDCR [31]. Postoperative adjustment of tube size or position was required frequently in patients who underwent external or endoscopic surgery. The authors have noted that endoscopically assisted CDCR is associated with a higher primary success rate than are procedures that are not assisted endoscopically. This likely reflects the enhanced visualization of intranasal landmarks and confirmation of satisfactory tube placement that are afforded by endoscopy.

The most common complication that is associated with Jones' tube placement seems to be tube migration. Internal movement of the tube may result in closure of the conjunctiva over the tube orifice. External migration may result in conjunctival or corneal inflammation. Pyogenic granuloma formation that interferes with tear drainage may occur with the tube in the desired position or with temporal tube migration. Internal migration of the tube may cause nasoseptal irritation or epistaxis, as well as poor tube function. In many cases, tube repositioning or replacement may be performed in the office setting using topical anesthesia. Once again, visual confirmation of appropriate tube positioning is achieved using the endoscope.

References

[1] Caldwell GW. Two new operations for obstruction of the nasal duct, with preservation of the canaliculi. Am J Ophthalmol 1893;10:189–92.

[2] West JM. A window resection of the nasal duct in cases of stenosis. Trans Am Ophthalmol Soc 1914;12(12):654.

[3] Mosher HP. Re-establishing intranasal drainage of the lacrimal sac. Laryngoscope 1921;31: 492–521.

[4] Toti A. Nuovo metodod conservatore di cura radicale delle suppurazioni croniche del sacco lacrimale (dacriocistorhinostomia). Clin Moderna 1904;10(10):385–7.

[5] Dupuy-Dutemps L, Bouquet M. Procede plastique de dacryocystorhinostomie et ses resulats. Ann D'Oculist 1921;158:241–61.

[6] Benger R, Forer M. Endonasal dacryocystorhinostomy–primary and secondary. Aust N Z J Ophthalmol 1993;21(3):157–9.

[7] Camara JG, Santiago MD. Success rate of endoscopic laser-assisted dacryocystorhinostomy. Ophthalmology 1999;106(3):441–2.

[8] Metson R, Woog JJ, Puliafito CA. Endoscopic laser dacryocystorhinostomy. Laryngoscope 1994;104(3 Pt 1):269–74.

[9] Metson R. The endoscopic approach for revision dacryocystorhinostomy. Laryngoscope 1990;100(12):1344–7.

[10] Migliori ME. Endoscopic evaluation and management of the lacrimal sump syndrome. Ophthal Plast Reconstr Surg 1997;13(4):281–4.

[11] Puxeddu R, Nicolai P, Bielamowicz S, et al. Endoscopic revision of failed external dacryocystorhinostomy. Acta Otorhinolaryngol Ital 2000;20(1):1–5.

[12] Tutton MK, O'Donnell NP. Endonasal laser dacryocystorhinostomy under direct vision. Eye 1995;9(Pt 4):485–7.

[13] Yung MW, Hardman-Lea S. Endoscopic inferior dacryocystorhinostomy. Clin Otolaryngol Allied Sci 1998;23(2):152–7.

[14] Mortimore S, Banhegy GY, Lancaster JL, et al. Endoscopic dacryocystorhinostomy without silicone stenting. J R Coll Surg Edinb 1999;44(6):371–3.

[15] Dolman PJ. Presented at the American Society of Ophthalmic Plastic and Reconstructive Surgery. Anaheim, California, November 13, 2003.

[16] Metson R. Endoscopic surgery for lacrimal obstruction. Otolaryngol Head Neck Surg 1991; 104(4):473–9.

[17] Rice DH. Endoscopic intranasal dacryocystorhinostomy results in four patients. Arch Otolaryngol Head Neck Surg 1990;116(9):1061.

[18] Sadiq SA, Hugkulstone CE, Jones NS, et al. Endoscopic holmium: YAG laser dacryocystorhinostomy. Eye 1996;10(Pt 1):43–6.

[19] Wormald PJ, Kew J, Van Hasselt A. Intranasal anatomy of the nasolacrimal sac in endoscopic dacryocystorhinostomy. Otolaryngol Head Neck Surg 2000;123(3):307–10.

[20] Chastain JB, Cooper MH, Sindwani R. The maxillary line: anatomic characterization and clinical utility of an important surgical landmark. Laryngoscope 2005;115(6):990–2.

[21] Javate R, Pamintuan F. Endoscopic radiofrequency-assisted dacryocystorhinostomy with double stent: a personal experience. Orbit 2005;24(1):15–22.

[22] Cokkeser Y, Evereklioglu C, Tercan M, et al. Hammer-chisel technique in endoscopic dacryocystorhinostomy. Ann Otol Rhinol Laryngol 2003;112(5):444–9.

[23] Ibrahim HA, Noble JL, Batterbury M, et al. Endoscopic-guided trephination dacryocystorhinostomy (Hesham DCR): technique and pilot trial. Ophthalmology 2001;108(12): 2337–45 [discussion 2345–6].

[24] Wormald PJ. Powered endoscopic dacryocystorhinostomy. Laryngoscope 2002;112(1): 69–72.

[25] Tsirbas A, Wormald PJ. Endonasal dacryocystorhinostomy with mucosal flaps. Am J Ophthalmol 2003;135(1):76–83.

[26] Massegur H, Trias E, Adema JM. Endoscopic dacryocystorhinostomy: modified technique. Otolaryngol Head Neck Surg 2004;130(1):39–46.

[27] Onerci M, Orhan M, Ogretmenoglu O, et al. Long-term results and reasons for failure of intranasal endoscopic dacryocystorhinostomy. Acta Otolaryngol 2000;120(2):319–22.

[28] Wormald PJ, Tsirbas A. Investigation and endoscopic treatment for functional and anatomical obstruction of the nasolacrimal duct system. Clin Otolaryngol Allied Sci 2004;29(4): 352–6.

[29] Yung MW, Hardman-Lea S. Analysis of the results of surgical endoscopic dacryocystorhinostomy: effect of the level of obstruction. Br J Ophthalmol 2002;86(7):792–4.

[30] Civantos FJ Jr, Yoskovitch A, Casiano RR. Endoscopic sinus surgery in previously irradiated patients. Am J Otolaryngol 2001;22(2):100–6.

[31] Trotter WL, Meyer DR. Endoscopic conjunctivodacryocystorhinostomy with Jones tube placement. Ophthalmology 2000;107(6):1206–9.

[32] Tripathi A, Lesser TH, O'Donnell NP, et al. Local anaesthetic endonasal endoscopic laser dacryocystorhinostomy: analysis of patients' acceptability and various factors affecting the success of this procedure. Eye 2002;16(2):146–9.

[33] Fayet B, Racey E, Assouline M. Complications of standardized endonasal dacryocystorhinostomy without unciformectomy. Ophthalmology 2004;111(4):837–45.

[34] Durvasula VS, Gatland DJ. Endoscopic dacrocystorhinostomy: long-term results and evolution of surgical technique. J Laryngol Otol 2004;118(8):628–32.

[35] Cokkeser Y, Evereklioglu C, Er H. Comparative external versus endoscopic dacryocystorhinostomy: results in 115 patients (130 eyes). Otolaryngol Head Neck Surg 2000;123(4): 488–91.

[36] Ibrahim HA, Batterbury M, Banhegyi G, et al. Endonasal laser dacryocystorhinostomy and external dacryocystorhinostomy outcome profile in a general ophthalmic service unit: a comparative retrospective study. Ophthalmic Surg Lasers 2001;32(3):220–7.

[37] Dolman PJ. Comparison of external dacryocystorhinostomy with nonlaser endonasal dacryocystorhinostomy. Ophthalmology 2003;110(1):78–84.

[38] Tsirbas A, Davis G, Wormald PJ. Mechanical endonasal dacryocystorhinostomy versus external dacryocystorhinostomy. Ophthal Plast Reconstr Surg 2004;20(1):50–6.

[39] Ben Simon GJ, Joseph J, Lee S, et al. External versus endoscopic dacryocystorhinostomy for acquired nasolacrimal duct obstruction in a tertiary referral center. Ophthalmology 2005; 112(8):1463–8.

ELSEVIER
SAUNDERS

Otolaryngol Clin N Am
39 (2006) 1019–1036

OTOLARYNGOLOGIC
CLINICS
OF NORTH AMERICA

Mechanical Endonasal Dacryocystorhinostomy with Mucosal Flaps

Angelo Tsirbas, MD[a],*, Peter John Wormald, MD[b]

[a]Department of Orbital and Ophthalmic Surgery, Jules Stein Eye Institute,
David Geffen School of Medicine at the University of California at Los Angeles,
100 Stein Plaza, Los Angeles, CA 90095, USA
[b]Department of Otolaryngology, 28 Woodville Road, Woodville, SA 5011, Australia

Initial surgical approaches to treating nasolacrimal duct obstruction (NLDO) were intranasal [1]. These attempts were made at the end of the nineteenth century but were abandoned because surgeons had difficulty visualizing the surgical site. In the twentieth century, external dacryocystorhinostomy (DCR) was described, and with a few modifications it has been the treatment most commonly used for the last 100 years [2–5]. In the 1980s the advent of endoscopic techniques revolutionized rhinologic procedures as precise mucosa-preserving surgical techniques were introduced with the aim of restoring nasal and sinus function. Since the first endoscopic DCR procedures in the late 1980s and early 1990s [6–8] there has been further improvement in instruments and endoscopes. In addition, the development of medical lasers also has allowed this technology to be used for lacrimal surgery.

The long-term success rate of external DCR in dedicated oculoplastic surgical centers is very high (90%–95%) [9–12]. These success rates have been replicated many times in centers around the globe. Until recently, the success rate of endonasal DCR had not matched that achieved with external DCR. As with any new surgical technique, however, endoscopic DCR has been modified and improved [13–17]. The authors believe that the key to

---

Portions of this article are reprinted from: Tsirbas A, Wormald PJ. Mechanical Endonasal Dacryocystorhinostomy. In: John J. Woog, Ed. Manual of Endoscopic Lacrimal and Orbital Surgery. Philadelphia: Butterworth/Heineman, 2004; with permission.

* Corresponding author. Jules Stein Eye Institute, David Geffen School of Medicine at the University of California at Los Angeles, 100 Stein Plaza, Box 957006, Room 2-267, Los Angeles, CA 90095.
E-mail address: angelotsirbas@hotmail.com (A. Tsirbas).

0030-6665/06/$ - see front matter © 2006 Elsevier Inc. All rights reserved.
doi:10.1016/j.otc.2006.07.007

oto.theclinics.com

improving the success rate of endonasal DCR is to attempt to replicate the external procedure as closely as possible. As such, the creation of a large bony rhinostomy and mucosal flaps is the key tenet of this mechanical endonasal DCR (MENDCR) procedure [18,19]. To achieve complete lacrimal sac exposure and correct siting of the rhinostomy, an understanding of the nasal anatomy and its relationship to the lacrimal sac is vital [20–23]. Research into the intranasal anatomy of the lacrimal sac has shown that the rhinostomy needs to be larger and higher on the lateral wall than previously thought [20,22]. To expose the lacrimal sac fully, a large rhinostomy is created. Creating this large rhinostomy requires removal of bone from the frontal process of the maxilla anterior to the middle turbinate, the lacrimal bone, as well as the bone above the insertion of the middle turbinate into the lateral nasal wall (the so-called "axilla" of the middle turbinate). This rhinostomy includes the agger nasi cell and extends posteriorly to the insertion of the uncinate, exposing the whole lacrimal sac. The size of this rhinostomy is similar to that created in external DCR. Another key factor in the MENDCR procedure is mucosal preservation. Previously described endonasal approaches involved the removal of both nasal mucosa and the mucosa of the medial lacrimal sac. MENDCR involves the conservation of nasal mucosa and the fashioning of lacrimal sac flaps to achieve mucosal apposition of the marsupialized sac and nasal mucosa. Experience in endoscopic nasal surgery is important to the success of this procedure, because the amount of bone removal and intranasal manipulation is greater than in most other endoscopic DCR techniques. Once expertise is gained, MENDCR can be used as a reproducible and successful way to treat NLDO.

Assessment before mechanical endonasal dacryocystorhinostomy

The preoperative assessment of patients who have epiphora is vital to the planning of a solution. In most cases seen in the clinic with a complaint of epiphora, the problem does not lie in a blockage in the nasolacrimal system. The balance of tear production and drainage is vital, especially in the older patient. In this article discussion is limited to patients in whom an assessment has revealed an obstruction to nasolacrimal drainage. It is important to be able to assess the level of obstruction of the nasolacrimal duct system and, if patent, to assess the function of the system. The authors' protocol, therefore, includes both a dacryocystogram (DCG) and lacrimal scintillography. The DCG allows anatomic assessment of the canaliculi, sac, and nasolacrimal duct, whereas scintillography allows functional assessment of the lacrimal pump and provides additional information on the level of functional obstruction of the nasolacrimal duct system if the system is anatomically patent. Part of the authors' protocol for preoperative assessment includes nasal endoscopy with a rigid nasal endoscope. This procedure allows septal deviation to be detected and any additional nasal or sinus pathologic conditions to be evaluated. If additional nasal or sinus abnormalities are present, other investigations, including a CT scan of the sinuses, may be performed. If indicated, sinus surgery may be performed at the same time as the MENDCR. Concomitant sinus surgery decreases intranasal inflammation and adhesions in the postoperative period and may improve nasal healing and the likelihood of success with endoscopic DCR. In addition, nasal endoscopy may allow other rare causes of epiphora (eg, intranasal tumor) to be identified. In revision DCR, the site of the previous surgical ostium can be evaluated endoscopically, and scarring, adhesions, or a septal deflection that may have contributed to the failure of the initial surgery may be identified. Observing the flow of fluorescein from the conjunctiva into the nose can identify sump formation in an incompletely marsupialized lacrimal sac.

Preparation for mechanical endonasal dacryocystorhinostomy

Instrumentation

Endoscopes and camera
Zero-degree and 30° endoscopes are required. An irrigating sleeve ("scope scrubber" to keep the end of the scope clear of blood) is a useful adjunctive tool that obviates the need for repeated removal of the scope from the nose for cleaning during surgery. A high-quality three-chip camera and video monitor provide excellent visualization even if the surgical field becomes bloody.

Endoscopic sinus surgery instrumentation
The standard equipment used in endoscopic sinus surgery should be available. The nasal flap can be cut using a scalpel or a sharp sickle knife. A suction Freer elevator (Martin, Tutltingen, Germany) helps lift the mucosal flap while keeping the surgical field free of blood. A forward-biting, 3- or 4-mm Hajek Koffler punch (Karl Storz, Tuttlingen, Germany) is used to remove bone. An angulation of 45° upwards on the punch can help remove bone anterosuperiorly in the ostium. The round knife (Karl Storz) and Bellucci scissors (Karl Storz) included in standard major ear trays are also used.

Powered microdebrider
A powered microdebrider with an angled (25°) rough diamond burr (2.7 mm) (Medtronic Xomed, Jacksonville, FL) should be included among the instruments. Cutting burrs can be used, but they tend to create damage and may even make a hole in the lacrimal sac if the burr contacts the sac. The microdebrider should have irrigation and suction on the burr.

Lacrimal sac instruments
Small instruments have been designed specifically to open the lacrimal sac. The spear and mini–right-angled sickle knives (Medtronic Xomed) are

used to open the sac. Bellucci scissors are used to cut the posterior flap. The mucosal flap is trimmed to size using a pediatric Blakesley through-biting (cutting) forceps (Medtronic Xomed). To keep this instrument sharp, it should be used only on the soft tissue in the nose, and it should be kept separate from the standard endoscopic sinus surgery instruments.

Intubation instrumentation

Lacrimal intubation can be undertaken with any of the commercially available silicone tubing sets. The spacer is a 4-mm, soft Silastic tube cut to a length of 8 to 10 mm. Ligar clips (Ethicon, Cincinnati, OH) are used to secure the tubes.

Positioning for surgery

The surgeon, patient's head, and monitor should be in a straight line (Fig. 1). A slim arm board is attached to the operating table to allow the surgeon to rest the elbow of the arm comfortably while holding the scope. The endoscope should always be held above any instrument in the nose, and the scope and instrument should never cross in the nasal cavity. The patient is placed in a 30°, head-up (reverse Trendelenberg's) position. Although surgery may be performed using local anesthesia, depending on the patient's and surgeon's preference, general anesthesia may be preferable.

Surgical team

At the authors' institution, the surgical team consists of an experienced endoscopic sinus surgeon (otolaryngologist) and an oculoplastic surgeon. Great benefit has been derived from having both surgeons present at lacrimal operations, because their skills are complementary. Although both surgeons are fully capable of performing all parts of the surgery, the sinus surgeon is able to deal with other intranasal and septal pathologic

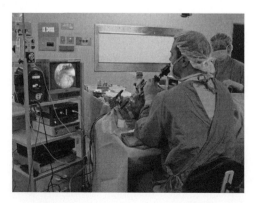

Fig. 1. Operating room setup for mechanical endonasal DCR.

conditions, and the oculoplastic surgeon has experience dealing with lid laxity, ectropion, entropion, and punctal and canalicular problems.

Intranasal anatomy of the lacrimal sac

Most early publications on endoscopic DCR described the lacrimal sac as a structure anterior to the middle turbinate on the lateral nasal wall [6,24–28] (Fig. 2). These early diagrams, which have been reprinted in most subsequent articles and texts, show the superior extent of the lacrimal sac as reaching just above the insertion of the middle turbinate on the lateral nasal wall, the so-called axilla of the middle turbinate. A recent study by Wormald and colleagues [21], using CT scans and DCGs, showed that the sac extends a significant distance (average of 8 mm) above the axilla of the middle turbinate.

If the bone anterior to the middle turbinate is removed, only the lower half of the sac will be exposed, and marsupialization of the sac is not possible (see Fig. 2). Therefore, an understanding of the anatomy is vital to a surgeon wishing to expose the entire sac with minimal loss of adjacent nasal mucosa, because that anatomic understanding allows the correct placement of the initial nasal mucosal incisions. Once all underlying bone is removed, the entire sac can be seen, and the sac marsupialized onto the lateral nasal wall with minimal bare bone remaining. This technique allows first-intention healing with minimal formation of granulation tissue and less scarring.

Surgical technique

The DCR procedure has been described previously [18,19]. It can be performed using either local or general anesthesia. Usually, if the surgery

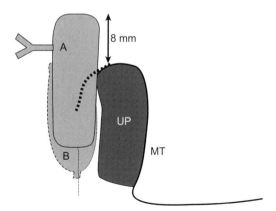

Fig. 2. Lacrimal sac position on the lateral nasal wall. The double-ended arrow indicates that the sac extends about 8 mm above the axilla (insertion of the middle turbinate on the lateral nasal wall) [21]. A, lacrimal sac position; B, previously described lacrimal sac position; MT, middle turbinate; UP, uncinate process.

is bilateral or if there is a major septal deviation that needs to be addressed, general anesthesia is preferred. General anesthesia is especially preferable for elderly patients, because it is difficult for them to lie still for more than an hour.

The nasal cavity is decongested using a mixture of 2 mL of 10% cocaine (in an adult), 1 mL of 1:1000 epinephrine, and 3 mL of saline . This solution is divided; half is kept on the sterile tray in case further decongestion or hemostasis is needed during surgery, and half is applied to six neurosurgical patties that are placed in the middle meatus, above the middle turbinate, and anterior to the middle turbinate. A solution consisting of 2 mL of 2% lidocaine and 1:80,000 Adrenalin (Astra Pharmaceuticals, Sydney, Australia) is infiltrated locally above and anterior to the middle turbinate. Any significant septal deviation is addressed before proceeding with any further surgery. In a recent modification to this technique the local anesthetic injection is given, and then the nose is packed. This packing helps compress any swelling of the mucosa caused by the injection of local anesthetic.

Step 1: mucosal incision

The mucosal incisions are made with a #15 scalpel blade. The superior incision is made 8 mm above the insertion of the middle turbinate on the lateral nasal wall (axilla). The incision is brought 8 mm anterior to the axilla of the middle turbinate and then run vertically down the frontal process of the maxilla about two thirds of the anterior length of the middle turbinate. It then is taken posterior to the insertion of the uncinate under the anterior edge of the middle turbinate (Fig. 3), creating a mucosal trapdoor hinged on a posterior base.

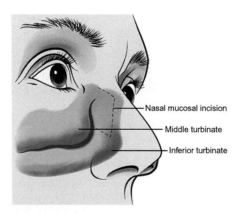

Fig. 3. Site of nasal mucosal incision on lateral nasal wall.

Step 2: flap elevation

A suction Freer elevator (Martin) is used to elevate the flap, keeping the tip of the instrument on the bone. This procedure is done along a broad base, and the flap is cleared of the surgical field by reflecting it over the head of the middle turbinate. Along the lower half of the flap, the soft lacrimal bone will be visible before the insertion of the uncinate (Fig. 4). The authors have found that there is always about 3 to 4 mm of thin lacrimal bone overlying the posteroinferior portion of the sac before the uncinate takes origin. This finding is contrary to the descriptions provided previously by other authors [29]. The flap also is raised above the axilla of the middle turbinate.

Step 3: bone removal with punch

The soft lacrimal bone is removed with a round knife from the ear instrument tray. A forward-biting, 3- or 4-mm Hajek Koffler punch (Karl Storz) is used to remove the frontal process of the maxilla anterior to the

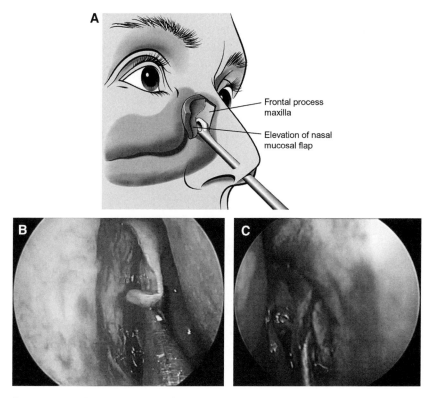

Fig. 4. (*A*) Elevation of the mucosal flap. (*B*) Endoscopic view of the flap elevation (right side). (*C*) Endoscopic view of the maxilla–lacrimal bone junction (left side).

soft lacrimal bone. This procedure exposes the lower half of the lacrimal sac (Fig. 5). If there is any doubt about the position of the lacrimal bone and frontal process of the maxilla, a DCR light pipe (Medtronic Xomed) or a 20-gauge vitreoretinal illuminator is introduced into the sac, and the sac is transilluminated. As the bone of the frontal process is removed superiorly, it gets thicker, and the punch cannot widen sufficiently to gain purchase on the bone.

Step 4: microdebriding

A 2.7-mm, 25°, curved, rough, diamond DCR burr (Medtronic Xomed) is used to continue bone removal upward to the superior mucosal incision (Fig. 6). As the bone above the axilla is removed, the agger nasi cell is exposed, and its mucosal lining is visualized. The agger nasi cell is a good guide to the fundus of the sac. In a very small percentage of patients, there is no agger nasi cell; in these patients, the bone above the axilla is thicker because of the absence of this cell. Bone removal is continued up to the original mucosal incisions. Bone is removed directly adjacent to the sac until the sac is entirely separate from the lateral nasal wall. The bony ostium should measure at least 15–20 mm. Thus, when the sac is opened, it is marsupialized and forms part of the lateral nasal wall. The ability to place the diamond burr in contact with the sac without damaging the sac wall helps facilitate complete bone removal from around the sac.

Step 5: cutting and marsupialization of the lacrimal sac

The inferior punctum is dilated, a Bowman's lacrimal probe (Visitec, Warwickshire, UK) or DCR light pipe is placed inside the lacrimal sac, and the medial wall of the sac is tented (Fig. 7). A specially designed DCR spear knife (Medtronic Xomed) is used to incise the sac vertically, as far posteriorly as possible, to create the largest possible, anteriorly based

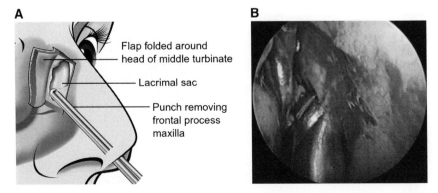

A

Flap folded around
head of middle turbinate

Lacrimal sac

Punch removing
frontal process
maxilla

B

Fig. 5. (*A*) Removal of the frontal process of the maxilla. (*B*) Endoscopic view of bone removal with punch.

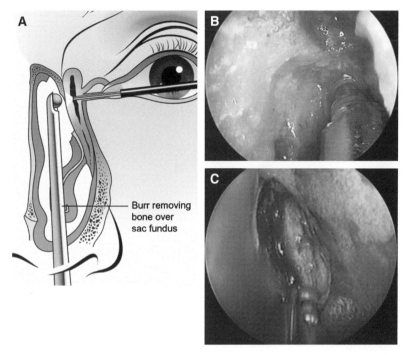

Fig. 6. (*A*) Removal of bone at the root of the middle turbinate to expose sac fundus. (*B*) Endoscopic view of the microdebrider at the middle turbinate root (right side). (*C*) Endoscopic view of the removal of the edges of the frontal process of the maxilla (left side).

flap. Just as effectively, a small-angled keratome such as that used in cataract surgery can be used to make this incision. The DCR mini-right-angled sickle knife (Medtronic Xomed) is used to cut horizontal releasing incisions in the anterior-based flap, and the flap is rolled out. Bellucci scissors (Karl Storz) are used to release the posterior flap (Fig. 8). The common

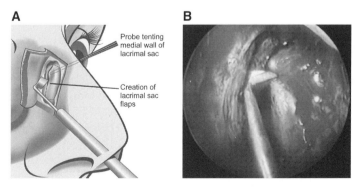

Fig. 7. (*A*) Vertical incision of the lacrimal sac to create anterior and posterior flaps. (*B*) Endoscopic view of sac incision.

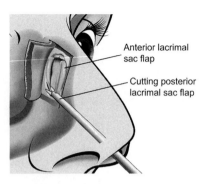

Fig. 8. Horizontal cuts are made to form the posterior sac flap.

canaliculus opening should be clearly visible in the lateral wall of the sac. If this is not the case, insufficient bone was removed above the axilla of the middle turbinate. The amount of raw bone superior, anterior, and inferior to the opened sac is estimated before the original mucosal flap is re-draped over the opened lacrimal sac. Usually, the raw bone superior to the opened sac measures approximately 3 mm. It is very important that the common canalicular opening is clear of any bone.

Step 6: nasal mucosal flaps

A pediatric, sharp, through-cutting Blakesley forceps (Medtronic Xomed) is used to trim the center of the original mucosal flap, leaving an appropriately sized upper limb of mucosa to cover the raw bone above and below the sac (Fig. 9). The flap is trimmed back until the posterior edge of the lacrimal sac and nasal mucosa are also in apposition. This trimming creates a C-shaped flap, the base of which is positioned posteriorly. Initially scoring these flaps at the start of the procedure may help in trimming. The mucosa of the agger nasi cell is incised and also is apposed to the posterosuperior edge of the lacrimal sac. In this way, mucosal apposition between the nasal and lacrimal mucosa is ensured.

Step 7: intubation

O'Donohue silicone lacrimal intubation tubes (Visitec) are placed, and a Silastic sleeve measuring 4 to 10 mm in length is slipped over the tubes and is advanced into the opened sac. An appropriate loop of Silastic tubing is pulled into the medial canthal region of the eye, and Ligar clips (Ethicon) are then placed below the Silastic tubing (Fig. 10A). Placing the clips ensures that there is no tension on the loop of the lacrimal tubes in the medial canthal region and reduces any risk of cheese wiring of the tubes through the puncta. The Silastic tubes are covered with Gelfoam (Pharmacia, Sydney, New SouthWales, Australia or Merocel (Medtronic Xomed), and the tubes are cut. The Gelfoam or Merocel is repositioned over the flaps after ensuring

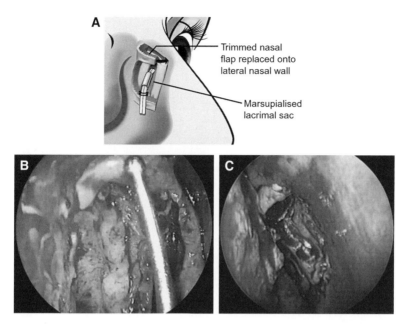

Fig. 9. (*A*) Formation of nasal mucosal flaps. (*B*) Superior and posterior nasal mucosal flaps are in place (right side). (*C*) Nasal mucosal flaps are in place around the open sac (left side).

that the flaps are rolled out and correctly positioned (Fig. 10B) to hold the flaps in place during the initial healing phase. A later modification has been incorporated in which the Gelfoam is soaked in triamcinolone, 50 mg per mL, before being placed. All patients receive broad-spectrum antibiotic therapy for 5 days and antibiotic eye drops for 2 weeks. Saline nasal spray is administered immediately after surgery and for 4 weeks postoperatively to aid in blood clot removal from the nasal cavity.

Complications

The major complications that can arise with MENDCR are the result of the surgeon's getting lost during the dissection and dissecting too far posteriorly, causing damage to the maxillary sinus drainage or frontal sinus drainage. Entry into the orbit also can occur posteriorly, resulting in orbital fat extrusion and possible injury to the ocular muscles [29]. In children, inappropriate superior dissection can potentially cause injury to the skull base with subsequent leakage of cerebrospinal fluid. The risk of such an injury in adults is very small. The other major complication is postoperative hemorrhage, which may require nasal packing and even hospitalization. In the authors' series of 163 consecutive patients, 3 patients experienced postoperative hemorrhage. All were treated successfully with nasal packing, and none required transfusion or hospitalization. This series thus had

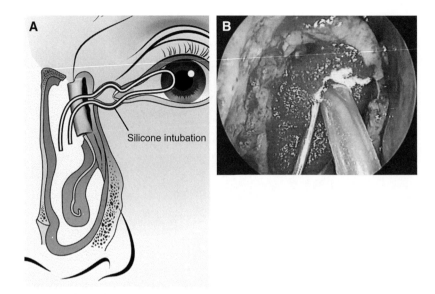

Fig. 10. (*A*) Intubated, marsupialized lacrimal sac. (*B*) A Gelfoam pack is in place with tubes.

a complication rate of less than 2%, which compares well both with previous endonasal studies [31] and with external DCR studies [31,32]. There were no cases of orbital fat exposure or frontal or maxillary sinusitis in this series. Because there is no dissection posterior to the sac with this technique, the risk is small. There is no need to perform an uncinectomy routinely to expose the lacrimal sac.

Results

The authors have undertaken a prospective interventional case series over the last 5 years. Follow-up periods range from 12 months to 4 years with a mean of 28 months. When examining the success rates of new endonasal procedures, it is important to set a definition for success. In the past, success has been determined either by postoperative anatomic patency of the naso-lacrimal duct system or by relief of epiphora [32–36]. The authors believe that both of these criteria should be met before surgery is declared success-ful. In their prospective case series, the authors use a definition that combines anatomic patency of the nasolacrimal duct system with total relief of symptoms. In the series, anatomic patency is assessed by placing a drop of fluorescein into the conjunctival sac and then endoscopically assessing flow of the fluorescein into the nasal cavity through the opened lacrimal sac. This procedure allows evaluation of both function [37] and patency of the lacrimal system as well as the morphology of the marsupialized lacrimal sac (Figs. 11 and 12) [38]. Patients' symptoms are assessed as being no better, somewhat better, or completely relieved. Only patients who are

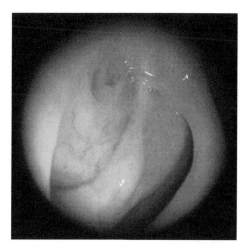

Fig. 11. The lacrimal sac is marsupialized into the lateral nasal wall.

asymptomatic (ie, whose symptoms have been relieved completely) are classified as having a successful surgical outcome. Patients are classified, according to the results of their preoperative assessment, into three groups: those undergoing (1) primary DCR, in whom the obstruction of the nasolacrimal duct is either anatomic or functional, (2) revision DCR (performed for anatomic obstruction), and (3) pediatric DCR, either primary or revision cases (performed for anatomic obstruction).

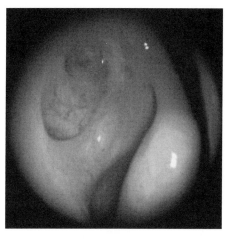

Fig. 12. Fluorescein drainage into the nose.

Primary dacryocystorhinostomy
(anatomic and functional nasolacrimal duct obstruction)

These patients had not undergone previous lacrimal surgery. From January 1999 to December 2001, 128 consecutive MENDCRs were performed. All patients had a minimum follow-up time of 12 months. A successful outcome (both anatomic and symptomatic) was reported in 115 cases (90%) (Table 1). In six cases there was a patent, well-marsupialized ostium with free fluorescein drainage, but the patient complained of some symptoms. The anatomic success rate, therefore, was 96% (121 cases). In 4% of cases, a scarred ostium was noted postoperatively, usually within the first 3 months. These patients were then classified according to their clinical findings and preoperative DCG and scintillography results as having either anatomic or functional NLDO. The success rate in patients who had confirmed anatomic obstruction was 95%, whereas the success rate in those who had functional NLDO was 81%. In this latter group, there was a 95% anatomic patency, but a number of patients still reported symptoms. This experience demonstrates that success in patients who have functional NLDO is not as high as in those who have anatomic NLDO, even though most of the so-called "failures" had an anatomically patent lacrimal ostium with free flow of fluorescein from the conjunctiva to the nose. Thus, from a symptomatic perspective, the prognosis is not as good in those who have functional NLDO as it is in patients who have anatomic NLDO. It is important to remember this discrepancy in outcome when counseling patients who have functional NLDO. In the authors' series, all patients who had functional NLDO who had anatomically patent lacrimal systems postoperatively considered themselves significantly improved as compared with their preoperative status. The anatomic success rate of MENDCR in the authors' series, then, is similar to the success rate of external DCR performed in other centers around the world [9,20,32,39]. An initial pilot study was conducted in which patients undergoing MENDCR were compared with a concurrent group of patients undergoing external DCR. This study showed similar success rates for the two groups at 3 years' follow-up [19].

Table 1
Results for primary, revision, and pediatric mechanical endonasal dacryocystorhinostomy

Result	Primary DCR (n = 128)	Revision DCR (n = 19)	Pediatric DCR (n = 16)
Total success	115 (90%)	13 (68%)	14 (88%)
Anatomic success (patent naso-lacrimal system)	121 (94.5%)	14 (74%)	14 (88%)
Failure	13	6	2
Anatomic	7	5	2
Functional	6	1	0
Septoplasty	60 (47%)	2 (11%)	1 (6%)

Abbreviation: DCR, dacryocystorhinostomy.

Septoplasty was required in approximately 46% of MENDCR cases. This rate is higher than seen with either external DCR [9] or other endonasal approaches [10,27,35,40]. The authors have a relatively low threshold for performing septoplasty, because adequate access to the lateral nasal wall is necessary if an appropriately sited large rhinostomy with mucosal flaps is to be achieved. Often with greater surgical experience the need for adjunctive septoplasty decreases. The exposure of the agger nasi cell also requires removal of part of the middle turbinate root; again, this removal is not necessary in other approaches that do not fully expose the lacrimal sac [10,30,33]. The ability to perform other intranasal surgery emphasizes the need for the team approach to these patients, with both an otolaryngologist and ophthalmologist being present. The requirement for accessory intranasal surgery can be assessed preoperatively in the clinic and the team assembled accordingly.

Revision dacryocystorhinostomy

With MENDCR, it is possible to remove bone at reoperation rather than simply opening the mucosa. The procedure is performed in exactly the same manner as the primary MENDCR. The frontal process of the maxilla is used as a guide. The incision should be brought forward until the hard bone of the frontal process can be felt under the scalpel. The suction Freer elevator is used to lift the mucosal flap off the bone, creating the correct surgical plane. As the scar tissue is encountered in the region of the previous osteotomy, a scalpel is used to stay in the plane created by the previous elevation of the flap. This technique allows the nasal mucosa to be separated from the underlying scarred sac. The bony ostium then is enlarged to the size of the mucosal incision with complete exposure of the sac. The operation proceeds as previously described.

The success rate (anatomic and symptomatic) in the authors' series of 19 revision MENDCRs was 74%. This success rate increased to 89% with a second operation. The MENDCR approach also allows treatment of very difficult cases in which no lacrimal sac mucosa remains after multiple previous surgeries. In one patient in this series who had undergone four previous DCRs, the agger nasi cell mucosa was removed and placed over the common canaliculus opening as a free mucosal autograft. Eighteen months after surgery, this patient remained asymptomatic, with an anatomically patent nasolacrimal duct system.

Pediatric dacryocystorhinostomy

The different anatomy of the middle meatus and nasal passages is an important factor to consider when performing MENDCR in children. In children, the turbinates and sinuses are less developed, and the superior meatus is small, so the anterior cranial fossa is in relatively close proximity to the axilla of the middle turbinate. The nasal cavity and nasal vestibule are much smaller than in the adult, making the procedure more difficult. Septal surgery is avoided in children, because it may affect future growth and appearance of the nose. The authors have performed 18 MENDCR procedures in children younger than age 10 years with a success rate (symptomatic and anatomic) of 88%. This rate is similar to the success rate reported for external DCR surgery [41–44] and other endoscopic surgical techniques [45–48] in children of this age group. Endonasal surgery, however, has the benefit of avoiding a facial incision, with preservation of the orbicularis oculi muscle and medial canthal tendon. This preservation may influence the function of the lacrimal pump in later life.

Learning curve in mechanical endonasal dacryocystorhinostomy

The authors believe that it is helpful to assemble a collaborative team of surgeons skilled in oculoplastic and ear, nose, and throat surgery before performing MENDCR. Such collaboration helps with the learning curve for surgeons unfamiliar with performing endoscopic surgery using a video monitor. The authors' initial 40 cases showed a success rate of 89%, which is similar to the overall success rate of their series (90%) [19]. The ability to manage associated nasal problems (deviated septum and sinus disease), both intraoperatively as well as in the clinic, is important, and the patient gains from skills offered by the surgical team. Removal of adhesions and granulations at postoperative visits can help decrease any fibrotic response in the nose and increases the success of endonasal approaches.

Summary: key points for mechanical endonasal dacryocystorhinostomy with mucosal flaps

The key to the success of the MENDCR procedure is to remove sufficient bone intranasally to expose the lacrimal sac completely [18,19]. The proven techniques of external DCR can be duplicated by the MENDCR approach. The lacrimal sac is fully exposed and marsupialized into the lateral nasal wall of the nose with nasal mucosa and lacrimal mucosa apposition [18,19]. This technique allows first-intention healing, rather than the formation of granulation tissue, to occur and lessens the risk of closure of the sac opening into the nose. The MENDCR approach also allows preservation of the lacrimal pump. No disruption of the orbicularis oculi muscle or medial canthal tendon occurs, resulting in preservation of the lacrimal pump action [10,37]. This advantage may be important for treating patients who have functional NLDO, although further research into this aspect is required.

Postoperative endoscopic assessment of the patient allows confirmation of anatomic patency by direct assessment of the lacrimal sac and drainage of fluorescein from the conjunctiva to the nose. It also allows the removal of granulations from the sac and may thus improve the success rate of the procedure.

Finally, the authors recommend that revision and pediatric MENDCR procedures be performed only by surgeons who have experience with adult primary MENDCR.

References

[1] Caldwell GW. Two new operations for obstruction of the nasal duct, with preservation of the canaliculi, and with an incidental description of a new lacrimal probe. Am J Ophthalmol 1893;10:189–93.

[2] Toti A. Nuovo metodo conservatore dicura radicale delle suppurazione croniche del sacco lacrimale (dacricistorhinostomia). Clin Mod (Firenza) 1904;10:385.

[3] Von Goethe JW. Aus meinem Leben. Dichtung and Wahrheit. Z. Theil. sechsles Buch. Goethe's stimtliche Werke, Bd. 22. P. Leipzig (Germany): Reclam jun; 1926. p. 136.

[4] Dupuy-Dutemp L, Bouguet M. Note preliminaire sur en procede de dacryocystorhinosto-mie. Ann Ocul (Paris) 1921;158:241.

[5] Jones LT. The cure of epiphora due to canalicular disorders, trauma and surgical failures on the lacrimal passages. Trans Am Acad Ophthalmol Otolaryngol 1962;66:506–10.

[6] McDonogh M, Meiring JH. Endoscopic transnasal dacryocystorhinostomy. J Laryngol Otol 1989;103:585–7.

[7] Massaro BM, Gonnering RS, Harris GJ. Endonasal laser dacryocystorhinostomy. A new approach to nasolacrimal duct obstruction. Arch Ophthalmol 1990;108:1172–86.

[8] Gonnering RS, Lyon DB, Fisher JC. Endoscopic laser-assisted lacrimal surgery. Am J Ophthalmol 1991;111:152–7.

[9] Tarbet KJ, Custer PL. External dacryocystorhinostomy. Surgical success, patient satisfaction and economic cost. Ophthalmology 1995;102:1065–70.

[10] Hartikainen J, Jukka A, Matti V, et al. Prospective randomised comparison of endonasal endoscopic dacryocystorhinostomy and external dacryocystorhinostomy. Laryngoscope 1998;108(12):1861–6.

[11] Ibrahim HA, Batterbury M, Banhegyi G, et al. Endonasal laser dacryocystorhinostomy and external dacryocystorhinostomy outcome profile in a general ophthalmic service unit: a comparative retrospective study. Ophthalmic Surg Lasers 2001;32(3):220–7.

[12] Hurwitz JJ, Merkur S, DeAngelis D. Outcome of lacrimal surgery in older patients. Can J Ophthalmol 2000;35(1):18–22.

[13] Bakri SJ, Carney AS, Downes RN, et al. Endonasal laser-assisted dacryocystorhinostomy. Hosp Med 1998;59(3):210–5.

[14] Lun Sham C, van Hasselt CA. Endoscopic terminal dacryocystorhinostomy. Laryngoscope 2000;110(6):1045–9.

[15] Javate RM, Campornanes BS, Nelson D, et al. The endoscope and the radiofrequency unit in DCR surgery. Ophthmalmic Plast Reconstr Surg 1995;11(1):54–8.

[16] Steadman MG. Transnasal dacryocystorhinostomy. Otolaryngol Clin North Am 1985;8(1):107–11.

[17] Muellner K, Bodner E, Mannor GE, et al. Endolacrimal laser assisted surgery. Br J Ophthalmol 2000;84:16–8.

[18] Wormald PJ. Powered endonasal dacryocystorhinostomy. Laryngoscope 2002;112:69–71.

[19] Tsirbas A, Wormald PJ. Mechanical endonasal DCR with mucosal flaps. Am J Ophthalmol 2003;135(1):79–86.

[20] Duffy MT. Advances in lacrimal surgery. Curr Opin Ophthalmol 2000;11:352–6.

[21] Wormald PJ, Kew J, van Hasselt CA. The intranasal anatomy of the naso-lacrimal sac in endoscopic dacryocystorhinostomy. Otolaryngol Head Neck Surg 2000;123:307–10.

[22] Rebeiz EE, Shapshay SM, Bowlds JH, et al. Anatomic guidelines for dacryocystorhinostomy. Laryngoscope 1992;102:1181–4.

[23] Unlu HH, et al. Anatomic guidelines for intranasal surgery of the lacrimal drainage system. Rhinology 1997;35:11–5.

[24] Hehar SS, Jones NS, Sadiq SA, et al. Endoscopic holmium: YAG laser dacryocystorhinostomy—safe and effective as a day-case procedure. J Laryngol Otol 1997;111:1056–9.

[25] Metson R. Endoscopic surgery for lacrimal obstruction. Otolaryngol Head Neck Surg 1991; 104:473–9.

[26] Linberg JV, Anderson RL, Busted RM, et al. Study of intranasal ostium external dacryocystorhinostomy. Arch Ophthalmol 1982;100:1758–62.

[27] Sprekelsen MB, Barberan MT. Endoscopic dacryocystorhinostomy: surgical technique and results. Laryngoscope 1996;106:187–9.

[28] Calhoun KH, Rotsler WH, Stiernberg CM. Surgical anatomy of the lateral nasal wall. Otolaryngol Head Neck Surg 1990;102:156–60.

[29] Fayet B, Racy E. Endonasal dacryocystorhinostomy (DCR) with protected drill. J Fr Ophthalmol 2000;23(4):321–6.

[30] Kong YT, Kim TI, Kong BW. A report of 131 cases of endoscopic laser lacrimal surgery. Ophthalmology 1994;101(11):1793–9.

[31] Tsirbas A, McNab AA. Secondary haemorrhage in dacryocystorhinostomy. Clin Exp Ophthalmol 2000;28(1):22–5.

[32] Welham RA, Wulc AE. Management of unsuccessful lacrimal surgery. Br J Ophthalmol 1987;71:152–7.

[33] Whittet HB, Shun-Shin AG, Awdry P. Functional endoscopic transnasal dacryocystorhinostomy. Eye 1993;7:545–9.

[34] Gleich LL, Rebeiz EE, Pankratov MM, et al. The holmium: YAG laser-assisted otolaryngologic procedures. Arch Otolaryngol Head Neck Surg 1995;121:1162–6.

[35] Pearlman SJ, Michalos P, Reib ML, et al. Translacrimal transnasal laser-assisted dacryocystorhinostomy. Laryngology 1997;107(10):1362–5.

[36] Woog JJ, Metson R, Puliafito CA. Holmium:YAG endonasal laser dacryocystorhinostomy. Am J Ophthalmol 1993;116:1–10.

[37] Becker BB. Nasal endoscopy in dye testing after dacryocystorhinostomy. Ophthalmic Plast Reconstr Surg 1990;6(1):64–7.

[38] Tsirbas A, Wormald PJ. Mechanical endonasal dacryocystorhinostomy with mucosal flaps. Br J Ophthalmol 2003;87(1):43–7.

[39] Woog JJ, Kennedy RH, Custer PL, et al. Endonasal dacryocystorhinostomy: a report by the American Academy of Ophthalmology. Ophthalmology 2001;108(12):2369–77.

[40] Szubin L, Papageorge A, Sacks E. Endonasal laser-assisted dacryocystorhinostomy. Am J Rhinol 1999;13(5):371–4.

[41] Nowinski TS, Flanagan JC, Mauriello J. Pediatric dacryocystorhinostomy. Arch Ophthalmol 1985;103:1226–8.

[42] Elder MJ. Paediatric dacryocystorhinostomy. Aust N Z J Ophthalmol 1992;20(4):333–6.

[43] Welham RAN, Hughes SM. Lacrimal surgery in children. Am J Ophthalmol 1985;99: 27–34.

[44] Hakin KN, Sullivan TJ, Sharma A, et al. Paediatric dacryocystorhinostomy. Aust N Z J Ophthalmol 1994;22(4):231–5.

[45] Cunningham MJ, Woog JJ. Endonasal endoscopic dacryocystorhinostomy in children. Arch Otolaryngol Head Neck Surg 1998;124(3):328–33.

[46] Doyle A, Russell J, O'Keefe M. Paediatric laser DCR. Acta Ophthalmol Scand 2000;78: 204–5.

[47] Wong JF, Woog JJ, Cunningham MJ, et al. A multidisciplinary approach to atypical lacrimal obstruction in childhood. Ophthal Plast Reconstr Surg 1999;15(4):293–8.

[48] VanderVeen DK, Jones DT, Tan H, et al. Endoscopic dacryocystorhinostomy in children. J Am Acad Pediatr Ophthalmol Surg 2001;5(3):143–7.

ELSEVIER
SAUNDERS

Otolaryngol Clin N Am
39 (2006) 1037–1047

OTOLARYNGOLOGIC
CLINICS
OF NORTH AMERICA

Endoscopic Management of Orbital Abscesses

Samer Fakhri, MD, FRCSC*,
Kevin Pereira, MD, MS(ORL)

*Department of Otolaryngology-Head and Neck Surgery, University of Texas Medical School
at Houston, 6410 Fannin Street, Suite 1200, Houston, TX 77030, USA*

Orbital complications of sinusitis have decreased steadily in the current antibiotic era. Nonetheless, sinusitis continues to be the most common cause of orbital inflammation and infection, especially in children. By far, the most common orbital complication of sinusitis is preseptal cellulitis. However, extension of an infectious process into the postseptal space of the orbit may occur. This condition, which is serious and requires prompt diagnosis and management, typically presents as a collection of purulence or inflammatory exudate in the subperiosteal space adjacent to the infected sinus. Less commonly, a collection may organize in the intraconal compartment of the orbit. The incidence of a subperiosteal abscess in orbital infections is about 15%. Unfortunately, about 15% to 30% of patients who have this complication will develop various visual sequelae, even with aggressive medical and surgical intervention [1]. Spread of orbital sepsis to the cavernous sinus and intracranial compartment (IC), although infrequent, can occur and is associated with a morbidity and a mortality rate of 10% to 20%, despite aggressive management [2,3].

Clinical presentation

The clinical signs of a postseptal infection include chemosis, proptosis, restriction of extraocular muscle movements, and, if untreated, progressive visual loss, which may be temporary or permanent. Damage to vision is caused by increased intraorbital pressure, optic neuritis, traction on the optic nerve, or retinal artery thrombosis. Residual visual sequelae are more

* Corresponding author.
E-mail address: samer.fakhri@uth.tmc.edu (S. Fakhri).

doi:10.1016/j.otc.2006.06.001

oto.theclinics.com

likely in patients who had a visual acuity of 20/60 or worse when treatment was initiated or those who did not undergo, or had delayed, surgery [4]. Hence, the management of these patients requires close cooperation between an otolaryngologist, ophthalmologist, and infectious disease specialist who is aware of the resistance patterns of the causative organisms in the area. The amount of information that can be obtained from an ophthalmologic examination varies from very limited in a febrile 2-year-old who has chemosis and proptosis, to detailed in a 14-year-old who has limited periorbital edema. Two pediatric studies of medial subperiosteal abscesses (SPA) in children reported that complete clinical examinations were possible in 57% and 62% of their subjects [5,6]. Diminished pupillary reflexes may not be seen until significant visual loss has occurred [7]. Being able to distinguish colors may be used as a guide to disease progression. Increasing intraorbital pressure causes loss of red/green perception before visual acuity deteriorates [1]. A recent study recommended visual acuity checks every 2 hours for 24 hours when awake, and every 4 hours when asleep. As clinical signs improve, acuity checks may be decreased to every 4 hours [6]. The ease of examination and certainty of objective clinical findings play a major role in guiding management.

Radiologic evaluation

CT scanning is the diagnostic imaging modality of choice in the management of patients who have postseptal complications of sinusitis. It is fast, widely available, and allows accurate assessment of both soft tissue and bony changes. In addition, it can be performed in children without the need for sedation, especially when using the spiral CT technique. Imaging may be repeated after 48 hours if the patient's condition does not improve. The paranasal sinuses and orbit present an area of highly contrasting densities with air, fat, and soft tissue, which increases the accuracy of the examination. Axial and coronal views of the orbits and sinuses with contrast should be obtained in both soft tissue and bone windows. Axial views better demonstrate the displacement of the medial rectus muscle and the abscess within the orbit, whereas coronals cuts are useful to delineate orbital and sinus anatomy. A medial subperiosteal abscess is seen on CT scans as a rim-enhancing mass within the orbit, next to the lamina papyracea displacing the medial rectus laterally. Edema and thickening of the medial rectus are also evident, when compared with the opposite side (Fig. 1). A recent study used lateral displacement of the medial rectus muscle of at least 2 mm as a diagnostic criterion for a subperiosteal abscess [6]. Intraconal involvement is not as well-defined and appears as a diffuse infiltration of orbital fat with a lack of clear visualization of the optic nerve and extraocular muscles. However, CT scans have their limitations in the diagnosis of sinonasal disease, especially in children. Mucosal changes tend to persist, despite the resolution of clinical disease, with one study reporting incidental

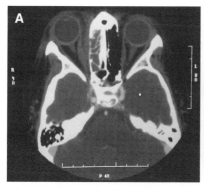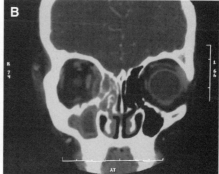

Fig. 1. Axial (A) and coronal (B) CT scans, soft tissue window with intravenous contrast, demonstrating a right subperiosteal abscess. Note ipsilateral ethmoid (A,B) and maxillary sinus opacification (B). Also note reactive thickening of the right medial rectus muscle.

soft tissue changes in up to 50% of subjects without sinus disease [8,9]. Additionally, CT scans have been found to correlate with surgical findings in only 84% of orbital complications of sinusitis, and can miss up to 50% of IC complications [3,10]. Using contrast while scanning the sinuses and brain enhances the ability to identify these complications.

MRI is the diagnostic study of choice for evaluating IC complications of sinusitis including cavernous sinus thrombophlebitis. MRI is superior to CT in identifying marrow space abnormalities such as edema or osteomyelitis, inflammation of the meninges, extra-axial empyemas, and early cerebritis [11]. It also provides superior soft tissue detail and does not expose the patient to radiation. However, an MRI study takes a lot longer than CT scanning, is sensitive to motion artifact, requires general anesthesia in younger children and sedation in older children. In patients who have orbital complications of sinusitis, MRI should be performed if fever recurs after an appropriate initial response to the antibiotic; if there are changes in the patient's mental status; or when CT findings suggest, but cannot confirm, IC spread of disease. Standardized orbital ultrasound has also been used in the diagnosis of intraocular pathology. It has the advantage of low cost and no radiation, and may be repeated at short intervals. It can be done at the bedside, and may be useful in monitoring the progress of an orbital infection. Its main disadvantage is its inability to detect a suppurative process in the posterior orbit [12].

Microbiology and antimicrobial therapy

The most common bacteria cultured from the postseptal space are streptococci (aerobic and anaerobic), staphylococci, and bacteroides. It has been observed that as a patient ages, multiple organisms are cultured and anaerobes tend to be the most common bacteria, followed by streptococci [6]. Whenever possible, middle meatal cultures should be obtained. Broad-spectrum intravenous antibiotic therapy that covers the above organisms, taking local resistance patterns into consideration, would be the reasonable initial management step. Augmented amino-penicillins such as ampicillin sulbactam would be an appropriate choice. Clindamycin is very effective against most bacteria causing intraorbital infections, but has the disadvantage of poor penetration of the blood brain barrier. Hence, it may not be a good choice if intracranial extension of the orbital suppurative process is suspected. The third-generation parenteral cephalosporin ceftriaxone is a highly effective gram-negative antibiotic that crosses the blood brain barrier and is very useful when combined with an antistaphylococcal drug. It can be used even for penicillin-resistant, pneumococcal infections.

Surgical indications for subperiosteal abscesses

Controversy exists about the optimal initial management of medial SPA in children. Some favor prompt drainage of the abscess, whereas others recommend a trial of medical management [5,6,2,13]. One study identified a subset of young subjects who had minimal restriction of ocular mobility and reported successful management with medical therapy alone [6]. Another prospective study claimed success with medical therapy alone in 27 of 29 subjects who had subperiosteal orbital abscesses. Inclusion criteria were: age below 9 years, absence of frontal sinusitis, medial location of the abscess, absence of gas in the abscess cavity, small abscess volume, nonrecurrent SPA, absence of acute optic nerve or retinal compromise, and a non-odontogenic infection. Surgical drainage was reserved for deterioration in visual acuity, appearance of an afferent pupillary defect, continuing fever after 36 hours, clinical deterioration after 48 hours, or no improvement after 72 hours of medical treatment [14].

Preoperative planning

A number of factors must be evaluated thoroughly, once the decision is made to proceed with drainage of a subperiosteal or intraorbital abscess. Clear communication between the ophthalmologist and the otolaryngologist (ENT) surgeon regarding the results of serial ophthalmologic examinations and their significance is critical and often time-sensitive. All relevant parameters of the ophthalmologic evaluation should be discussed, including status of the optic nerve and extraocular muscles, degree of proptosis, and orbital pressures. This information is crucial to planning both the timing and extent of the surgical intervention. For example, in a patient who has an intraorbital abscess and high orbital pressures, the surgeon must be prepared to perform a wide orbital wall decompression, in addition to incising the periorbita and draining the abscess. In this case, failure to recognize the high orbital pressures or to decompress the orbit may result in persistently elevated pressures and, ultimately, an unfavorable outcome. The intraoperative availability of an ophthalmology colleague is extremely helpful and, in fact, encouraged, especially when dealing with an intraorbital abscess.

Careful preoperative review of the CT scan in both the coronal and axial planes is imperative, and provides a road map for the surgical procedure. Most SPAs are located medially within the orbit, but many could extend superiorly or inferiorly, especially when associated with frontal and maxillary sinusitis, respectively. The surgeon should study carefully the bony anatomy of the sinonasal cavity and the skull base to recognize variant configurations and minimize intraoperative complications.

Objectives

The objectives of the surgical management of a subperiosteal or intraorbital abscess include draining the orbital collection, addressing the offending sinuses, and obtaining intraoperative cultures. In addition, decompression of one or more orbital walls may be necessary if intraoperative orbital pressures continue to be elevated, despite an adequate drainage procedure.

Choice of surgical approach

The surgeon should weigh the advantages and disadvantages of the different surgical approaches available to achieve the above-stated objectives. Surgical approaches to drain medial orbital abscesses can be divided into open, transnasal endoscopic, or combined approaches. The traditional approach for draining medial orbital collections has been through the external ethmoidectomy incision. However, the past 20 years have witnessed a tremendous expansion in the applications of rigid endoscopes as surgical tools in the treatment of disorders of the sinonasal cavity, anterior skull base, and orbit. The transnasal endoscopic approach to draining orbital abscesses has become a widely accepted and well-established alternative to the traditional open approach. The endoscopic approach offers several advantages. It provides unsurpassed and magnified visualization of the surgical field, including the sinonasal cavity and medial orbital wall. Also, angled telescopes can be used to visualize laterally and around corners into the orbit, especially in the case of an intraorbital abscess. In addition, the endoscopic approach allows comprehensive treatment of the orbital abscess and the offending paranasal sinuses. Finally, the endoscopic approach obviates the need for facial incisions. Manning [15] published the first case review in 1993, wherein he reported the successful endoscopic treatment of SPA in 5 pediatric subjects. Since then, multiple studies have shown that the endoscopic technique yielded similar success rates, when compared with the traditional open approach, and led to shorter hospitalization and less postoperative edema

[16–18]. For these reasons, the endoscopic drainage of orbital collections is the approach of choice in many institutions, including the authors'.

The main limitation of the endoscopic approach is related to the bleeding potential of the acutely inflamed mucosa, which may compromise visualization seriously, especially if operating within the confines of a pediatric nose. Even for experienced endoscopists, significant bleeding and poor visualization may compromise the safety and completeness of the procedure. Measures to improve hemostasis (see later discussion) and enhance visualization may not always be successful, and, therefore, the surgeon should always be prepared to convert to an external approach if the need arises. This eventuality should always be discussed preoperatively with the patient or the family and included in the informed consent.

Endoscopic approach: operative technique

The operation is performed under general anesthesia with orotracheal intubation. The patient is placed on the operating table supine or in a slight reverse trendelenburg position. The eye should be left uncovered, but corneal exposure should be avoided. The nose is decongested with 1% oxymetazoline hydrochloride on cotton pledgets placed in the nasal cavity. This procedure should be done in the least traumatic way to avoid mucosal lacerations and unnecessary bleeding. The mucosa of the lateral nasal wall is infiltrated with 1% lidocaine with 1:100,000 epinephrine. Multiple mucosal stabs should be avoided, considering the bleeding potential of an acutely inflamed mucosa.

Typically, the authors elevate the head slightly and ask the anesthetist to maintain the lowest mean arterial pressure that is safe for the patient. Often, frequent and sequential decongestion is required to achieve optimal visualization as the surgeon proceeds deeper into the sinonasal cavity. Sometimes, the mucosa in the anterior nasal cavity is severely edematous and friable, and responds poorly to decongestion. If this is the case, and visualization of the middle turbinate and middle meatus cannot be achieved, the surgeon should consider converting to an external approach. In the authors' experience, this is rarely necessary. Additional measures to improve hemostasis or enhance visualization should be considered. Lens-cleaning devices, such as Endo-Scrub (Medtronic Xomed, Jacksonville, Florida), are often very helpful, but they add to the diameter of the telescope and, therefore, their use may become problematic in pediatric noses. Microdebriders, with their concurrent suction and fast tissue removal, are terrific tools to enhance visualization and expedite the surgical procedure. However, they should be used cautiously to avoid complications and unnecessary mucosal injury.

The authors use the 4-mm telescopes in all adult cases and in most pediatric noses. The 0-degree telescope is used to perform the uncinectomy, ethmoidectomy, and sphenoidotomy, if the latter is indicated. The 30-degree telescope is used to perform the maxillary antrostomy and to drain the orbital abscess. Rarely, a frontal recess dissection and frontal sinusotomy are necessary and require visualization with 30-degree and 70-degree telescopes. Angled telescopes afford significant surgical advantages, but they also add to visual distortion; their use should be reserved to experienced surgeons.

1. At the beginning of the procedure, any purulence in the middle meatus should be collected in a sterile fashion and the specimen sent for cultures. The results are used to guide postoperative antimicrobial therapy.
2. The initial maneuver is to remove the uncinate process and identify the natural ostium of the maxillary sinus.
3. If there is no disease, or if there is minimal mucosal thickening in the maxillary sinus, a formal maxillary antrostomy may not be necessary, and the maxillary sinus outflow tract is best left undisturbed.
4. The bulla ethmoidalis is then penetrated and removed with through-cutting instruments or with a microdebrider. Care should be taken to avoid injury to the middle turbinate and medial orbital wall, especially when using powered instrumentation. The blade of the microdebrider should be pointing perpendicular to the medial orbital wall. The lamina papyracea is then skeletonized with through-cutting instruments in preparation for the drainage of the orbital abscess. Sometimes, pus can be seen streaming from the orbit at the completion of the ethmoidectomy, usually occurring through a natural dehiscence or a crack in the lamina papyracea, especially when orbital pressures are elevated. Purulence should be collected and sent for cultures.
5. Drainage of the orbital collection is initiated by cracking the lamina papyracea with a Cottle or freer elevator. This step is omitted if there is spontaneous drainage of pus from the orbit. The 30-degree telescope may be used to perform this maneuver.
6. Bone from the lamina papyracea is elevated gently with a Cottle or freer elevator and removed until adequate drainage of a subperiosteal abscess into the middle meatus is achieved. Complete drainage of the abscess may be confirmed by placing gentle pressure on the eye.
7. The nasal cavity is then irrigated with normal saline. If the middle turbinate is sitting in a lateral position and there is a risk of scarring to the decompressed orbit, a middle-turbinate medialization technique may be performed. Alternatively, a piece of gelfilm or gelfoam may be placed. Nasal packing is avoided.

Additional steps

1. Posterior ethmoidectomy is indicated if there is significant posterior ethmoid disease and extension of the abscess toward the orbital apex. It may also be necessary to achieve wide exposure and decompression of the medial orbital wall, especially if the orbital pressures continue to

be elevated substantially. This step is sometimes necessary when dealing with intraorbital abscesses, but is needed rarely in subperiosteal abscess drainage. Posterior ethmoidectomy begins with perforating the basal lamella on its superior and lateral aspect back to the face of the sphenoid. The medial orbital wall is skeletonized and elevated carefully. In the case of a subperiosteal abscess, care should be taken not to violate the periorbita.

2. Presence of isolated sphenoid or frontal sinus disease in patients who have orbital abscesses is extremely rare, especially in the pediatric population. Therefore, sphenoidotomy and frontal sinusotomy are undertaken only on rare occasions.

3. Incision of the periorbita is usually necessary to drain an intraorbital abscess (Fig. 2). The authors use a sickle knife under the guidance of the 30-degree telescope. The tip of the knife should remain superficial; the incision is made from posterior to anterior. This maneuver usually affords good drainage of most extraconal abscesses. Drainage of intraconal abscesses is best achieved through a combined approach and should never be attempted without the active participation of ophthalmologic colleagues. The intraoperative measurement of orbital pressures is extremely helpful and often dictates the extent of orbital decompression.

Postoperative care

In adults, postoperative care is performed as in routine sinus surgery. Patients are instructed to perform twice-daily nasal saline irrigations. Endoscopic debridement is performed after 1 week, to remove debris and crusts,

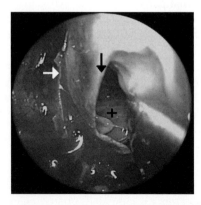

Fig. 2. Endoscopic view of a left extraconal intraorbital abscess that was drained using the transnasal endoscopic approach. The lamina papyracea (*white arrow*) has been widely decompressed. The periorbita (*black arrow*) has been incised to expose and drain an extensive intraorbital collection (+).

and may be repeated as needed. In pediatric patients, office or bedside endoscopic debridement obviously is not easily tolerated. The authors individu-
alize the decision regarding the need for a second-look procedure, based on
the extent of surgery and mucosal trauma, the position of the middle turbinate, and the amount of dissolvable packing used. Depending on the age
of the patient, nasal saline irrigations or nasal saline mist may be used.
All patients continue to receive systemic, culture-directed antibiotics
postoperatively.

Role of computer-aided surgery

During the past 2 decades, the availability of computer-aided surgery
(CAS) technology has enhanced the ability and confidence of the endoscopic
sinus and skull base surgeon in addressing complex pathology in difficult
and vital anatomic areas. Disease processes involving or abutting the orbit
provide an elegant example of CAS applications. Common examples include
tumors and mucoceles of the sinonasal cavity involving the orbit. However,
there is a paucity of data in the literature about the application of CAS in
the management of orbital abscesses [19]. There are several reasons for
this. First, the diagnosis of an orbital collection is usually based on routine
CT scan protocols not suited for CAS. Second, the radiation exposure risks
of obtaining a repeat CT scan for the purposes of CAS may not be acceptable, especially considering that most patients are in the pediatric age group.
Third, surgical management of orbital collections may sometimes be time-
sensitive (eg, deteriorating visual acuity), precluding any further tests.
Fourth, many surgeons do not feel that CAS enhances the outcome of the
drainage procedure, considering the limited scope of the intervention. Fifth,
ENT surgeons performing the endoscopic drainage may not be familiar or
comfortable with CAS technology, considering the often nonelective nature
of the surgical management. Finally, expenses incurred from a repeat scan
for the purposes of CAS may not be justifiable to insurance carriers. The advantages gained from using CAS technology in frontal sinus and skull base
pathology also apply to the surgical management of orbital abscesses. Preoperative CT review using this modality allows the surgeon to develop
a three-dimensional appreciation of relevant anatomy and the location
and extent of orbital collections. Simultaneous viewing of a single point
of interest in axial, coronal, sagittal, and three-dimensional model reconstruction provides the surgeon with critical anatomic information simply
not afforded by static films. Intraoperatively, surgical navigation provides
the surgeon with a depth dimension and allows him to correlate CT images
with the two-dimensional and often bloody anatomy provided by the telescopes. This advantage, along with the high localization accuracy of CAS,
may increase the precision, completeness, and safety of the procedure.
The use of CAS should not be a substitute for thorough knowledge of the
endoscopic anatomy. CAS technology has its limitations, and operational

errors may not be recognized by the unsuspecting surgeon unless the accuracy of the system is confirmed periodically against known anatomic landmarks. Failure to recognize these errors may place the patient at risk for devastating complications.

The guidelines for using CAS technology remain general, reflecting the absence of consensus on whether CAS is considered standard of care. The American Academy of Otolaryngology–Head and Neck Surgery [20] has the following policy statement regarding the intraoperative use of CAS:

> The American Academy of Otolaryngology – Head and Neck Surgery endorses the intraoperative use of computer-aided surgery in appropriately select cases to assist the surgeon in clarifying complex anatomy during sinus and skull base surgery... examples of indications in which use of computer-aided surgery may be deemed appropriate include...disease abutting the skull base, orbit, optic nerve or carotid artery.

Because of the difficulty of obtaining evidence to support the role of CAS, the merit of this technology in the surgical management of orbital abscesses is currently based on surgeon preference and expert consensus opinion. Compounding the problem is the recent move of some insurance providers to label CAS as experimental, and therefore deny reimbursement for the use of this technology.

Summary

Optimal management of orbital abscesses requires a multidisciplinary approach. Surgical management is indicated in most cases where orbital collections are present. Clear communication between the ophthalmologist and the ENT surgeon is critical to guide the timing and extent of the surgical intervention. The endoscopic approach to the medial orbit offers significant advantages over the traditional external approach, but may have some limitations in an acutely inflamed and bloody surgical field. The preoperative and intraoperative use of CAS technology may be a useful adjunct in the endoscopic management of orbital abscesses.

References

[1] Osguthorpe JD, Hochman M. Inflammatory sinus diseases affecting the orbit. Otolaryngol Clin N Am 1993;26:657–71.
[2] Herrmann BW, Forsen JW. Simultaneous intracranial and orbital complications of acute rhinosinusitis in children. Int J Pediatr Otorhinolaryngol 2004;68:619–25.
[3] Nathoo N, Nadvi SS, van Dellen JR, et al. Intracranial sybdural empyemas in the era of computed tomography: a review of 699 cases. Neurosurgery 1999;44:529–36.
[4] Schramm V, Curtin H, Kenneerdell JS. Evaluation of orbital cellulites and results of treatment. Laryngoscope 1982;92:723–38.
[5] Pereira KD, Mitchell RB, Younis RT, et al. Management of medial subperiosteal abscess of the orbit in children – a 5 year experience. Int J Pediatr Otorhinolaryngol 1997;38:247.

[6] Brown CL, Graham SM, Griffin MC, et al. Pediatric medial subperiosteal orbital abscess: medical management where possible. Am J Rhinol 2004;18:321–7.

[7] Patt BS, Manning SC. Blindness resulting from orbital complications of sinusitis. Otolaryngol Head Neck Surg 1991;104:789–95.

[8] Vazquez E, Creixell S, Carreno JC, et al. Complicated acute pediatric bacterial sinusitis: imaging updated approach. Curr Probl Diagn Radiol 2004;33:127–45.

[9] Glasier CM, Ascher DP, Williams KD. Incidental paranasal sinus abnormalities on CT of children: clinical correlation. AJNR Am J Neuroradiol 1986;7:861–4.

[10] Clary RA, Cunningham MJ, Eavy RD. Orbital complications of acute sinusitis: comparison of computed tomography and surgical findings. Ann Otol Rhinol Laryngol 1992;101: 598–600.

[11] Kronemer KA, McAlister WH. Sinusitis and its imaging in the pediatric population. Pediatr Radiol 1997;27:837–46.

[12] Kaplan DM, Briscoe D, Gatot A, et al. The use of standardized orbital ultrasound in the diagnosis of sinus induced infections of the orbit in children: a preliminary report. Int J Pediatr Otorhinolaryngol 1999;48:155–62.

[13] Rahbar R, Robson CD, Petersen RA, et al. Management of orbital subperiosteal abscess in children. Arch Otolaryngol Head Neck Surg 2001;127:281–6.

[14] Garcia GH, Harris GJ. Criteria for nonsurgical management of subperiosteal abscess of the orbit: analysis of outcomes 1988–1998. Ophthalmology 2000;107:1454–6.

[15] Manning SC. Endoscopic management of medial subperiosteal orbital abscess. Arch Otolaryngol Head Neck Surg 1993;119(7):789–91.

[16] Arjmand EM, Lusk RP, Muntz HR. Pediatric sinusitis and subperiosteal orbital abscess formation: diagnosis and treatment. Otolaryngol Head Neck Surg 1993;109(5):886–94.

[17] Page EL, Wiatrak BJ. Endoscopic vs external drainage of orbital subperiosteal abscess. Arch Otolaryngol Head Neck Surg 1996;122(7):737–40.

[18] Froehlich P, Pransky SM, Fontaine P, et al. Minimal endoscopic approach to subperiosteal orbital abscess. Arch Otolaryngol Head Neck Surg 1997;123(3):280–2.

[19] White JB, Parikh SR. Early experience with image guidance in endoscopic transnasal drainage of periorbital abscesses. J Otolaryngol 2005;34(1):63–5.

[20] American Academy of Otolaryngology–Head and Neck Surgery. Intra-operative use of computer aided surgery. Available at: http://www.entlink.net/practice/rules/image-guiding. cfm. Accessed February 27, 2006.

ELSEVIER
SAUNDERS

Otolaryngol Clin N Am
39 (2006) 1049–1057

OTOLARYNGOLOGIC
CLINICS
OF NORTH AMERICA

Endoscopic Orbital Fracture Repair

Yasaman Mohadjer, MD*, Morris E. Hartstein, MD

*Department of Ophthalmology, Saint Louis University School of Medicine,
1755 South Grand Boulevard, St. Louis, MO 63104, USA*

Orbital fracture is a common occurrence in patients who have facial trauma. Blowout fractures involving the inferior and medial walls of the orbit occur most frequently. Indications for the repair of orbital fractures include entrapment of extraocular muscles or the other surrounding soft tissues causing diplopia. Cosmetically significant enophthalmos or hypoglobus, with or without diplopia, may necessitate surgical intervention (Figs. 1–3) [1].

The primary goal of fracture repair is to remove all herniated tissues from the site of the fracture. Visualization of all edges of the fracture is imperative before an implant is placed. Traditional approaches to the orbital floor include transconjunctival or subciliary incisions. Often, isolated medial wall fractures are approached through a caruncular incision. However, visualization of the posterior aspect of the fracture is often challenging with these approaches because of the posterosuperior angulation of the orbital floor, relative to the anteroinferior orbital rim. Thus, fractures involving the middle or posterior third of the orbital floor are the hardest to visualize with traditional surgical approaches.

With increased interest in minimally invasive surgery, in the hopes of reducing recovery time and minimizing aesthetic concerns, endoscopic-guided orbital fracture repair has become an increasingly popular approach to assist with visualization. The authors have previously described endoscopic examination of the orbital floor through an antrostomy or ethmoidoscopy [2]. The endoscopic method is a superior method to assure that all surrounding tissues have been elevated from the fracture site and that they remain so after orbital implant placement. Besides better visualization, advantages include increased illumination; video projection for the rest of the surgical

This study was supported in part by an unrestricted departmental grant from Research to Prevent Blindness.
* Corresponding author.
E-mail address: mohadjery@yahoo.com (Y. Mohadjer).

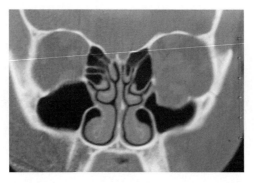

Fig. 1. A coronal CT scan of the orbits, revealing a large left posterior orbital floor fracture secondary to blunt trauma.

team and for documentation and recording; confirmation of correct implant placement; and, most important, precise and complete reduction of herniated orbital soft tissues.

Surgical procedure

General anesthesia is recommended for orbital fracture repair. At the beginning of the procedure, cotton pads soaked in oxymetazoline hydrochloride or 4.0% cocaine hydrochloride are placed inside the nose for decongestion. An injection of 1.0% xylocaine with 1:100,000 epinephrine is given to the lateral nasal mucosa using endoscopic visualization.

A transconjunctival approach with lateral canthotomy and cantholysis, as described by McCord and Moses [3], allows a broad exposure to the inferior orbital rim. A 4-0 silk traction suture is placed just below the insertion of the inferior rectus muscle. An incision in the periorbita is made just anterior to the orbital rim in the inferior fornix; the periorbita is then elevated posteriorly, allowing exploration of the floor and assessment of the extent of

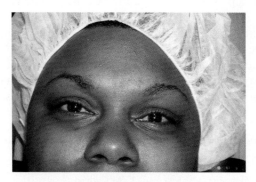

Fig. 2. Preoperative external photograph of the same patient as in Fig. 1, demonstrating significant enophthalmos left eye.

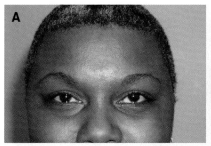
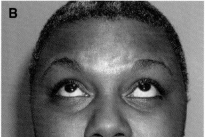

Fig. 3. Postoperative photograph after standard transconjunctival approach of the same patient as in Figs. 1 and 2 showing improved enophthalmos (*A*), and no upgaze limitation (*B*).

the fracture. Bony fragments are removed and saved for potential replacement at the end of the procedure.

The patient is placed in 20 to 30 degrees of reverse Trendelenburg position. A straight 4-mm endoscope is then introduced. The uncinate process is resected. The maxillary ostium is identified and enlarged. A side-biting forceps allows anterior extension of the opening. A telescope is then advanced easily into the maxillary ostium. In patients who have more complex fractures, such as tripod fractures involving the maxilla and zygoma, a 30-degree angled telescope may be useful for further lateral visualization. In these cases, ostium enlargement may not be necessary if the telescope can be passed through the pre-existing maxillary fracture.

The fracture site is identified and all soft tissues are elevated carefully (Fig. 4A). An implant of choice (titanium, supramyd, silicone, or Medpor) is fashioned appropriately and introduced by way of the initial inferior fornix incision. The endoscope is used to guide the implant into the proper position and to ensure that it is resting on stable bone on all sides, especially posteriorly (Figs. 4B, 5A, and 5B). Care is taken to ensure that no soft tissue

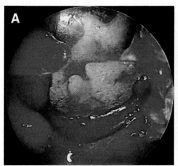
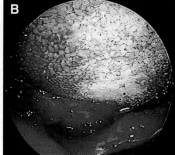

Fig. 4. (*A*) Endoscopic view from below of a large fracture of the orbital floor with a malleable elevating the periorbital tissues out of the fracture site. (*B*) Endoscopic view of a Medpor sheet resting on a secure ledge of bone.

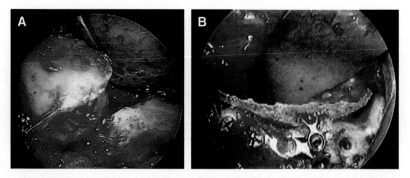

Fig. 5. (*A*) Endoscopic view of large inferior orbital rim step-off fracture and orbital floor fracture. (*B*) Endoscopic view after repair of the inferior orbital rim (plate) and orbital floor (Medpor channel implant).

is trapped under the implant, and that the implant itself is not compromising other structures posteriorly, such as the annulus of Zinn or the optic nerve. The inferior rectus traction suture is pulled in a series of gentle tugs, and the orbital floor is observed from below to confirm that all tissues have been repositioned properly. The implant is then secured appropriately in place and the incision is closed.

In medial orbital wall fracture repair, an additional 4-0 silk traction suture is used to tag the medial rectus muscle. A limited endoscopic ethmoidectomy allows for appropriate visualization. The fragments of bone impinging on the medial rectus are then removed.

Discussion

A transconjunctival inferior fornix incision is the authors' method of choice in inferior orbital wall fracture repair. However, a subciliary approach may be used with similar exposure, but has the added disadvantages of an external incision, potential scarring, and a greater chance of postoperative lid retraction. The limitations of both approaches, however, include incomplete visualization of the posterior aspect of the fracture, further hindered by the superior angulation of the orbital floor from rim to apex. Furthermore, imperfect view during posterior dissection increases the risk of damage to the optic nerve and other posterior structures. A cadaveric study of the orbits showed a wide variance in the anatomy of the orbital wall, based on gender and ethnicity, implying that there may be no "safe" area of dissection to ensure no damage to these posterior structures [4]. Because of this, many surgeons may limit posterior dissection, which may cause residual entrapped tissue posteriorly or improper implant positioning leading to continued or recurrent enophthalmos. The endoscope is a vital tool to visualize and prevent damage to the optic nerve and other vital structures, while allowing proper surgical dissection.

Maxillary sinus approaches to the orbit have been well documented. Ducic [5] reported the use of the endoscope in small orbital floor fractures. He used a 30-degree rigid endoscope, introduced by way of a gingivobuccal access incision, and a maxillary sinus approach, which allowed for continuous visualization in suspected trapdoor fractures of the inferior orbital floor with entrapment of inferior rectus or oblique muscles. The endoscope is useful and efficient in those cases not requiring implant placement, compared with a more invasive and time-consuming periorbital approach.

Alternative endoscopic approaches to the floor for larger fractures have been described without a concurrent subconjunctival approach [6–8]. Persons and Wong [6] described a transantral approach by way of a transoral incision to expose the anterior maxillary wall. An antral bone flap was created and a 30-degree endoscope introduced. Orbital floor fractures were identified, orbital contents were reduced, and the fracture was repaired using resorbable plates. No fixation was necessary in cases with stable orbital shelves. In the five cases reported, there were no cases of postoperative enophthalmos, and the three cases of diplopia resolved. One subject who had preoperative entrapment had restoration of full motility. The investigators described the clear benefit of enhanced visualization without risk of injury to the lower eyelid, along with elimination of external incisions.

Strong [7] used a similar approach to the orbital floor by way of a sublabial (Caldwell-Luc) incision with the creation of a maxillary antrostomy. He described the added benefit of endoscopy to evaluate the need for surgical repair of the orbital floor. In some cases of complex zygomaticomaxillary fracture repair, there may be an increased displacement of a concurrent orbital floor fracture after reduction of the zygoma. The endoscope is beneficial in these cases in exploring the orbital floor through the maxillary face fracture, to decide whether floor repair is necessary. Endoscopic access also may be useful in certain cases to eliminate globe retraction, often required in traditional open maneuvers, which may be important to prevent further bleeding and complications in cases with concurrent hyphemas [7,8].

A combination of endoscopic orbital floor fracture repair and balloon catheter technique for tissue reduction has been described by several investigators [9,10]. Ikeda and colleagues [9] also described a purely endoscopic approach in orbital blowout fractures. An endonasal approach is used to enlarge the maxillary ostium and an angled endoscope is used to visualize as bony fragments are identified and removed. When forced ductions have improved, a ureteral balloon catheter is introduced into the maxillary sinus and inflated with saline until all orbital contents are elevated out of the fracture site. The balloon is removed 2 to 3 weeks after surgery. This approach is best applied to more anterior fractures. In a series of 29 consecutively treated subjects, Miki and colleagues [10] described a similar method of balloon reduction in orbital floor fractures, but using a 1.5-cm gingival-buccal incision and standard Caldwell-Luc approach. Postoperatively, all 20 cases of enophthalmos and 93% of all diplopia resolved within 3 months of surgery. Neither diplopia nor enophthalmos recurred during an average 23-month follow-up period.

In the authors' experience, using the nasal telescope may limit or even eliminate the need for a Caldwell-Luc incision if an intranasal maxillary antrostomy is used instead. A large anterior antrostomy can be avoided, because this approach may be associated with soft tissue herniation and facial depression. Superb visualization of the posterior orbital floor may be noted with intranasal maxillary antrostomy; this is often the most difficult area to view through a transconjunctival approach. Good postoperative drainage of the maxillary sinus is an added benefit.

Complications of maxillary sinus antrostomy may include prolonged bleeding, loss of vision, cerebrospinal fluid leak, and a longer operative time. These complications have not occurred in the authors' experience, but may occur more often with open incisions. In fact, endoscopic approaches may shorten operating time by eliminating large open incisions and closures [9]. The technique described herein may enhance the safety and efficacy of orbital fracture repair by using a small or pre-existing opening for direct visualization of the orbital tissues and the orbital implant (if necessary), in relation to the fracture edges. The stability of the fracture repair may be viewed more easily, and vital posterior structures avoided more clearly.

Very anterior fractures may be visualized and repaired easily using standard transconjunctival and subciliary approaches, without endoscopic assistance. However, the endoscope becomes most useful for visualization and to prevent damage to adjacent structures in those cases where fractures extend to the middle and posterior portions of the orbital floor (Figs. 6A, 6B, and 7). Endoscopic guidance becomes very helpful in cases of extensively delayed fracture repair or in secondary repair when tissue scarring becomes a significant concern, and to ensure proper fracture reduction and implant placement.

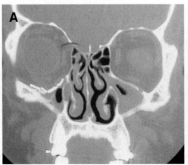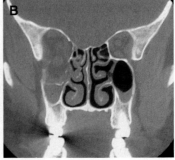

Fig. 6. (*A*) Postoperative CT scan of the orbits demonstrates good anterior implant placement. (*B*) More posterior CT views demonstrate residual fracture causing enophthalmos. This patient underwent successful repair with correction of enophthalmos using a combined transconjunctival and endoscopic approach.

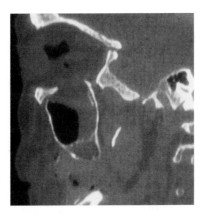

Fig. 7. CT scan demonstrates large blowout fracture of the orbit, extending posteriorly. Difficult to visualize through standard external approaches, the posterior extent of this fracture may be visualized more easily using the endoscope.

Isolated medial orbital wall fractures may occur more frequently and may be a more severe and frequent cause of enophthalmos than inferior floor fractures [11]. Several investigators have described their use of endonasal endoscopic reduction of medial wall blowout fractures [12–14]. Jin and colleagues [12] described 14 out of 16 subjects with complete resolution of symptoms, with the other two subjects requiring transorbital implant placement. Yamaguchi and colleagues [13] reported good results using this technique, with reduced enophthalmos and improved or resolved diplopia in all 12 of their cases. H.M. Lee and colleagues [14] reported that 15 of their 16 cases had complete resolution of their symptoms postoperatively. The remaining symptomatic subject had persistent diplopia, although no soft tissues remained herniated postoperatively. No complications were reported in any of these cases. Benefits of the endonasal endoscopic approach include direct access to the surgical site, reduced bleeding, and lack of an external scar.

M.J. Lee and colleagues [15] described their technique of transnasal endoscopy for medial orbital wall fractures using a balloon catheter and Merocel (Medtronic, Mystic, Connecticut). Seventeen subjects were operated on for enophthalmos greater than 2 mm, diplopia, or muscle restriction. A transnasal endoscope was used to reduce soft tissue and bone fragments and then supported by a balloon catheter or Merocel packing, which was then left in place for 1 to 3 weeks. Large defects of the medial orbital wall were grafted with the resected uncinate process. The average length of surgery was 50 minutes. Postoperative CT scans were used to adjust balloon inflation in cases of over- or undercorrection of the orbital wall reduction. This procedure provided good symptomatic results, with improved enophthalmos and diplopia, no increased morbidity, and no external scar. This technique may be most useful in isolated cases of medial wall fracture with significant symptoms.

Naraghi and Kashfi [16] used an endonasal endoscopic approach to medial orbital fracture repair by way of rotational repositioning of the bony fragments to eliminate the need for grafting or implants. A subject who had lateral gaze diplopia and medial wall fracture was treated with endonasal endoscopic reduction of the medial rectus muscle. A 30-degree endoscope was used to reposition soft tissues and to rotate the largest segment of bony fragments 45 degrees sagittally over the horizontal axis. Diplopia was assessed intraoperatively in their awake subjects, and was mostly resolved by the end of the repositioning. A cutaneous scar was avoided, and repositioning of bony fragments obviated the need for synthetic implant materials, eliminating the risks of infection, migration, and inflammation. The investigators did state that the technique has limitations, including the availability of a large bony fragment (50% of the fracture area), minimal to no enophthalmos, and a primary indication of diplopia. In select cases, however, the endoscopic rotational repositioning of large bony fragments may produce excellent surgical results.

Summary

Based on these multiple reports, it is clear that the endoscope provides an efficient method to visualize and manage orbital wall fractures. It has shown to be especially important in reducing operative time, soft tissue manipulation, and hemorrhage. The potential for external scarring may be eliminated completely. Visualization and illumination is enhanced for the surgeon and his/her entire operating team. Morbidity is reduced and hospitalization time may be decreased significantly. The authors' experience suggests that the endonasal endoscopic approach is a useful adjunct to the transconjunctival approach, and may eliminate potential complications associated with transantral-Caldwell-Luc approaches, such as recurrent sinusitis, papillomas, and possibly infraorbital hypesthesia [17,18]. The endoscope is especially useful in the treatment of posterior fractures or secondary repairs for residual enophthalmos. The disadvantages are few, but may include a requirement of special equipment and a steeper learning curve in the beginning.

References

[1] Hartstein ME, Roper-Hall G. Update on orbital floor fractures: indications and timing for repair. Facial Plast Surg 2000;16(2):95–106.
[2] Woog JJ, Hartstein ME, Gliklich R. Paranasal sinus endoscopy and orbital fracture repair. Arch Ophthalmol 1998;116:688–91.
[3] McCord CD Jr, Moses JL. Exposure of the inferior orbit with fornix incision and lateral canthotomy. Ophthalmic Surg 1979;10:53–63.
[4] Nguyen PN, Sullivan P. Advances in the management of orbital fractures. Clin Plat Surg 1992;19:87–98.

[5] Ducic Y. Endoscopically assisted repair of orbital fractures. Plast Reconstr Surg 2001; 108(7):2011–8.
[6] Persons BL, Wong GM. Transantral endoscopic orbital floor repair using resorbable plate. J Craniofac Surg 2002;13(3):483–8.
[7] Strong BE. Endoscopic repair of orbital blow-out fractures. Otolaryngol Head Neck Surg 2004;20(3):223–30.
[8] Strong EB, Kim KK, Diaz RC. Endoscopic approach to orbital blowout fracture repair. Otolaryngol Head Neck Surg 2004;131:683–95.
[9] Ikeda K, Suzuki H, Oshima T, et al. Endoscopic endonasal repair of orbital floor fracture. Arch Otolaryngol Head Neck Surg 1999;125:59–63.
[10] Miki T, Wada J, Haraoka J, et al. Endoscopic transmaxillary reduction and balloon technique for blowout fractures of the orbital floor. Minim Invasive Neurosurg 2004;47(6): 359–64.
[11] Whitehouse RW, Batterbury M, Jackson A, et al. Prediction of enophthalmos by computed tomography after 'blow out' orbital fracture. Br J Ophthalmol 1994;78(8):618–20.
[12] Jin HR, Shin SO, Choo MJ, et al. Endonasal endoscopic reduction of blowout fractures of the medial orbital wall. J Oral Maxillofac Surg 2000;58(8):847–51.
[13] Yamaguchi N, Kim C, Ma Y, et al. Endoscopic endonasal technique of the blowout fracture of the medial orbital wall. Op Tech Otolaryngol Head Neck Surg 1992;2:269–74.
[14] Lee HM, Han SK, Chae SW, et al. Endoscopic endonasal reconstruction of blowout fractures of the medial orbital walls. Plast Reconstr Surg 2002;109(3):872–6.
[15] Lee MJ, Kang YS, Yang JY, et al. Endoscopic transnasal approach for the treatment of medial orbital blow-out fracture: a technique for controlling the fractured wall with the balloon catheter and Merocel. Plast Reconstr Surg 2002;110(2):417–26.
[16] Naraghi M, Kashfi A. Endonasal endoscopic treatment of medial orbital wall fracture via rotational repositioning. Am J Otolaryngol 2002;23:312–5.
[17] Barzilai G, Greenberg E, Uri N. Indications for the Caldwell-Luc approach in the endoscopic era. Otolaryngol Head Neck Surg 2005;132(2):219–20.
[18] Carrasco JR, Castillo I, Bilyk JR, et al. Incidence of infraorbital hypesthesia and sinusitis after orbital decompression for thyroid-related orbitopathy: a comparison of surgical techniques. Ophthal Plast Reconstr Surg 2005;21(3):188–91.

ELSEVIER
SAUNDERS

Otolaryngol Clin N Am
39 (2006) 1059–1074

OTOLARYNGOLOGIC
CLINICS
OF NORTH AMERICA

Endoscopic Management of Pediatric Nasolacrimal Anomalies

Michael J. Cunningham, MD[a,b,*]

[a]Harvard Medical School, Boston, MA, USA
[b]Massachusetts Eye and Ear Infirmary, 243 Charles Street, Boston, MA 02114, USA

Dacryocystocele (nasolacrimal duct cyst)

Etiology

The nasolacrimal drainage system begins development in the third fetal month from a cord of epithelium found between the maxillary and fronto-nasal recesses [1]. Canalization of this cord occurs uniformly throughout its entire length, and final communication with the inferior nasal meatus usually occurs by the sixth fetal month. If complete canalization fails to occur, it most commonly leaves a membranous barrier between the nasolacrimal duct and the nasal cavity at the level of the valve of Hasner. This membranous barrier may last up to or beyond the time of birth and is the most common cause of nasolacrimal drainage obstruction in infants.

A congenital dacryocystocele occurs when there is both an imperforate nasolacrimal duct distally and a valvelike obstruction at the junction of the common canaliculus and lacrimal sac proximally [2]. Fluid accumulates, and the nasolacrimal duct system becomes distended. The proximal obstruction is attributed to distention of the sac compressing the canalicular system, causing a functional trapdoor-type block. The presence of such a functional obstruction often can be substantiated by the absence of an anatomic barrier on nasolacrimal probing as well as by the common finding of a partially patent nasolacrimal drainage system on irrigation or dacryocystogram evaluation [3]. These latter findings confirm a functional proximal obstruction and in some cases suggest a partial distal obstruction, possibly attributable to a redundancy of membranous tissue at the valve of Hasner, that impedes

Portions of this article are reprinted from: Cunningham MJ. Endoscopic Techniques in the Management of Pediatric Nasolacrimal Anomolies. In: John J. Woog, Ed. Manual of Endoscopic Lacrimal and Orbital Surgery. Philadelphia: Butterworth/Heineman, 2004; with permission.

* Correspondence address. 243 Charles Street, Boston, MA 02114.
E-mail address: michael_cunningham@meei.harvard.edu

doi:10.1016/j.otc.2006.07.004

but does not completely obstruct tear outflow. Chronic distention of the nasolacrimal system in the setting of partial distal obstruction also may adversely affect lacrimal pump function, further compromising tear drainage.

Amnioticocele and amniocele were terms originally used to describe these lesions because of the misconception that they represented embryologic cysts containing amniotic fluid. The term "mucocele" began to be used when evaluation of the cyst fluid revealed it actually to consist of mucus and tears [4]. The more descriptive and appropriate terms are "congenital dacryocystocele" or "nasolacrimal duct cyst," which reflect the lesion's true origin.

Clinical presentation

Congenital dacryocystoceles have a significant demonstrable female preponderance [5–8]. They also seem to be more common in whites than in other racial groups [5,7]. These observations suggest a genetic predilection. Familial cases have been described only sporadically, however [5,7].

Congenital dacryocystoceles may be either unilateral or bilateral. Although bilateral symptomatic presentations are infrequent, asymptomatic pathologic changes in the contralateral nasolacrimal drainage system may be present and often can be confirmed by radiologic or endoscopic investigation [7,9,10].

Congenital dacryocystoceles typically present at birth or become apparent within the first few weeks of life as tear production increases. Epiphora is the most common manifestation. In many affected infants, a cystic mass of bluish coloration is noted in the medial canthal region (Fig. 1). Manual

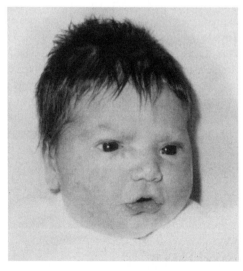

Fig. 1. The external presentation of a congenital dacryocystocele is typically a bluish cystic medial canthal mass.

compression of this cystic mass usually fails to result in the reflux of tears through the lacrimal puncta [11].

Infants who have congenital dacryocystoceles are at increased risk for secondary infection. This predisposition is attributable to the absence in very young children of the well-defined fascial layer present in older children and adults that isolates the lacrimal sac from the orbit. In fact, acute dacryocystitis, periorbital cellulitis, or orbital cellulitis in the neonatal age group should raise suspicion of the potential existence of this congenital anomaly (Fig. 2) [7,12].

As can be predicted by its embryologic development, a dacryocystocele should have a nasal component. The clinical association between congenital dacryocystocele and an ipsilateral intranasal cyst has been confirmed by several studies with a near 100% correlation when nasal endoscopy is used [7,8]. In some infants the dacryocystocele expansion may occur only intranasally, and the child may present solely with nasal congestion. Other children, alternatively, may present with both an external medial canthal and an intranasal mass.

Respiratory distress is commonly associated with congenital dacryocystocele with nasal extension because infants are obligate nasal breathers [9,13,14]. Bilateral nasolacrimal duct cysts can cause life-threatening airway obstruction akin to that seen in infants who have choanal atresia. Large, unilateral, nasolacrimal duct cysts can likewise cause airway compromise attributable to the dacryocystocele completely obstructing one nasal passage while the normal, cyclic, vascular congestion of the nasal mucous membranes obstructs the contralateral nasal passage.

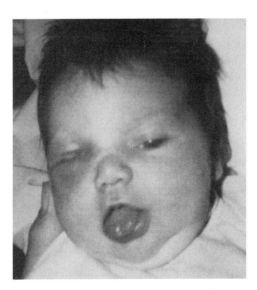

Fig. 2. Orbital cellulitis in the neonatal age group may reflect the presence of an underlying dacryocystocele.

All children who are suspected of having a dacryocystocele require a thorough nasal examination with flexible or rigid nasal endoscopy. Both nares should be examined, focusing on the inferior meatus. The application of a topical decongestant such as oxymetazoline hydrochloride to the nasal mucous membranes before endoscopy enhances visualization. A cystic mass arising from the undersurface of the inferior turbinate is sought (Fig. 3); at times, only redundant mucosa without an obvious cyst is apparent. If a mass is present, it will be soft and compressible when palpated with a nasal probe or suction.

A large intranasal dacryocystocele obstructing the nasal cavity needs to be differentiated from other cystic soft tissue masses, most significantly encephaloceles or meningoencephaloceles. Nasal dermoid cysts and nasal gliomas also are included in the differential, although these lesions tend to have a comparatively much firmer consistency.

Although not routinely indicated for diagnosis when an intranasal dacryocystocele presents in its classic inferior meatus location, radiologic imaging can distinguish between these various lesions. The characteristic radiologic findings of a congenital dacryocystocele with nasal extension include the triad of a medial canthal cystic mass, a dilated ipsilateral nasolacrimal duct, and an intranasal cystic mass, all in continuity (Fig. 4) [15]. The intravenous administration of iodinate contrast agents may demonstrate a slight rim of enhancement of these dilated cystic structures [16]. CT provides excellent detail of the surrounding osseous nasal anatomy. MRI offers additional soft tissue delineation that is useful if there is any question of an alternative diagnosis with contiguous intracranial communication.

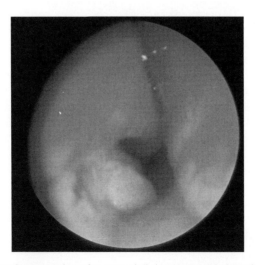

Fig. 3. The intranasal presentation of a congenital dacryocystocele is typically a cystic mass arising from the inferior meatus.

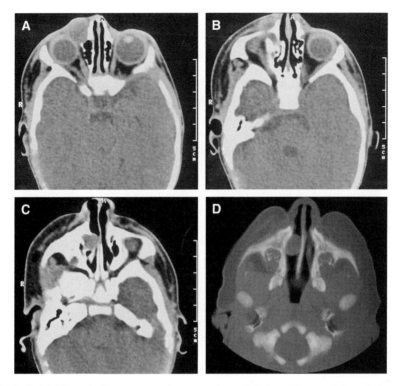

Fig. 4. Axial CT study demonstrates, from superior to inferior, (A) a medial canthal mass, (B) dilation of the nasolacrimal duct, (C) lacrimal canal, and (D) an intranasal mass.

Management

From a management standpoint, congenital dacryocystoceles are best divided into uncomplicated and complicated categories based on clinical presentation. Surgical intervention is clearly indicated if a dacryocystocele presents with associated acute or chronic dacryocystitis; if the external medial canthal cyst is large and visually obstructive, causing corneal astigmatism with risk of amblyopia; or if an intranasal cyst causes respiratory distress [2,5]. The natural history and optimal treatment of uncomplicated congenital dacryocystocele is less well defined. There is evidence to suggest that spontaneous dacryocystocele resolution may occur [5]. The frequency of such resolution and the timing of intervention if spontaneous resolution fails to occur are uncertain.

In the absence of complicating factors, initial treatment may be conservative [5,7]. Warm compresses and lacrimal massage are advocated to enhance nasolacrimal drainage. Topical antibiotics may be used to prevent secondary conjunctivitis. Lacrimal probing is proposed if spontaneous resolution does not occur. Such probing, to be effective, needs to relieve both the functional proximal obstruction and the complete or incomplete distal obstruction of the nasolacrimal drainage system. Probing actually may be quite difficult because pressure or swelling at the junction of the lacrimal sac and common canaliculus can effectively close the valve of Rosenmuller [5,11]. Transcutaneous needle or incisional aspiration of the dilated lacrimal sac has been used alternatively. This approach, however, does not treat the underlying problem and carries risk of lacrimocutaneous fistula formation [11].

A joint otolaryngologic and ophthalmologic approach to the treatment of congenital dacryocystocele is recommended [3,7,8]. Such an approach is advocated even when there is no evident intranasal cyst because the removal of redundant mucosa from the lateral inferior meatal wall in the presumed region of the valve of Hasner effectively treats the distal obstruction. When there is an identifiable intranasal cyst, marsupialization with endoscopic excision of the medial cyst wall is preferred over simple cyst puncture with decompression. Endoscopic cyst marsupialization is best performed in instrumental fashion using appropriately sized biting forceps and other endoscopic sinus surgical instruments (Fig. 5). Laser mucosal vaporization is an alternative approach but adds unnecessary time and cost without improved effectiveness. Anesthesia and intraoperative preparation arrangements are identical to those described in the following section on pediatric endonasal endoscopic dacryocystorhinostomy (DCR).

Concomitant nasolacrimal probing and irrigation are necessary to ascertain nasolacrimal system patency [3]. Typically, after the nasolacrimal sac has been decompressed distally, the proximal one-way valve of Rosenmuller

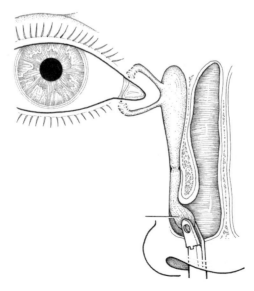

Fig. 5. Endoscopically guided marsupialization/excision of the intranasal dacryocystocele component is the recommended treatment.

will be able to function normally. Silicone intubation of the lacrimal outflow system may be performed, although it is not necessarily required.

The therapeutic approach described also provides tissue for confirmatory histopathologic examination [17]. Congenital dacryocystoceles with nasal extension are lined by pseudostratified, ciliated, columnar nasal mucosa on one side and by nasolacrimal duct epithelium within the cyst cavity; the latter is composed of nonciliated, pseudostratified, columnar epithelial cells with scattered secretory goblet cells (Fig. 6).

Pediatric endonasal endoscopic DCR

Indications and patient selection

Symptomatic congenital obstruction of the nasolacrimal system is a common clinical problem, estimated to be present in approximately 5% to 6% of newborns [18]. Clinical signs and symptoms depend upon the nature and anatomic level of the obstruction. Most commonly, the obstruction is distal at the level of the valve of Hasner, between the nasolacrimal duct and nasal cavity. More proximal obstruction involving the canaliculi, common canaliculus, or lacrimal sac occurs less frequently. Additional congenital nasolacrimal anomalies associated with tear flow obstruction include dacryocystoceles, as described earlier; agenesis of the puncta or canalicular structures; congenital lacrimocutaneous fistula; and nasolacrimal obstruction secondary to craniofacial dysmorphism [19].

Between 85% and 95% of children who have uncomplicated congenital nasolacrimal obstruction experience spontaneous resolution by 1 year of age [20]. Most of the children who have distal nasolacrimal duct obstruction who remain symptomatic respond to a single probing and irrigation; only a small percentage of children require repeat probing, with or without silicone intubation of the nasolacrimal system [21]. For the few children who have persistent distal nasolacrimal obstruction that is refractory to such

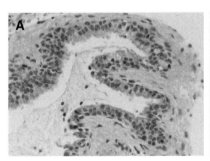 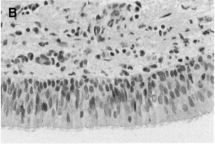

Fig. 6. (*A*) A low-power photomicrograph demonstrates a nasolacrimal duct cyst lined by (*B*) nonciliated, pseudostratified, double-layered epithelium evident on high-power magnification.

treatment measures, and for those children who have more proximal naso-lacrimal system obstruction, additional surgical correction in the form of DCR is indicated [22]. The exception to this rule is the dacryocystocele, which can be managed, as previously discussed, in an alternative surgical fashion. Early surgical intervention by means of DCR is often advocated for children whose congenital nasolacrimal obstruction becomes compli-cated by chronic or recurrent dacryocystitis. The prognosis after probing and nasolacrimal intubation in such children is relatively poor, perhaps ow-ing to inflammation-induced canalicular scarring or chronic lacrimal sac dis-tension [23].

The role of external DCR as a safe and effective procedure in the pediat-ric population is well established. Overall success rates between 83% and 96% are reported for both primary and revision external DCR procedures performed in this age group [23–25]. The higher rates of success are achieved after primary procedures for uncomplicated congenital nasolacrimal ob-struction; children who have acquired nasolacrimal obstruction secondary to trauma or prior canaliculitis do comparatively less well.

An endonasal operative approach to the lacrimal system was first de-scribed by Caldwell [26] in 1893, was modified by West [27] in 1910, and was advocated by Mosher [28] in 1921. The endonasal approach fell into disfavor, mainly because of limited transnasal visualization complicated by bleeding. Jokinen and Karja [29] revived the endonasal approach from a contemporary standpoint in 1974. The subsequent application of the operating microscope [30] and, eventually, endoscopic telescopes [31] to transnasal lacrimal surgery provided the illumination and magnification necessary to solve the visualization problem.

With the advent of new instrumentation and techniques for endoscopic sinus surgery, several authors were able to demonstrate that endonasal DCR could be performed safely in adults with success rates equal to those achieved with the traditional external approach [32–38]. Several of these adult series included a child among their successful cases [32,36]. Cunningham and Woog [39] first reported on four children undergoing endonasal endoscopic DCR in 1988. In 1999, Wong and colleagues [19] further expanded on this series in a retrospective review of eight children who had a wide variety of lacrimal outflow anomalies. Subsequent reports have confirmed the value of transnasal endoscopic DCR as a highly successful alternative to external DCR in children who have persistent distal naso-lacrimal system obstruction [40–42].

Surgical technique

Endonasal endoscopic DCR is facilitated by a joint otolaryngologic and ophthalmologic team approach. General anesthesia typically is necessary in children. The child is positioned in standard sinus surgical fashion and draped so that both the nose and affected eye are included in the operative field. Confirmatory lacrimal probing and irrigation, as well as intraoperative dacryocystography, may be performed before DCR when indicated.

Both the 4.0-mm and 2.7-mm endoscopic telescopes with 0° and 30° viewing angles should be available for intraoperative use. Operative intervention with the 4.0-mm telescopes is preferred because of their better illumination and wider field of vision. The narrow anatomic dimensions of the young child's nasal airway may dictate the use of the 2.7-mm telescopes in certain cases. Use of a video monitor display is suggested to enhance participation by all members of the surgical team.

Hemostasis is important for adequate intraoperative visualization. Initial topical vasoconstriction is performed with 0.05% oxymetazoline hydrochloride solution, followed by submucosal infiltration of the lateral nasal wall (and middle turbinate, if necessary) with 1% lidocaine with 1:100,000 epinephrine. Topical 4% cocaine solution (maximum, 1 mg/kg) may also be required once tissue disruption commences, particularly in revision cases with extensive soft tissue scarring.

An extremely important step in the successful performance of endonasal DCR is proper identification of the lacrimal sac. The maxillary line is a valuable anatomic landmark in this regard; the lacrimal sac is located lateral to the maxillary line at its superior aspect [43]. Identification of the lacrimal sac is enhanced further by the passage of a rigid fiberoptic light probe through the superior or inferior punctum into the lacrimal sac (Fig. 7). The transilluminated lacrimal sac can be visualized readily through the lateral nasal

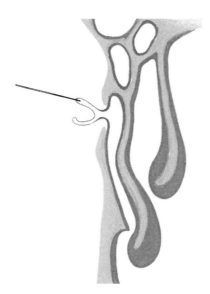

Fig. 7. The passage of a fiberoptic endoilluminator into the superior canaliculus facilitates endonasal identification of the lacrimal sac.

wall. The sac's position determines whether a partial anterior middle turbinectomy is necessary for adequate surgical access.

The rhinotomy portion of the endonasal DCR consists of the separate removal of nasal mucosa and nasal bone. An area of anterosuperior nasal mucosa approximately 2.0 cm in diameter is excised under guidance by the light probe. The nasal mucosa is incised initially in trapdoor fashion with a #15 blade, sickle knife, or angled keratotomy knife (Fig. 8). A mucosal flap is elevated in an anterior-to-posterior direction with an otologic canal wall elevator and then is stripped with a Blakesley forceps. Others have reported the use of the radiofrequency desiccation [36] or laser ablation for this purpose [35].

Removal of the underlying lacrimal bone is more easily performed posteriorly, where it is thinner, but is more safely performed anteriorly to avoid the possibility of orbital disruption. Guidance with the fiberoptic light probe significantly decreases this risk. The goal is to achieve a large bony ostium 1.0 cm to 1.5 cm in diameter. High-speed drilling, using a posteriorly hooded tip burr, is an effective means of initial bone removal. Angled neurosurgical microrongeurs and otologic curettes then may be used to enlarge the initial opening to the desired size. An alternative osteotomy technique is the use of a laser applicable to bone ablation such as the holmium:YAG laser [33].

The dacryocystostomy is performed next. The medial wall of the lacrimal sac can be "tented" with the fiberoptic light or with a standard lacrimal probe to facilitate initial sac incision (Fig. 9). The sac wall can be quite thick secondary to previous inflammation. The sac is incised, preferably with an

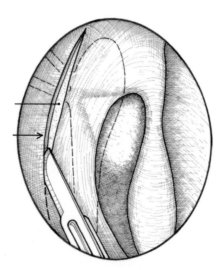

Fig. 8. The rhinotomy portion of endonasal DCR begins with incision of the nasal mucosa with a #15 blade, sickle knife, or angled keratotomy knife.

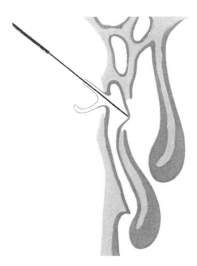

Fig. 9. The lacrimal sac mucosa is "tented" medially with a fiberoptic endoilluminator to facilitate the dacryocystostomy.

angled keratotomy knife, a sickle knife, or a myringotomy knife (Fig. 10); alternately, a radiosurgical electrode or laser may be used. Surgical incision of the lacrimal sac is favored, because ideally the lacrimal sac flaps so created can be anastomosed to the adjacent nasal mucosa [44,45]. Such flap anastomosis is not always technically possible in children, however. Alternatively, angled endoscopic biting forceps are used to create a lacrimal sac opening of approximately 1.0 cm in diameter.

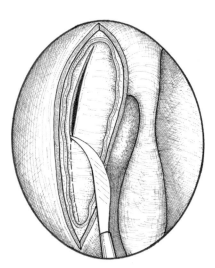

Fig. 10. The lacrimal sac mucosa is incised with a sickle knife, a myringotomy knife, or an angled keratotomy knife.

After the endonasal DCR is completed, patency is confirmed by lacrimal irrigation. Bicanalicular silicone tubing intubation of the nasolacrimal system through the surgically created nasolacrimal fistula is then performed. The ends of the tubing are knotted so that there is one continuous loop through the inferior and superior canaliculi, common canaliculus, nasolacrimal sac, and intranasal ostium (Fig. 11). This knot is secured to the lateral nasal wall with a single suture. A Gelfilm nasal stent (Pharmacia & Upjohn Company, Kalamazoo, MI) is placed between the lateral nasal wall and middle turbinate only if it is necessary to medialize an unstable turbinate remnant. No packing is used. The nostril is filled with clindamycin phosphate topical gel. Ophthalmic antibiotic steroid drops are applied topically.

Endonasal DCR procedures typically are performed as ambulatory procedures with patients being discharged to home the same day. Prophylaxis with systemic antibiotics is continued for approximately 1 week after surgery or until nasal stenting, if used, is removed. Use of ophthalmic antibiotic steroid drops is continued for 1 to 2 weeks after surgery. Intranasal saline and topical steroid sprays are used if the age of the patient allows ease of administration.

The subsequent postoperative removal of nasolacrimal silicone tubing usually can be completed in an outpatient office setting in cooperative older children but may require the use of general anesthesia in young children. Both an endoscopic examination of the nares and an assessment of nasolacrimal patency should be performed at that time.

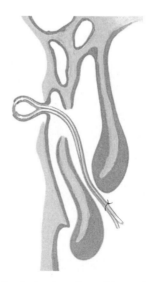

Fig. 11. Bicanalicular silicone intubation is performed in continuous loop fashion through the surgically created nasolacrimal fistula.

Results and complications

The primary surgical failure rate after external DCR in children approximates 10% [23–25]. Subsequent scarring within the nasolacrimal drainage system and obstructive intranasal pathology are the predominant causes. Complications related to the external incision, such as wound infection, bleeding, and cutaneous scar hypertrophy, are relatively infrequent.

The principal advantages of endonasal DCR over external DCR include the absence of a facial incision, the preservation of the integrity of the orbicularis oculi muscle and the medial palpebral ligaments that constitute the functional pump mechanism of tearing, and comparatively reduced morbidity during the immediate postoperative course [38]. The endonasal endoscopic approach also allows a detailed examination of the intranasal and sinus anatomy, with potential correction of any intranasal pathologic conditions that may contribute to DCR failure [46].

Disadvantages associated with endoscopic endonasal DCR include anatomic limitations in small children, the need for meticulous hemostasis, the requirement for specialized training in endoscopic sinus surgical technique, and the need for appropriate instrumentation.

Although there is no external incision with endonasal DCR, nasal vestibule abrasion secondary to drill shaft rotation with the potential subsequent development of hypertrophied scar has been reported [39]. This problem has been resolved by the use of powered instrumentation in which the shaft does not rotate for lacrimal bone removal.

Whether DCR is performed by external or endonasal technique, some children experience problems related to silicone tubing intubation of the nasolacrimal system [47]. The purpose of such nasolacrimal stenting is to

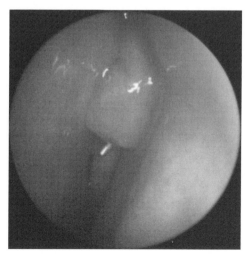

Fig. 12. Granuloma formation at the intranasal ostium is a potential complication contributing to endonasal DCR failure.

maintain DCR ostium patency during the expected period of wound con-
tracture. There is evidence, however, that the presence of silicone tubing
itself may increase rather than decrease the incidence of DCR failure by
inciting granuloma formation at the nasolacrimal fistula site (Fig. 12) [48].
For this reason, earlier removal of nasolacrimal tubing is advocated, as
soon as 3 to 6 weeks after the operation in primary endonasal DCR cases.
Revision procedures may require a more prolonged period of tubal stenting.
The intraoperative application of adjuvant topical chemotherapeutic agents
such as mitomycin C [49] and the postoperative intranasal administration of
topical nasal steroid sprays also may help decrease the risk of granulation
tissue formation.

In summary, the use of endonasal endoscopic DCR in children is evolving. Although their smaller anatomic dimensions pose a technical challenge,
this joint ophthalmologic-otolaryngologic approach to nasolacrimal obstruction in children offers several key advantages. These advantages include
the elimination of a cutaneous incision, the limited medial canthal dissection, the concomitant detailed examination of intranasal anatomy, and
decreased immediate postoperative morbidity.

References

[1] Sevel D. Development and congenital abnormalities of the nasolacrimal apparatus. J Pediatr
    Ophthalmol Strabismus 1981;18:13–9.
[2] Hepler KM, Woodson GE, Kearns DB. Respiratory distress in the neonate: sequela of a con-
    genital dacryocystocele. Arch Otolaryngol Head Neck Surg 1995;121:1423–5.
[3] Calcaterra EE, Annino DJ, Carter BL, et al. Congenital nasolacrimal duct cysts with nasal
    obstruction. Otolaryngol Head Neck Surg 1995;113:481–4.
[4] Hulka GF, Kulwin DR, Weeks SM, et al. Congenital lacrimal sac mucoceles with intranasal
    extension. Otolaryngol Head Neck Surg 1995;113:651–4.
[5] Mansour AM, Cheng KP, Mumma JV, et al. Congenital dacryocele: a collaborative review.
    Ophthalmol 1991;98:1744–51.
[6] Paoli C, Francois M, Triglia JM, et al. Nasal obstruction in the neonate secondary to naso-
    lacrimal duct cysts. Laryngoscope 1995;105:86–9.
[7] Levin AV, Wygnanski-Jaffe T, Forte V, et al. Nasal endoscopy in the treatment of congenital
    lacrimal sac mucoceles. Int J Pediatr Otorhinolaryngol 2003;67:255–61.
[8] Shashy RG, Durairaj VD, Holmes JM, et al. Congenital dacryocystocele associated with
    intranasal cysts: diagnosis and management. Laryngoscope 2005;113:37–40.
[9] Berkowitz RG, Grundfast KM, Fitz C. Nasal obstruction of the new-born revisited: clinical
    and subclinical manifestations of congenital nasolacrimal duct obstruction presenting as
    a nasal mass. Otolaryngol Head Neck Surg 1990;103:468–71.
[10] Holzberg N, Ward RF. Bilateral congenital dacryocystoceles. Otolaryngol Head Neck Surg
    1993;109:1074–7.
[11] Boynton JR, Drucker DN. Distention of the lacrimal sac in neonates. Ophthalmic Surg 1989;
    20:103–7.
[12] Campolattaro BN, Lueder GT, Tychsen L. Spectrum of pediatric dacryocystitis: medical
    and surgical management of 54 cases. J Pediatr Ophthalmol Strabismus 1997;34:143–53.
[13] Mazzara CA, Respler DS, Jahn AF. Neonatal respiratory distress: sequela of bilateral naso-
    lacrimal duct obstruction. Inter J Pediatr Otorhinolaryngol 1993;25:209–16.

[14] Yee SW, Seibert RW, Bower CM, et al. Congenital nasolacrimal duct mucocele: a cause of respiratory distress. Int J Pediatr Otorhinolaryngol 1994;29:151–8.

[15] John PR, Boldt D. Bilateral congenital lacrimal sac mucoceles with nasal extension. Pediatr Radiol 1990;20:285–6.

[16] Rand PK, Ball WS, Kulwin DR. Congenital nasolacrimal mucoceles: CT evaluation. Radiol 1989;173:691–4.

[17] Silva AB, Hotaling A, Raslan W. Pathologic quiz case 2: nasolacrimal duct cyst. Arch Otolaryngol Head Neck Surg 1994;120:888–92.

[18] MacEwen CJ, Young JDH. Epiphora during the first year of life. Eye 1991;5:596–600.

[19] Wong JF, Woog JJ, Cunningham MJ, et al. A multidisciplinary approach to atypical lacrimal obstruction in childhood. Ophthal Plast Reconstr Surg 1999;15:293–8.

[20] Petersen RA, Robb RM. The natural course of congenital obstruction of the nasolacrimal duct. J Pediatr Ophthalmol Strabismus 1998;15:246–50.

[21] Paul TO, Shepherd R. Congenital nasolacrimal duct obstruction: natural history and the timing of optimal intervention. J Pediatr Ophthalmol Strabismus 1994;31:362–7.

[22] Yeatts RP. Current concepts in lacrimal drainage surgery. Curr Opin Ophthalmol 1996;7:43–7.

[23] Hakin KN, Sullivan TJ, Sharma A, et al. Pediatric dacryocystorhinostomy. Aust N Z J Ophthalmol 1994;22:231–5.

[24] Welham RAM, Hughes SM. Lacrimal surgery in children. Am J Ophthalmol 1985;99:27–34.

[25] Nowinski TS, Flanagan JC, Mauriello J. Pediatric dacryocystorhinostomy. Arch Ophthalmol 1985;103:1226–8.

[26] Caldwell GW. Two new operations for obstructions of the nasal duct with preservation of the canaliculi. Am J Ophthalmol 1893;10:189.

[27] West J. A window resection of the nasal duct in cases of stenosis. Trans Am Ophthalmol Soc 1910;12:659.

[28] Mosher HP. Mosher-Toti operation on the lacrimal sac. Laryngoscope 1921;31:284–6.

[29] Jokinen K, Karja J. Endonasal dacryocystorhinostomy. Arch Otolaryngol 1974;100:41–4.

[30] Heermann J, Neues D. Intranasal microsurgery of the paranasal sinuses, the septum and the lacrimal sac with hypotensive anesthesia. Ann Otol Rhinol Laryngol 1986;95:631–8.

[31] McDonough M, Meiring JH. Endoscopic transnasal dacryocystorhinostomy. J Laryngol Otol 1989;103:585–7.

[32] Gonnoring RS, Lyon DB, Fisher JC. Endoscopic laser-assisted lacrimal surgery. Am J Ophthalmol 1991;111:152–7.

[33] Woog JJ, Metson R, Puliafito CA. Holmium:YAG endonasal laser dacryocystorhinostomy. Am J Ophthalmol 1993;116:1–10.

[34] Weidenbecher M, Hosemann W, Buhr W. Endoscopic endonasal dacryocystorhinostomy: results in 56 patients. Ann Otol Rhinol Laryngol 1994;103:363–7.

[35] Kong WT, Kim TI, Cong BW. A report of 131 cases of endoscopic laser lacrimal surgery. Ophthalmology 1994;101:1793–800.

[36] Javate RM, Campomanes BSA Jr, Co ND, et al. The endoscope and the radiofrequency unit in DCR surgery. Ophthal Plast Reconstr Surg 1995;11:54–8.

[37] Wormald PJ. Powered endoscopic dacryocystorhinostomy. Laryngoscope 2002;112:69–72.

[38] Tsirbas A, Davis G, Wormald PJ. Mechanical endonasal dacryocystorhinostomy versus external dacryocystorhinostomy. Ophthal Plast Reconstr Surg 2004;20:50–6.

[39] Cunningham MJ, Woog JJ. Endonasal endoscopic dacryocystorhinostomy in children. Arch Otolaryngol Head Neck Surg 1998;124:328–33.

[40] Vandrveen DK, Jones DT, Tan H, et al. Endoscopic dacryocystorhinostomy in children. J AAPOS 2001;5:143–7.

[41] Berlucchi M, Staurenghi G, Brunori PS, et al. Transnasal endoscopic dacryocystorhinostomy for treatment of lacrimal pathway stenoses in pediatric patients. Int J Pediatr Otorhinolaryngol 2003;67:1069–74.

[42] Kominek P, Cervenka S. Pediatric endonasal dacryocystorhinostomy: a report of 34 cases. Laryngoscope 2005;115:1800–3.
[43] Chastain JB, Cooper MH, Sindwani R. The maxillary line: an anatomic characterization and clinical utility of an important surgical landmark. Laryngoscope 2005;115:990–2.
[44] Tsirbas A, Wormald PJ. Endonasal dacryocystorhinostomy with mucosal flaps. Am J Ophthalmol 2003;136:579–80.
[45] Tsirbas A, Wormald PJ. Mechanical endonasal dacryocystorhinostomy with mucosal flaps. Br J Ophthalmol 2003;87:43–7.
[46] Nussbaumer M, Schreiber S, Yung MW. Concomitant nasal procedures for endoscopic dacryocystorhinostomy. J Laryngol Otol 2004;118:267–9.
[47] Allen K, Berlin AJ. Dacryocystorhinostomy failure: association with nasolacrimal silastic intubation. Ophthal Surg 1989;20:486–9.
[48] Anderson RL, Edwards JJ. Indications, complications and results with silicone stents. Ophthalmol 1979;86:1474–87.
[49] Kao SC, Liao CL, Tseng JH, et al. Dacryocystorhinostomy with intraoperative mitomycin C. Ophthalmology 1997;104:86–91.

ELSEVIER
SAUNDERS

Otolaryngol Clin N Am
39 (2006) 1075–1079

OTOLARYNGOLOGIC
CLINICS
OF NORTH AMERICA

Index

Note: Page numbers of article titles are in **boldface** type.

0030-6665/06/$ - see front matter © 2006 Elsevier Inc. All rights reserved.
doi:10.1016/S0030-6665(06)00134-4

Moving?

Make sure your subscription moves with you!

To notify us of your new address, find your **Clinics Account Number** (located on your mailing label above your name), and contact customer service at:

E-mail: elspcs@elsevier.com

800-654-2452 (subscribers in the U.S. & Canada)
407-345-4000 (subscribers outside of the U.S. & Canada)

Fax number: 407-363-9661

Elsevier Periodicals Customer Service
6277 Sea Harbor Drive
Orlando, FL 32887-4800

*To ensure uninterrupted delivery of your subscription, please notify us at least 4 weeks in advance of move.

United States Postal Service

Statement of Ownership, Management, and Circulation

1. Publication Title	2. Publication Number	3. Filing Date
Otolaryngologic Clinics of North America	4 6 6 - 5 5 0	9/15/06

4. Issue Frequency	5. Number of Issues Published Annually	6. Annual Subscription Price
Feb, Apr, Jun, Aug, Oct, Dec	6	$205.00

7. Complete Mailing Address of Known Office of Publication (Not printer) (Street, city, county, state, and ZIP+4)

Elsevier Inc.
360 Park Avenue South
New York, NY 10010-1710

Contact Person
Sarah Carmichael

Telephone
(215) 239-3681

8. Complete Mailing Address of Headquarters or General Business Office of Publisher (Not printer)

Elsevier Inc., 360 Park Avenue South, New York, NY 10010-1710

9. Full Names and Complete Mailing Addresses of Publisher, Editor, and Managing Editor (Do not leave blank)

Publisher (Name and complete mailing address)

John Schrefer, Elsevier Inc., 1600 John F. Kennedy Blvd., Suite 1800, Philadelphia, PA 19103-2899

Editor (Name and complete mailing address)

Joanne Husovski, Elsevier Inc., 1600 John F. Kennedy Blvd., Suite 1800, Philadelphia, PA 19103-2899

Managing Editor (Name and complete mailing address)

Catherine Bewick, Elsevier Inc., 1600 John F. Kennedy Blvd., Suite 1800, Philadelphia, PA 19103-2899

10. Owner (Do not leave blank. If the publication is owned by a corporation, give the name and address of the corporation immediately followed by the names and addresses of all stockholders owning or holding 1 percent or more of the total amount of stock. If not owned by a corporation, give the names and addresses of the individual owners. If owned by a partnership or other unincorporated firm, give its name and address as well as those of each individual owner. If the publication is published by a nonprofit organization, give its name and address.)

Full Name	Complete Mailing Address
Wholly owned subsidiary of	4520 East-West Highway
Reed/Elsevier Inc., US holdings	Bethesda, MD 20814

11. Known Bondholders, Mortgagees, and Other Security Holders Owning or Holding 1 Percent or More of Total Amount of Bonds, Mortgages, or Other Securities. If none, check box ► ☐ None

Full Name	Complete Mailing Address
N/A	

12. Tax Status (For completion by nonprofit organizations authorized to mail at nonprofit rates) (Check one)
The purpose, function, and nonprofit status of this organization and the exempt status for federal income tax purposes:
☐ Has Not Changed During Preceding 12 Months
☐ Has Changed During Preceding 12 Months (Publisher must submit explanation of change with this statement)

(See Instructions on Reverse)

PS Form **3526,** October 1999

13. Publication Title	14. Issue Date for Circulation Data Below
Otolaryngologic Clinics of North America	June 2006

15. Extent and Nature of Circulation		Average No. Copies Each Issue During Preceding 12 Months	No. Copies of Single Issue Published Nearest to Filing Date
a. Total Number of Copies (Net press run)		3,550	3,200
b. Paid and/or Requested Circulation	(1) Paid/Requested Outside-County Mail Subscriptions Stated on Form 3541. (Include advertiser's proof and exchange copies)	1,705	1,492
	(2) Paid In-County Subscriptions Stated on Form 3541 (Include advertiser's proof and exchange copies)		
	(3) Sales Through Dealers and Carriers, Street Vendors, Counter Sales, and Other Non-USPS Paid Distribution	995	992
	(4) Other Classes Mailed Through the USPS		
c. Total Paid and/or Requested Circulation [Sum of 15b. (1), (2), (3), and (4)]	►	2,700	2,484
d. Free Distribution by Mail (Samples, complementary, and other free)	(1) Outside-County as Stated on Form 3541	178	194
	(2) In-County as Stated on Form 3541		
	(3) Other Classes Mailed Through the USPS		
e. Free Distribution Outside the Mail (Carriers or other means)			
f. Total Free Distribution (Sum of 15d. and 15e.)	►	178	194
g. Total Distribution (Sum of 15c. and 15f.)	►	2,878	2,678
h. Copies not Distributed		672	522
i. Total (Sum of 15g. and h.)	►	3,550	3,200
j. Percent Paid and/or Requested Circulation (15c. divided by 15g. times 100)		93.82%	92.76%

16. Publication of Statement of Ownership
☐ Publication required. Will be printed in the **October 2006** issue of this publication. ☐ Publication not required

17. Signature and Title of Editor, Publisher, Business Manager, or Owner

John Fanucci – Executive Director, Subscription Services   Date 9/15/06

I certify that all information furnished on this form is true and complete. I understand that anyone who furnishes false or misleading information on this form or who omits material or information requested on the form may be subject to criminal sanctions (including fines and imprisonment) and/or civil sanctions (including civil penalties).

Instructions to Publishers

1. Complete and file one copy of this form with your postmaster annually on or before October 1. Keep a copy of the completed form for your records.
2. In cases where the stockholder or security holder is a trustee, include in items 10 and 11 the name of the person or corporation for whom the trustee is acting. Also include the names and addresses of individuals who are stockholders who own or hold 1 percent or more of the total amount of bonds, mortgages, or other securities of the publishing corporation. In item 11, if none, check the box. Use blank sheets if more space is required.
3. Be sure to furnish all circulation information called for in item 15. Free circulation must be shown in items 15d, e, and f.
4. Item 15h., Copies not Distributed, must include (1) newsstand copies originally stated on Form 3541, and returned to the publisher, (2) estimated returns from news agents, and (3), copies for office use, leftovers, spoiled, and all other copies not distributed.
5. If the publication had Periodicals authorization as a general or requester publication, this Statement of Ownership, Management, and Circulation must be published; it must be printed in any issue in October or, if the publication is not published during October, the first issue printed after October.
6. In item 16, indicate the date of the issue in which this Statement of Ownership will be published.
7. Item 17 must be signed.

Failure to file or publish a statement of ownership may lead to suspension of Periodicals authorization.

PS Form **3526,** October 1999 (Reverse)